Meeting the Challenge of Chronic Illness

Meeting the Challenge of Chronic Illness

Robert L. Kane, M.D.

Reinhard Priester, J.D.

Annette M. Totten, Ph.D.

Division of Health Services Research and Policy,
University of Minnesota School of Public Health,
Minneapolis, Minnesota

Foreword by
Edward Wagner, M.D., M.P.H.

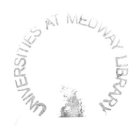

The Johns Hopkins University Press / Baltimore

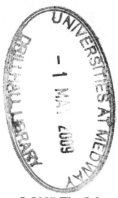

The Johns Hopkins University Press
2715 North Charles Street
Baltimore, Maryland 21218-4363
www.press.jhu.edu

Library of Congress Cataloging-in-Publication Data

Kane, Robert L., 1940–
    Meeting the challenge of chronic illness / Robert L. Kane, Reinhard Priester,
Annette M. Totten.
        p. ; cm.
    Includes bibliographical references and index.
    ISBN 0-8018-8209-5 (hardcover : alk. paper)
    1. Chronic diseases.
    [DNLM: 1. Chronic Disease—economics.   2. Chronic Disease—nursing.
3. Caregivers—psychology.   4. Long-Term Care—organization & administration.
5. Socioeconomic Factors.]   I. Priester, Reinhard.   II. Totten, Annette M. 1964–
III. Title.
    RA644.5.K36 2005
    616′.044—dc22   2004030319

A catalog record for this book is available from the British Library.

Contents

Foreword

We are living in the midst of a pervasive, relentless, but silent worldwide epidemic. The number of people with one or more major chronic illnesses is increasing dramatically. This surge is partly the result of increased risks from smoking, obesity, and other lifestyle and environmental factors. But, principally, the epidemic is a consequence of steady increases in longevity. People in both the developed and the developing world (other than sub-Saharan Africa) are living longer as a result of breakthroughs in the prevention and treatment of infectious diseases and in public health. People who develop chronic disease are also living longer as a consequence of increasingly effective treatments for their illnesses. Despite the advances in therapy, mounting evidence documents that one-half or more of chronically ill Americans are not receiving the care they need. Until very recently the epidemic of chronic illness has attracted little attention from providers and policymakers. To this day, it remains largely invisible to the public despite the well-documented deficiencies in quality of care, double-digit cost inflation, and potentially devastating impacts on medical care. The Institute of Medicine labeled the quality problem a "chasm." This is an apt metaphor because a chasm is a deep cleft or divide, in this case, separating usual care from optimal care.

We have long needed a comprehensive analysis of this epidemic—its causes, its effect on people and families, its impact on health care delivery and costs, and the various remedies that have been proposed. This book serves that need extraordinarily well. It views the issues from the perspectives of patients and families and of professional caregivers and policymakers. Unlike many discussions of chronic illness care, it considers the entire spectrum of chronic illness, from fully functional individuals trying to control their illness and prevent complications to frail, older people in need of ongoing supportive services. In addition to analyzing current problems and proposals, the book assures the reader that major improvements in the care and lives of people with chronic illness are within our grasp.

We now have a substantial evidence base from trials comparing usual and enhanced care that demonstrates the size of the quality chasm and ways to cross it. For major chronic illnesses like diabetes, depression, congestive heart failure, or asthma, the chasm, the consequences of improvement, appears to be quite wide—major reductions in diabetic complications like heart attacks and blindness, lower mortality and fewer hospitalizations for heart failure, fewer symptoms and school absences for kids with asthma, and many more recoveries from major depression. Common sense suggests that differences in health status of this magnitude must result in differences in job or school productivity and health care costs, yet debate persists as to whether there is a "business case" for chronic illness quality improvement. Those arguing that a business case for quality improvement does not exist apparently must feel that there is a business case for mediocre care, unhappy patients and professionals, and double-digit inflation—the status quo.

This book correctly identifies the culprit as the mismatch between the care needs of the chronically ill and our current approaches to delivering and financing health care, which evolved decades, perhaps centuries ago when acute, infectious disease and injuries prevailed. For those conditions, the time course of ill health is short, terminating in recovery or death within days or weeks. Patients initiate the interactions with medical care in response to acute problems, and the diagnosis and treatment of the immediate problem dominate the visit. Decisions are left to the professionals, who expect patients to follow instructions. Although the nature of the health problems confronting health care has changed dramatically, little has changed in the way sick people access the system or the system responds. In the words of the Institute of Medicine, "current care systems cannot do the job."

The trials that documented the width of the quality chasm also provide evidence suggesting how the quality chasm can be crossed. Nearly one hundred years ago, Paul Ehrlich coined the term "magic bullet" to describe single compounds that would target particular virulent organisms and toxins. The intellectual (and practicable) allure of the magic bullet persists in medicine to this day as we search for single gene mutations and therapies. Similarly, many seek a magic bullet capable of crossing the quality chasm for chronic illness care, with electronic health records and financial incentives receiving the most attention. Although growing evidence affirms that chronic illness care can be improved, unfortunately, there is no magic bullet. Rather, major improvements in care follow the comprehensive redesign of care delivery. This should not surprise us given the mismatch described here. Is radical practice change possible for busy delivery systems? In fact, many delivery organizations have demonstrated that they can change their systems and meet the needs of the chronically ill. This has been especially true in large systems like the Veteran's Health Administration and Kaiser Permanente.

Major obstacles still must be overcome if we are to improve chronic care for all Americans, especially for the great majority of patients who are cared for by smaller practices lacking the resources available to large systems. The book thoroughly discusses the challenges of an inadequately trained medical workforce, unengaged patients and families, elusive and disorganized patient information, and counterproductive reimbursement schemes. Although the public at large has not yet gone to the barricades to protest the current situation, many purchasers and health care professionals are beginning to advocate change and try new ways to improve care. Many of these new approaches to redesigning practice, using computer technology to improve the quality and accessibility of patient information, or changing financial incentives hold real promise for improving the lives of the chronically ill and the professionals caring for them.

Unfortunately, diffusion has been slow and measurable improvement has been spotty. It must accelerate or we may well see a serious erosion of frontline American health care. Practitioners, especially in primary care, are struggling to care for an older population with complex health needs with antiquated office and reimbursement systems and are leaving practice at an alarming rate. Fewer and fewer new trainees are choosing to take their place. Frustrated by stagnant performance and accelerating cost increases, legislators, purchasers, and health plans have turned to commercial disease management companies, thus further fragmenting care. But there is hope based on the growing evidence about what needs to be done. For most people with chronic illness, we have proven clinical, preventive, behavioral, and rehabilitative interventions that will prolong and improve their lives. We also have models and tools to create care delivery and financing systems that can cross the quality chasm. What we lack at the population level is concerted leadership and a central nervous system that understands the health care enterprise, can integrate and support its disparate parts, and guarantee the necessary infrastructure to improve the care of patients. In the absence of federal health care reform, the best hope will be regional efforts.

We have needed a thoughtful, comprehensive examination of the evidence and issues in caring for individuals and families with chronic illness. Now we have one.

Edward Wagner, M.D., M.P.H.,
Director, MacColl Institute for Healthcare Innovation,
Seattle, Washington

Acknowledgments

The authors wish to acknowledge the assistance that we received from many individuals and organizations in writing this book. This book grew out of a two-year series of meetings with a wide range of university faculty to discuss aspects of chronic disease. We thank our colleagues on the University-wide Committee on Chronic Illness Care for their valuable insights into both the shortcomings of our current health care system and the opportunities for improving chronic illness care. Members of the committee, all on the faculty at the University of Minnesot a, were: Margaret Artz, Donna Bliss, Richard DiFabio, Sandra Edwardson, Stan Finkelstein, James Gambucci, Celia Gershenson, Leslie Grant, Patricia Hart, Kenneth Hepburn, Jeremy Holtzman, Merrie Kaas, Anne Kane, Rosalie Kane, Alice Larson, Terry Lum, Teresa McCarthy, Anne Murray, Dean Neumann, John Nyman, Mary Beth O'Connell, James Pacala, Edward Ratner, Hanna Bloomfield Rubins, Patricia Schaber, Gary Schwitzer, LaDora Thompson, Gregory Vercellotti, Jean Wyman, Shirley Zimmerman, and Greg Arling (a visiting professor from the University of Missouri).

We benefited from presentations by guests invited to meetings of the University-wide Committee on Chronic Illness Care. Dr. Richard Della Penna, Director of the Kaiser Permanente Aging Network of The Permanente Federation, updated us on the various chronic care initiatives throughout the Kaiser Permanente system. Dr. Mary Mundinger, Dean of the Columbia University School of Nursing, spoke to the committee about the changing roles and responsibility of advanced practice nurses to better meet the needs of patients with chronic conditions. Dr. Ian Philp, National Director for Older People's Services in the United Kingdom's National Health Service, discussed efforts to improve chronic illness care in the United Kingdom. Dr. Edward Wagner, Director of the MacColl Institute of Healthcare Innovation at the Center for Health Studies, Group Health Cooperative in Seattle, keynoted the Center on Aging's conference on chronic care and outlined strategies for refocusing the health care system to one that is proactive and focused on keeping a person as healthy as possible. The presenters' contributions of time and knowledge are appreciated.

We would also like to thank the following people with whom we met to discuss their respective organization's initiatives to improve chronic illness care: John Mach (Evercare, UnitedHealth Group); Steven Eisenberg (Blue Cross and Blue Shield of Minnesota); Terry Crowson (HealthPartners); Lois Quam (UnitedHealth Group); Robin Whitebird (HealthPartners Research Foundation); Richard Bringewatt (Chronic Care Consortium); Peter Wyckoff (Minnesota Senior Federation); Gayle Hallin (Minnesota Department of Health); Barbara Kind, Kenneth Riff, and Steven LaPort (Medtronic); Tom Plocher and Sue Mae Richardson (Honeywell).

We are grateful to Gay Bloom and Katherine Kegan, who each wrote a personal vignette for the book—Gay Bloom, from the perspective of a person with a chronic illness; Katherine Kegan, from the perspective of a daughter caring for her parents with chronic conditions. These first-person accounts vividly illustrate the broad impact of chronic conditions on the persons with the condition and the family members who care for them. We also thank Gary Schwitzer, assistant professor of journalism at the University of Minnesota, who wrote an essay on why journalists struggle with the chronic illness story (App. A). Ian Philp, David Colin-Thome, and Sue Roberts, all national clinical directors with the National Health Service, contributed an essay on lessons from the United Kingdom (App. B). Teresa McCarthy, Macaran Baird, Jayne Penney, David Lyon, Richard Della Penna, Jan Smolowitz, William Doherty, and Tai Mendenhall wrote exhibits on existing programs and strategies that help link the book's topics to real-world examples.

We would like to acknowledge a number of people in the University of Minnesota's Center on Aging who provided support and assistance. Aaron Kual, a graduate research assistant, conducted the initial literature review. Sheryl Papp, Lorri Todd, and Krystal Wiesenberg provided administrative assistance, assuring the accuracy of the references and developing the tables and figures in the book. Finally, we thank Marilyn Eells, whose superb management of the Center on Aging's office facilitated this project and ensured that all our requests for assistance were promptly and capably filled.

Financial support for the project came from the Merck Institute of Aging and Health, but none of the content reflects their policies. The authors alone are responsible for the content of this book.

Introduction

The time is out of joint.

HAMLET, Act 1, sc. 5, l. 189–90

We live with a health care system that is out of step with current demographic realities. Sophisticated and complex, this system represents a large share of the national economy. The United States now spends nearly $1.5 trillion a year on a health care system that is world class in trauma, transplantation, and other high-tech care. But the majority of people who use the system need something else. They come with chronic illnesses that require ongoing, long-term attention and management. For these people the system often provides care that is insufficient and ineffective.

This misalignment has been recognized by many parties, but the task of turning the medical care ocean liner to a radically new course is difficult. Well entrenched and powerful interests have a heavy investment in the status quo. These invested parties include both the providers of care, who constitute the medical industrial complex that has made health care one of America's major economic investments, as well as the consumers of care, who have come to expect technologically sophisticated care at each encounter and believe in the promises of more to come. Previous harbingers have largely gone unheard and certainly unheeded. Diagnoses and recommendations from the Institute of Medicine (Institute of Medicine, 2001; Kohn, Corrigan, & Donaldson, 2000), dire warnings about the effects of not changing the health care system to accommodate chronic disease, and new care proposals from leading experts like Edward Wagner (Wagner, 2001; Wagner, Austin, & Von Korff, 1996b) and David Lawrence (Lawrence, 1997, 2002) have prompted only modest changes in the way care is provided.

For most infectious diseases, injuries, and other acute conditions, prompt diagnosis and treatment—often carried out during a single encounter by a solo clinician—are sufficient to restore the patient's health. Most chronic conditions, in contrast, require a much broader set of health and supportive services spanning assessment, diagnosis, prevention of exacerbations, rehabilitation, and monitoring—often provided by many different clinicians over a long period of time—to maintain health, slow decline, and mitigate the condition's impact on the patient's life. Chronic conditions such as arthritis, heart disease, and Parkinson disease are more than an isolated failure of a person's body or organ; they threaten the integrity of a person's being and transform personal, intimate, and family relationships. Like the conditions themselves, the care required is complex and dynamic. Far too frequently, however, the care provided is fragmented, uncoordinated, or incomplete as components of the many services needed for optimal care are overlooked, or inadequately linked, or in conflict with each other.

Care for persons with chronic conditions requires a much more sophisticated, integrated, interdisciplinary, and individualized approach than our current acute health care system is able to provide. Improving this system to better meet the needs of people with chronic conditions is the predominant health care challenge of the new century. Already, nearly half of all patients seeking care have one or more chronic conditions and their care consumes three-fourths of our health care dollars. Forecasts based on the aging of the population, continued advances in medicine, and other demographic and technological changes project increases in both the number of people with chronic conditions and the share of health care expenditures devoted to their care. Given these facts and trends, improving the system is not a choice but a necessity. And, since chronic illnesses affect nearly everyone—those (currently) without a chronic condition themselves almost surely love and provide assistance to a family member or friend who has a chronic condition—reorganizing the health care system to be more responsive to chronic conditions would benefit all.

However, changing the health care system to fit the population's contemporary needs is no easy task. Nor is there widespread active demand for such a shift. Although the faults and limitations have been observed repeatedly, and although major national organizations have identified the need for substantial redesign, there is no groundswell of cries for major reforms. People complain about some aspects of health care, but not about the system's technological sophistication. The dramatic lifesaving effects of acute interventions capture all the attention, even though chronic care is the predominate problem for the majority of ill persons in this country. No TV shows and few magazine covers or evening news stories celebrate chronic care.

As a society, we must recognize that our health care system must be made more responsive. Without a concerted effort, combining consumer pressure with demonstrations of what is possible and financial incentives to reinforce adoption of these innovations, change will come slowly, if at all. With this book we hope to convince readers that changing the system to meet the needs of people with chronic conditions is necessary and to outline some of the elements of this essential reform.

Scope of the Book

This book is intended to draw together some of the arguments in favor of change and to suggest directions that need to be pursued. We lay no claims to being the first to discover these truths. Indeed, we build heavily on the work of others and have tried to acknowledge those resources whenever possible. We view this book as an amalgamation of much of what is known about managing chronic disease and as a guide to the challenges yet to be mastered

In the United States and many other high-income countries, the health care system is organized to respond to acute but short-term diseases and injuries. Reorganizing these systems to provide better chronic care calls for a sustained, integrated approach involving all stakeholders and all segments of the health care system. Reflecting the need for such a broad perspective, this book emphasizes the commonalities that cut across chronic conditions rather than the characteristics that are unique to specific conditions. It provides an overview of the problem of chronic illness in the United States, the components of a health care system capable of providing better chronic care, and the opportunities and barriers to developing such a system. Though we focus our attention on the United States, we also consider the exciting efforts that are occurring in the United Kingdom, where it may be possible to use some of the principles of managed care more successfully since the system operating under the National Health Service is less influenced by the pressures of market-driven health care.

This book concentrates on chronic conditions among the nation's adult population and the infrastructure changes needed for improving chronic care for this population. Two topics are notably absent. Care for chronic conditions in children and chronic mental illness are both important dimensions of the problem of chronic illness.[1] Addressing these areas of care requires somewhat different approaches because they interact with different elements of our social structure. They also merit more in-depth study than was possible in this project. Hopefully others will tackle these important topics.

Reforming Chronic Illness Care

The effective management of chronic conditions is gradually being recognized as the greatest challenge to our health care system. In contrast to a hundred years ago, chronic conditions are now by far the most important cause of all mortality, premature mortality, morbidity, and potential life years lost. They are the leading causes of disability, loss of productivity, and deterioration in the quality of life. And they are responsible for the vast majority of health care expenditures. Yet the implications of the massive change in the nature of the diseases that affect most patients have not permeated the structures of health care. Therein lies the great paradox of today's health care system: although we now live in a world dominated by chronic conditions, health care is still structured much the same as it was at the start of the twentieth century, organized around events that reflect a commitment to acute care. The contemporary health care establishment is prepared to fight the wrong kind of war. It is lined up to respond to acute events and brief encounters even though the majority of illnesses require more sustained contact and observation. The challenge is how best to deal with the shift from the primacy of acute illnesses to the predominance of chronic conditions.

Much work has already been done and many of the elements for reorganizing chronic care already exist—including clinical knowledge about how to effectively manage chronic conditions, proven strategies for improving the delivery of chronic care, and models of successful chronic care programs. A host of innovative ideas for reforming chronic illness care have been promoted. A leading example is the Chronic Care Model (CCM) developed by Edward Wagner and his colleagues, a widely used design incorporating "essential elements of a system that encourages high-quality chronic disease management" (Wagner, Austin, & Von Korff, 1996b).[2] Numerous successful demonstration projects, using the CCM or based on similar ideas, have been implemented, but significant barriers remain. Though elements of the CCM have been shown to improve health outcomes and reduce costs, the complete model has not yet been rigorously evaluated (Bodenheimer, Wagner, & Grumbach, 2002b). (The Chronic Care Model is further discussed in chapter 11.) By and large, chronic care demonstration projects, whether using the CCM or other approaches, have remained just that, demonstration projects, and have yet to become mainstream by overcoming the strong social forces that reinforce the status quo.

Progress has been agonizingly slow. The generally conservative health care industry presents formidable barriers to the changes in infrastructure needed to provide better chronic care. As one author argues, a business case does not yet exist for good chronic disease care (Coye, 2001). Moreover, although many pieces exist, the mosaic is still incomplete. In addition, a diverse set of issues, from accountability to cost containment to new roles for primary care, will complicate efforts at chronic care reform, regardless of the pace and ultimate direction of change. Our society's challenge is to address these issues and combine what is already known into a coherent approach for reforming the health care system to more effectively and efficiently meet the needs of people with chronic conditions.

Whether improving chronic illness care in our health care system will increase or decrease total health care expenditures cannot yet be determined. In theory, better management of problems earlier should prevent subsequent expensive hospital care; but there are simply too many variables and too many unknowns to accurately predict if a health care system that meets the needs of people with chronic conditions will require more resources, or if such a system will create efficiencies that result in lower overall health care expenditures. However, even if more resources are needed, more money, by itself, is not a complete solution. The answer lies not simply in transforming the payment system (although that step is central to achieving sustained reform); it requires fundamental changes in the basic structure of medical care, including changing the payment system to providers to provide incentives for doing the right things. Nonetheless, even if all the financial barriers to timely and effective chronic illness care were eliminated, the challenge of providing optimal chronic illness care would still be with us.

In addition to a redistribution of resources, a revolution in thinking is needed to bring the health care system into alignment with the epidemiological reality of chronic illness. Responding to chronic illness means changing the way we think about health care. Instead of the paradigm of medical treatment for acute conditions as they occur, we must think in terms of long-term health care and supportive services for persons with one or more chronic illnesses. We must recognize that most of these illnesses are both lifelong (at least the rest of our lives once we get them) and often life changing. They are far more than isolated biological malfunctions. Thus, to respond to these challenges, we must better understand how and why the health care system fails to adequately meet the needs of people with chronic conditions. We must then develop and implement strategies to ensure that our health care system effectively and efficiently provides them with the full range of services they need.

This book does not purport to offer "the solution"; indeed, a single solution to the challenge of chronic illness care probably does not exist. Instead, it focuses on the underlying principles and essential components of a health care system that provides optimal chronic care. It takes a broad look at chronic care from a variety of perspectives. The overall goal is to describe the current status and the challenges of chronic illness care, to analyze some of the major factors that must be addressed in creating a more appropriate and responsive health care system, and to look forward to what can be accomplished and how to achieve it.

Structure of the Book

The first of three sections examines current deficiencies in chronic illness care. The opening chapter contrasts acute care with chronic care, arguing that, although the two are fundamentally connected, chronic care needs a significantly different system because chronic conditions are substantially different from acute conditions. Compared with acute care, chronic care has different goals, timelines, and patient and provider roles. Chapter 1 defines the terms that are central to a discussion of chronic care reform. Chapter 2 presents the magnitude and dimensions of chronic illness in the United States and how it affects individuals, families, and society. Chapter 3 describes how the current system fails in providing effective chronic illness care. The core problem is that the health care system uses the wrong model of care: it is structured primarily to respond to acute conditions and thus ignores the fundamentally different approach that is needed to care for people with chronic conditions. Other deficiencies in the system's structure and function, payment systems, and workforce development further hinder providing optimal chronic illness care.

The five chapters in the second section explore ways for improving chronic illness care. Chapter 4 reviews several specific strategies for reorganizing chronic care that have been implemented and evaluated: patient self-management, disease management, case management, group visits, interdisciplinary team care, and geriatric evaluation and management. These strategies are among the "building blocks" for a reconfigured health care system. The next two chapters focus on formal and informal (i.e., paid and unpaid) caregivers, respectively. Chapter 5 explores the current health education enterprise and delineates changes needed to ensure a professional workforce capable of providing optimal chronic care. Chapter 6 then considers the roles for patients in managing their own chronic conditions and appropriate roles and responsibilities of family members. The final three chapters in this section concentrate on other essential elements of an improved health care system for chronic illness care: the use of health care technology in chronic care (chapter 7); preventing the onset of disease, the progression of chronic conditions, and iatrogenic complications (chapter 8); and changes in the payment for health care needed to provide comprehensive chronic illness care (chapter 9).

The third section considers the prospects for reforming chronic care. If the public is to demand better chronic disease care it must know and understand what is possible. Chapter 10 offers a brief review of recent health reform initiatives, concluding that, although chronic illness and chronic care have been largely ignored in reform efforts over the past 40 years, these topics must now be put at the forefront of the health reform agenda. It also explores the barriers that hinder efforts to improve chronic illness care. Chapter 11 delves into the future, speculating about what is on the immediate horizon and what are the essential next steps.

We have included two appendixes that provide useful insights. One might hope that the media would serve as a vehicle to educate the public about the realities of chronic disease. The first appendix explores the media's failure to actively address chronic disease topics and its almost exclusive focus on acute care issues, such as the SARS epidemic. The media's fascination with acute care reflects the prominence the health care system itself gives to such care. The next appendix provides a report on efforts to redesign chronic care in the United Kingdom, which is facing many of the same chronic care challenges as the United States, although in the context of a markedly different health care system. In many respects, the United Kingdom provides an opportunity to test many of the attractive features of managed care without the shadow of proprietary interests, and its experience may hold lessons for our own country's efforts to reorganize chronic care.

PART I

Caring for People with Chronic Illness

1. What's So Special about Chronic Illness Care?

ACUTE CARE VIGNETTE

♣ "Call an ambulance!" screams a woman in the Los Angeles convention hall audience. Stan Jones, the owner of a small construction company in Athens, Georgia, has just slumped over in his chair with sharp, piercing chest pain. The emergency medical technicians recognize Mr. Jones' symptoms as a potential heart attack (myocardial infarction) and take him to the emergency room (ER) of a large urban hospital three miles from the convention site. The ER physician assesses Mr. Jones, confirms that he was experiencing a heart attack, starts thrombolytic therapy, and transfers him to the hospital's cardiac intensive care unit (CICU), which is fully equipped with the latest technology.

A member of the CICU's interprofessional staff completes a brief medical history. Stan is 61 years old, divorced with two children, without any drug allergies, a life-long smoker, and 30 pounds overweight; he has no family history of heart disease. Stan confesses that his physician, a family practitioner, has repeatedly encouraged him to stop smoking, lose weight, and strive to reduce work-related stress and other heart attack risk factors.

The ER physician tells Stan that tests indicate he will need immediate surgery to remove blockage in three of his heart arteries. Bypass surgery is scheduled for the next day. The hospital's physicians, nurses, and support staff who operate on Mr. Jones, have conducted, as a team, hundreds of heart procedures a year. The procedure is uneventful and Mr. Jones is quickly returned to the CICU for recovery. Before the surgery, the cardiac surgeon explained the procedure to him. A cardiac nurse had then spoken at length with him, answering all his questions and allaying his fears. Other than these encounters, Mr. Jones had never met any of the cardiac team members before they performed his surgery.

After one day in the CICU, Mr. Jones is transferred to the hospital's newly remodeled cardiac recovery unit for five more days. He is then discharged from the hospital, with the appropriate medications and a comprehensive rehabilitation plan, to the care of his sister, who had moved to Los Angeles with her husband in 1973. During the next two weeks he returns to the hospital several times for rehabilitation therapy. At the end of the two

3

weeks, Mr. Jones goes back to Georgia, where he first returns to work part-time and within a month resumes his normal life.

The full records of Mr. Jones's hospital stay are forwarded to his primary physician in Georgia. This physician refers Mr. Jones for follow-up cardiac care to a cardiologist in the same multispecialty clinic. Neither Mr. Jones nor his Georgia physicians have any further contact with the health care professionals in Los Angeles who cared for him during his heart attack. Within two months, Mr. Jones receives the bills for the hospitalization and physician services. Of a total cost of $30,000 for the entire heart attack episode, his out-of-pocket costs are $1,500.

(This case is hypothetical. Any resemblance to persons living or dead is purely coincidental.)

CHRONIC CARE VIGNETTE

♣ Bill McCormick, a 61-year-old divorced truck driver who lives in Chicago, was diagnosed with type 2 (non-insulin-dependent) diabetes 12 years ago. Overweight for most of his adult life, he now weighs 225 pounds with a 32 body mass index, or BMI (a BMI of 30 is the threshold for obesity). He also has high blood pressure and low back pain that has grown steadily worse during the past two years. Within the past few months Mr. McCormick has begun to experience eyesight problems, causing him to take wrong exits and experience close calls. (Once he misread a sign and narrowly missed wedging his semi-trailer truck under a low-clearance bridge.) For fear of losing his job, he has kept this problem from both his physician and his employer.

Ever since the younger of his two daughters, Mary Margaret, moved out of the home six years ago, Mr. McCormick has tried hard to keep up his Chicago house and to meet all his day-to-day needs. When he is overwhelmed, Mary Margaret (who lives in the same neighborhood) helps with cooking, cleaning, or other household chores. But Mr. McCormick is reluctant to ask for her assistance, knowing that with a young family of her own she, too, is struggling to make ends meet.

In addition to his primary-care physician, who has known him as a patient for almost 20 years, Mr. McCormick has seen, with referrals, four other clinicians during the past year, including a cardiologist, endocrinologist, orthopedic surgeon, and diabetes nurse-educator. Each of these clinicians works in a specialty care clinic, independent of each other and of the primary care physician. Their care is limited to the specific problem Mr. McCormick presents and, according to Mr. McCormick, they show little interest in any of his medical problems that lie outside their immediate expertise. Even his primary care physician does not always have time during his brief visits with Mr. McCormick to thoroughly review or coordinate his patient's multiple conditions and overall health. As a result, for example, he was unaware that last week Mr. McCormick's cardiologist prescribed a new blood pressure medication that would interact with one of Mr. McCormick's diabetes drugs. Mr. McCormick feels that even with so many clinicians involved (or perhaps *because* so many are involved), no one has the time or wants to take overall responsibility for his care.

His clinicians share a similar confusion about where their own responsibilities end and someone else's begin. Consequently, some routine services are missed. For instance, it had been more than twelve months since a clinician examined Mr. McCormick's feet (annual foot examinations are recommended for all patients with type 2 diabetes). A foot examination was not performed until Mr. McCormick complained of open sores.

Unhappy with some of his care, in particular, the inability to identify the cause of or to resolve his back pain, Mr. McCormick took the advice of his neighbor and visited a chiropractor, an acupuncturist, and a naturopath during the past year. Except for the visit to the chiropractor, Mr. McCormick has not told his primary care physician about these visits or about the natural remedies that he is taking on the advice of these practitioners. Mr. McCormick is also reluctant to tell his primary care physician that he simply cannot afford the physician's recommended diet (heavy on fresh vegetables and unprocessed food). He feels as if his physician blames him for his inability to lose weight.

Mr. McCormick's clinicians want him to take more control over his own care. Though he agrees with this goal, he often is not given the necessary information and tools. For instance, a diet and exercise program that included bimonthly group meetings with a diabetes nurse-educator held at his diabetes clinic was replaced recently with an on-line program administered by a national disease management firm. But Mr. McCormick does not own a computer.

Mr. McCormick's multiple health conditions have been difficult to control. When he cannot afford the costly drugs that are not covered by his insurance, he sometimes skips taking them. Although he monitors his blood sugar at home and reports "normal" readings to his physician, he is not sure if he is doing the at-home testing correctly. He has never been shown how to use the device properly and now feels reluctant to ask for assistance.

He worries intensely about his future. Mr. McCormick is unsure how he will obtain and pay for all the services he needs, particularly if his eyesight continues to deteriorate. Full-time work has become difficult. Although his employer has allowed him to cut back on his behind-the-wheel hours, lately any amount of driving exacerbates his back pain. He fears that if he loses his job he will be without health insurance because his multiple chronic conditions would make him "uninsurable."

Mr. McCormick is currently insured through his employer. However, the 50-person trucking company is facing double-digit premium increases for the third year in a row and has several older employees such as Mr. McCormick who are in poor health. As a result, the company will likely have to reduce benefits again to continue to provide insurance coverage for its employees. Among the services already reduced or cut altogether are home health care, outpatient prescription drugs, physical therapy, and other services that are potentially of greatest benefit to people, such as Mr. McCormick, who have chronic conditions. Changes in his insurance plan have raised Mr. McCormick's annual out-of-pocket costs for health care to above $6,000, nearly 15% of his income.

(This case is hypothetical. Any resemblance to persons living or dead is purely coincidental.)

The neatly packaged, fast-paced episodes of Hollywood's popular medical shows on broadcast TV are a more accurate reflection of the U.S. health care system than you imagine. With all the elements of a pithy television script, America's health care system is designed first and foremost to treat acute conditions that exhibit a predictable beginning, middle, and end. Like actors on a Hollywood set, millions of clinicians in countless hospitals and clinics throughout the country stand ready to respond to injuries and illnesses as they occur. A person in need of prompt medical attention for an infectious disease, accident, or other acute condition (and who is insured) typically receives care that is second to none. Health care professionals marshal resources from an array of technology to diagnose and treat the patient's condition. Typically, as in the example of Mr. Jones, the encounter between a patient and the health care system mirrors the tightly written television storyline—a brief and straightforward performance that restores the patient back to health. For these "contained crisis" encounters, the system performs admirably, albeit expensively and with occasional errors.

For the 125 million Americans with chronic illnesses, however, this "ER" experience is often just a chimera. Although individuals with a chronic condition, such as Mr. McCormick, receive care from the same clinicians in the same facilities as people with acute conditions, they need and use health care very differently. Their needs stretch over long periods of time, requiring ongoing management of their chronic conditions that is punctuated by only periodic interactions with their clinicians or other health care providers. For them, what occurs away from health care settings—off the set—is at least as, if not more important than, what takes place while they are in the hospital, clinic, or clinician's office. But our health care system, focused as it is on clear-cut encounters, frequently fails to connect the dots. As a result, people with chronic conditions too often receive inadequate care.

Chronic illness care is the predominant challenge facing America's health care system. Although significant progress in research has helped medical professionals better identify the origins of disease and treat illnesses, the number of individuals with chronic infirmities continues to increase. By 2020, 157 million people in the United States, nearly half the total population, are projected to have at least one chronic condition. The cost of caring for people with chronic conditions will continue to increase as well, from an estimated 75% of total health care expenditures in 2000 to nearly 80% in 2020 (Wu & Green, 2000).

Acute and Chronic Conditions

Chronic conditions differ from acute conditions on a variety of important dimensions. In general, acute conditions have a sudden onset. They last for only a short time and usually are stopped with the appropriate care or end spontaneously, without requiring ongoing treatment. They usually end with cure but sometimes with death. The National Center for Health Statistics defines an "acute condition" as a condition that has lasted less than three months and has involved either a physician visit (medical attention) or restricted activity. Acute conditions include, for instance, the common cold; communicable diseases such as chicken pox; illnesses due to *Escherichia coli*, the West Nile, or other viruses; injuries with short recovery periods; and appendicitis or other conditions requiring prompt medical or surgical interventions but not necessarily requiring continued care.

In general, an illness or condition is considered chronic if it has persistent or recurring health consequences lasting for a substantial period of time (variously identified as at least three months, six months, or longer), is not self-limiting, waxes and wanes in terms of severity, and typically cannot be cured. The essential aspect of a chronic condition is its lengthy duration. (*Chronic* is derived from the Greek, *khronos*, meaning "time".) A chronic condition is enduring and is not simply a series of disconnected complaints.

In addition to differences in duration, the sudden onset of most acute conditions contrasts with the progressive nature of many chronic conditions. People "come down" with an acute illness, whereas they "develop" a chronic condition. Also in contrast to acute conditions, chronic conditions tend to have multiple causes and can occur long after the causative exposure or behavior. For example, a person's exposure to carcinogens such as asbestos fibers can lead to a chronic lung condition several decades later. Acute and chronic conditions also differ markedly in their impact on a person's health and life. In acute conditions the threat to a person's health is discrete and relatively brief. In chronic conditions the threat is ongoing, long lasting, and global—affecting the social, physical, psychological, and economic aspects of the person's life.

Nonetheless, the boundaries between acute and chronic conditions blur at times. A chronic condition can evolve from an acute disease. A person with a chronic condition such as asthma may experience an acute attack, or exacerbation, that is resolved with a dose of medication or an urgent-care visit. Likewise, a person who had a heart attack is viewed and treated as acutely ill, but the underlying heart disease may require continued monitoring and behavior changes over a period of months or even years. Less obvious, but also important are the points where chronic and acute conditions overlap. In some cases a chronic condition can affect the nature of an acute illness. A relatively benign case of the flu, for example, may be more serious if the person affected has diabetes and cannot take over-the-counter medications. Influenza in patients with congestive heart failure or chronic obstructive pulmonary disease may be enough to destabilize their already compromised health status. The overlap of acute and chronic conditions also presents a challenge in treatment. Surgical interventions to repair an injury may not be viable options for a patient with heart disease or for a diabetic patient with nerve damage. Despite such overlap, however, the differences between acute and chronic conditions, as summarized in table 1.1, are relatively clear-cut.

Chronic conditions are not only distinguishable from acute conditions but are themselves dissimilar. Although chronic conditions share many commonalities, they include a broad spectrum of illnesses and impairments that vary significantly from one another in their impact on a person's life and activity and in their underlying causes, symptoms, progression, and modes of treatment (Jennings, Callahan, & Caplan, 1988). They can be of a physical or mental nature and the age of onset can range from before birth to late in a person's life. Illnesses such as Parkinson disease, Alzheimer disease, and multiple sclerosis pose very high risk of disability and can significantly limit a person's activities, whereas other chronic illnesses, such as hypertension, can usually be controlled (even if their underlying causes cannot be eliminated) and present a low risk of activity limitation. Some chronic conditions, such as heart disease and cancer, are life threatening; many others, such as arthritis and hearing impairments, are not. Chronic conditions, such as cystic fibrosis and spina bifida, have distinct genetic causes; in contrast, the eti-

TABLE 1.1.
Differences between Acute and Chronic Conditions

Acute Conditions	Chronic Conditions
Short duration	Last more than 6 months; often lifelong
Usually curable or self-limiting	Typically not curable; not self-limiting
Discrete threat to patient's health	Global impact on patient's health and life; with significant social, psychological, and economic consequences
Sudden onset	Progressive onset
Distinct, identifiable cause	May have multiple causes
Examples	Examples
• Common cold	• Diabetes
• Chicken pox	• Parkinson disease
• Appendicitis	• Arthritis
• Pneumonia	• Hypertension
• Broken bones	• Coronary artery disease
• Most injuries	• Depression

ologies of emphysema, cancer, and heart disease are varied, complex, and, to a significant degree, still unknown.

Chronic conditions also vary greatly in their developmental course. Most are progressive, with no clear distinctive onset. Some occur suddenly with long-lasting residual impairment, and still others can remain in long-term remission with an absence of symptoms. Finally, some chronic conditions improve over time. Although the vast majority of chronic illnesses are not amenable to cure, treatments can lead to complete recovery for some, such as treatment for stomach ulcers or rehabilitation for a mild stroke. In addition, some chronic conditions disappear, as when persons "grow out of" illnesses such as asthma.

Acute and Chronic Care

Just as acute conditions differ from chronic conditions, so too do the appropriate responses to these two categories of ailments. In an acute care system the patient presents for treatment and provides a history of the event; the clinician examines the patient, makes a diagnosis, and performs a procedure or prescribes a treatment. All this happens in a single encounter, be it a visit to the clinician's office or a hospital admission. The encounter may occasionally require several visits to complete, as was true for Mr. Jones's heart attack, but it is usually short-lived.

Contrast that scenario to what happens in the context of chronic illness. For people such as Mr. McCormick, their chronic condition is diagnosed, sometimes only after symptoms accumulate over a long period of time, and a course of treatment is prescribed. They experience and are affected by the condition daily, sometimes for the rest of their lives. The challenge is to manage the condition so as to minimize complications, above all, the catastrophic events that lead to hospitalizations. This type of management requires continual monitoring. For people who have multiple chronic conditions, such as Mr. McCormick, this may require tracking a variety of vital signs (e.g., blood sugar and body weight), analyzing the information, and modifying care as needed. In between the periodic visits to a clinician, the responsibility for monitoring and management rests largely with the patients themselves. Addressing chronic conditions thus requires rethinking the relationship between, and the respective roles of, clinicians and patients.

Although care for acute conditions differs from care for chronic conditions, the two are fundamentally connected. As noted, both types of care are usually provided by the same clinicians in the same health care facilities. Like all other patients, chronically ill patients will require services to prevent, diagnose, and treat their diseases, that is, the pathological changes in their bodies. However, because these types of acute care services focus on immediate symptoms and cure, they do not necessarily address the long-term impairments associated with chronic conditions. Treating and managing chronic conditions entails moving beyond episodic, symptomatic acute care services that treat only the patient's medical problems. In addition to surgical, medical, and pharmaceutical interventions, people with chronic conditions may need services to address their functional problems and the psychosocial aspects of living with chronic illness. These services include long-term monitoring; counseling; social and other supportive services; assistance with diet, exercise, and other lifestyle issues; education about and support in managing their illness; and long-term care. Such additional services target the myriad ways in which chronic conditions affect patients' functioning and in which they affect patients' lives and the lives of those who care for them. A full spectrum of health care and supportive services may thus be needed to address the many ways in which chronic conditions can affect patients. The specific services appropriate for any particular patient will, of course, depend on the patient's chronic condition(s) and his or her circumstances.

What Is Different about Chronic Illness Care?

The same system that works well for discrete acute events does not work well for continuous chronic conditions. A new approach, indeed a new philosophy of care, is needed. The new approach must differ from the old in several important elements:

- The goals of care are different. Acute care strives for cures; chronic care aims to manage the condition and help the patient cope with its impact. Preventing or even slowing the rate of decline represents a victory in chronic illness care. The goals of chronic care can change over time, adjusting to changes in the patient's condition and circumstances.

- The timeframe is different. In the acute care system events are experienced in the present. Success is measured by relatively immediate improvement. In the world of chronic illness, the future plays a big role. Efforts are undertaken now to realize benefits later.

- The roles of patients and clinicians are different. For acute conditions, patients seek and clinicians provide a diagnosis and treatment. Chronically ill patients, in contrast, live with their condition 24 hours a day, 7 days a week. Clinicians see the patients only occasionally for brief visits. Patients must play a vital role in managing their condition. Clinicians and patients must share responsibility for care decisions and outcomes.

To illustrate these differences, consider Mr. Jones and Mr. McCormick in the two vignettes. Mr. Jones's prompt and aggressive care restored his health. The clinicians successfully repaired his blocked arteries and, after a brief rehabilitation, he was able to resume his former life with only minor changes, although he may be motivated to change his lifestyle to prevent a recurrence. For Mr. McCormick, the goals are both more modest and more difficult to achieve. Successfully managing his multiple conditions will likely only slow the inexorable decline in his health and functioning. This will require vigilant monitoring and frequent adjustments in his treatment and care. Mr. Jones's encounter with the health care system was over in a matter of weeks. Since returning to work, he views the heart attack and the bypass surgery as discrete events in his past. In contrast, Mr. McCormick's experiences with diabetes and his other conditions are ongoing and ever-present; they profoundly influence his daily life and also his future—both in terms of his prognosis and in how he thinks about his life and his own plans for the future. Much of his daily care is done with an eye toward reducing the risk of complications that may not occur for another 10 or 15 years. Finally, Mr. Jones's surgeons performed the bypass surgery on him. Though he gave his informed consent to the procedure, he had little input into how, when, and by whom the surgery was performed. He was a passive recipient of the surgery team's professional services. Only after his brief rehabilitation therapy ended was Mr. Jones expected to assume some responsibility for reducing his risk factors for heart problems. Mr. McCormick, on the other hand, has to actively manage his chronic conditions. He is responsible for the day-to-day management of his conditions, bridging the time between his brief—albeit relatively frequent—visits with his clinicians.

Different Goals of Care

Acute care aims to cure. In contrast, managing a degenerative condition to mitigate functional limitations and maximize quality of life is the central aim of chronic illness care. Although it is easy to talk about the differences between curing a condition and managing its impact, it is harder to accept the consequences of that distinction. We live in a world that celebrates success and expects triumphs. Emergency medicine is lauded because people come in seriously injured or sick and often live. Such an experience requires no statistics to be seen as a success. If someone who seems about to die is saved, the results of care are apparent.

In the world of chronic care, successes are far less dramatic and often hidden. Frequently, the most effective care means nothing happens. No exacerbations occur. No one is rushed to the emergency room or hospitalized. No new symptoms develop. Managing chronic illnesses is not seen—by either clinicians or the public—to be as exciting as replacing a diseased organ or saving the life of an injured victim. We are not nearly so good at celebrating the types of success possible in chronic illness care. In many instances we do not even know how to measure them.

This difficulty in defining and measuring success in chronic care derives, in part, from the multiplicity of goals. One goal of chronic care is to avoid (or at least minimize) the frequency and extent of exacerbations and thereby slow the inevitable decline over time. Chronic conditions are generally progressive, although the clinical course may have remissions and exacerbations. For chronically ill patients, who are typically on a downward clinical trajectory, success must be measured by comparing what happened as a result of care with what would otherwise have happened without care. In essence, the key to assessing the success of chronic care is to compare the patient's actual clinical course with the expected course. This is difficult to measure because for much of chronic care, success lies not so much in changing the direction of the course (i.e., moving from decline to improvement) as in slowing the rate of decline. That slowing is invisible; it is apparent only when contrasted to the alternative clinical course.

Figure 1.1 presents a simple graphic display of the effects of good chronic care. The solid line shows the actual clinical course with good care. The patient's condition is getting worse over time. That is the picture the patient and the clinician see; despite good efforts, the condition is worsening. However, the figure also shows a dotted line, which represents the clin-

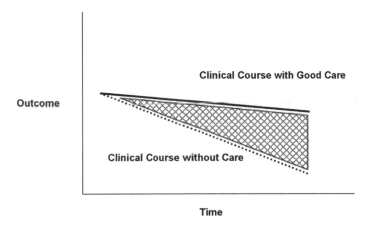

FIGURE 1.1.

Clinical course for chronic condition.

ical course without treatment. The hatched area between those lines represents the gains achieved by good care. Unfortunately these benefits are invisible unless we have the ability to estimate the difference between the two lines. In the absence of such data, both patients and clinicians can become disheartened, and good care can go unappreciated.

Another goal of chronic care is to maintain patients' sense of normality, while allowing them to adjust to the reality of having an often serious problem. Although chronic care should not deny the reality of the chronic condition—which may be life shaping, changing even the way in which patients view themselves—it should encourage patients to not let the condition dominate their lives any more than is necessary. Chronic care should similarly allow patients to assume an active role in managing their illness, without letting this task overwhelm their life. Finally, chronic care should integrate health care with other aspects of patients' lives without medicalizing those aspects. Maintaining such balance, however, is notoriously difficult.

Delineating the goals of chronic care for an individual patient is no easy task. It may involve defining and also distinguishing between short-term and long-term agendas. It may require choosing between competing outcomes (for example, reducing pain or improving function). Such a process does not come about easily. It requires facilitation and structure, but few clinicians are taught even the rudiments of such decision counseling. The process becomes even more complex when families are involved. Often opinions vary among family members or between patients and their families and long-standing conflicts may emerge.

Different Timelines

The very concept of chronicity implies a different meaning of time. Moving from individual visits between patient and clinician and other discrete health care *encounters* for acute conditions to *episodes* of chronic illness is like switching from a series of photographs to a movie. For chronic care, the change in a person's illness is more important than a single observation at any given point in time. Assessing and evaluating such changes requires, at a minimum, having a continuous stream of information that can detect alterations in a person's status. Effective chronic illness care must then respond to such changes, providing ongoing monitoring and management of the chronic condition and prompting responses to any unexpected events.

Because chronic care is long-term, patient-clinician encounters are best viewed as part of an ongoing planning and review process, continually subject to revision and adjustment to deal with changes over time. At the periodic encounters that punctuate this process, the clinician and patient will need to consider what has changed in the patient and his or her environment, how the patient has responded to the treatment prescribed, and what alterations in the patient's behavior or treatment regimen may need to be made. As part of a larger process, the encounter itself has no definitive beginning or end. Information gained from monitoring the patient's condition and questions the patient or clinician plan to ask of each other are brought into the visit, while any prescribed changes in the patient's treatment or behavior serve to pull the visit into the future, even after the face-to-face visit has ended.

Even under the best of circumstances, good clinical decision making takes time, but the current medical care system seems to be structured to provide little time for such contemplation. Decisions about surgery are often made literally under the knife. Hospital discharge plans, which may affect the course of the rest of a person's life, are expected to be made in less than 24 hours. Without structure and preplanning it is unlikely that the brief clinician-patient encounters, today lasting on average about 18 minutes, are long enough to permit good clinical decisions for patients with chronic conditions (Mechanic, McAlpine, & Rosenthal, 2001). Better decision making will require adequate time, adequate information, and a structure that ensures clinicians and patients (and often their families) will have the opportunity for careful thought concerning each component of the encounter—the preparation for the encounter, the encounter itself, and any follow-up.

Different Patient and Provider Roles

Traditionally, clinical decisions have been made by health care professionals, who then turn to the patient for concurrence. Effective chronic illness care will require an inversion, or at a minimum an adjustment, in the balance of power between clinician and patient. Such care may also demand a reallocation of tasks. The very term "patient" may need to be replaced because it implies a need to wait in some subordinate role. Because patients are the ones who live with chronic illness, they must play an active role in its management. This means they must be involved in making decisions about their care at all levels. Patients are also the logical source for much information about their conditions, including the impact on their lives and any changes in their health that occur between visits with their clinicians. They will therefore need to become more educated about what to look for and how to respond to changes.

The idea of patients playing an active role in managing their illnesses is hardly new. Some diabetics have been doing just this for years. They are initially taught the symptoms of low and high blood sugar, how to measure their blood sugar levels, and how to respond to them, for example, by adjusting their insulin doses and carefully controlling everyday food intake, and then often becoming experts in their own unique responses. These types of tasks and responsibilities need to be carried over to other chronic illnesses. The challenge lies in how to encourage patients to play an active role in their care without making their illnesses the dominant aspects of their lives.

If patients are to play a real role in decision making regarding the management of their chronic conditions, they will need to have access to the same information as their clinicians. Indeed, if patients are to assume more responsibility for decisions about their own care, the clinician's role may become one of information collector and purveyor. To make truly informed decisions, patients may need to identify the outcomes they most want to maximize and the risks they most want to avoid. Their clinicians, in turn, may need to provide their own insights, drawn from science and experience, about the extent of those risks and benefits. Patients and their clinicians would then jointly develop the care management plans most likely to achieve the patients' goals.

If patients are to become partners in decision making, they must also be prepared to share the responsibility for the consequences of those decisions. Our society has not yet come to grips with how to operationalize such sharing. Ours is a litigious society. We will need to separate responsibility for poor delivery of services, or poor accomplishment of procedures, from poor decisions about the necessity of those actions. The new roles and responsibilities of clinicians are discussed in chapter 5; issues related to the patients' role in managing their own chronic conditions are further discussed in chapter 6.

Defining the Territory

Chronic illness care is a vast and complex concept; clear at the center, but increasingly imprecise as you approach the margins. Examining the terms that are central to "chronic illness care" will illuminate the scope of both the concept itself and of this book. This is easier said than done, however, because there are multiple definitions and little consensus on the meaning of relevant terms. In addition to the common-usage meanings in everyday speech and writings, terms such as "chronic illness" and "disability" are defined by a variety of private and public agencies and organizations concerned with health and disability issues. But these agencies and organizations do not share common, unambiguous definitions of the terms. Health insurance companies, for example, define some of the terms with great precision to regulate access to and payment for services, but the definitions vary considerably across insurers. Many of the terms are also defined in a variety of state and federal statutes. Here, too, the definitions vary; even within the same jurisdiction a single term may be defined differently. At the federal level, for example, "disability" under the Social Security Act is defined narrowly with reference to a person's inability to work, whereas the term under the Americans with Disabilities Act (ADA) focuses more broadly on a person's inability to engage in the normal activities of daily living.

How the central terms are defined is important, for the definitions not only delineate, for example, what is and is not a disease, but also directly and indirectly influence the health care system's responses and our individual and societal attitudes. Again using "disability" as an example, the term may be defined, for instance, as a physical or mental impairment that is directly caused by disease, trauma, or other health condition and that interferes with or prohibits an individual from performing the normal activities of daily life. In this view, a disability would typically require medical care in the form of individual treatment provided by health care professionals. The goal of the care would be to alleviate the disability or to help the individual adjust and modify his or her behavior. Alternatively, disability may be defined not solely as an attribute of an individual but with reference to external factors as well, including the individual's social and physical environment. According to this latter definition, a disability would not result only from the person's impairment or functional limitation but would arise in combination with the social and physical environment that fails to meet the person's needs and from the ways other people perceive disabilities. The interaction of a person's impairment with social and environmental factors, not the impairment alone, determines whether the person has a disability. In other words, a person's disability would be seen not just as a physical condition, but as a social issue as well (Pope & Tarlov, 1991).

Disease

One perspective, using the biological model of disease, defines "disease" narrowly, with reference to changes in a person's body. Disease is a value-free concept, rooted in biology and chemistry, and refers to any abnormality or deviation from what is normal, species-typical functioning (Caplan, Englehardt, & McCartney, 1981). Diseases thus mark the presence of biological malfunction and indicate pathological (i.e., abnormal) changes in the body.

Another perspective uses the social model of disease and adopts a normative or value-laden approach. With this model, the concept of disease is culture dependent and its definition depends on sociological, culturally determined value judgments (Englehardt, 1995). Describing the status of a person's body or mind or the functional output of an organ or organ system is not enough to say whether the person has a disease. Thus, although a pathological change in the body or a deviation from the norm is necessary, it does not by itself indicate the presence of disease. Instead, in the social model of disease, "the only way to transform a biological fact into a disease ascription is by assessing the biological fact in the light of functions, capacities, abilities, and powers that are considered desirable or undesirable, useful or useless, good or bad" (Caplan, Englehardt, & McCartney, 1981). The existence of a disease requires both an empirical fact (i.e., a pathological change in the body) and a value judgment regarding that fact.

Because the value judgments that indicate the presence of a disease can vary across cultures (and over time within a given culture), what is a disease in one context or social setting may not be so in another. In cultures where certain conditions are very common, they are accepted as normal, much as we view the changes associated with aging. For example, in some developing nations people generally do not seek (nor do health care professionals offer) treatment for cataracts until the condition is relatively advanced. Because neither the public nor health care professionals recognize early stages of cataracts as a problem in need of medical attention, early-stage cataracts would not be identified as a "disease." In contrast, in the United States, early-stage cataracts are viewed as undesirable and in need of medical attention and thus characterized as a disease. Indeed, we may screen for these to address them earlier. With the biological model, in contrast, whether early-stage cataracts are or are not a disease would be answered solely with an appeal to biology and "normal species-typical functioning."

Illness

To some, "disease" and "illness" are nearly synonymous and any distinctions between these concepts are without a meaningful difference. Most people agree, however, that it is important to distinguish between them. Disease is the biological cause of a person's malady and is defined primarily in terms of the body and its systems. In contrast, illness embraces the person's experience of the disease, including its symptoms as well as the more complex and difficult-to-measure consequences such as pain, distress, and suffering. Accordingly, illness is a broader concept that, from the patient's perspective, encompasses both the disease processes and the experience of the disease's impact on his or her body, existence, and life. A disease is something you have; an illness is an altered state of being. One person with a chronic condition captured this broader dimension by writing about her chronic illness in terms of her experience of "illness-as-lived:"

> Illness is fundamentally experienced as a loss of wholeness. This loss is the perception of bodily impairment, not so much a simple recognition of the specific impairment but a loss of a sense of bodily integrity . . . The body can no longer be taken for granted or ignored. It has seemingly assumed an opposing will of its own, beyond the control of the self. Rather then functioning effectively at the bidding of the self, the body-in-malfunctioning thwarts plans, impedes choices, renders actions impossible. Illness disrupts the fundamental unity between the body and self. Illness is experience not only as a threat to the body but to the self. (Toombs, 1987)

The distinction between disease and illness is crucial for chronic care. Care that treats only the disease itself, relieving its signs and symptoms and aiming to cure the body, will not effectively respond to all dimensions of a chronic condition. Rather, effective chronic care must also address the impact of the disease on the person, by relieving the pain and suffering of the person who is experiencing the disease, seeking to minimize functional limitations, and responding to other subjective experiences that result from or accompany the disease.

Chronic Illness, Chronic Conditions

Some use "chronic condition" and "chronic illness" interchangeably. Others, however, distinguish between the two and use "chronic condition" as an umbrella term encompassing chronic illness as well as impairments, where the latter term refers to all losses of function or physiological, psychological, or anatomical abnormalities (e.g., hearing loss). In this book, we use "chronic illnesses" and "chronic conditions" as synonyms, where both terms include losses or abnormalities that are due to active pathology (e.g., blindness due to glaucoma) as well as developmental disorders (e.g., cerebral palsy, autism) and conditions caused by injuries (e.g., spinal cord injuries).

Disability

Disability refers to the functional consequences of a patient's impairment or disease. It can be defined broadly as any limitation in a person's usual activity or more narrowly as a physical or mental impairment that substantially limits one or more of the major life activities of an individual (Americans with Disabilities Act). While there is considerable overlap, not all people with disabilities have a chronic condition and the majority of people with chronic conditions have no disability (fig. 1.2). For example, although many people with hypertension (one of the most common chronic conditions) are not

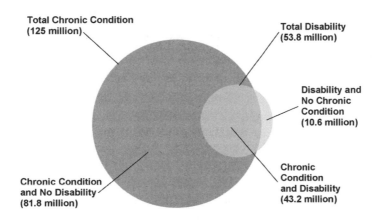

FIGURE 1.2.

Overlap of chronic conditions and disability among noninstitutionalized Americans, 2000.

Data from Anderson and Knickman, 2001.

limited in their activity in any meaningful way, people with dyslexia or a similar learning disability do not have a chronic condition.

Handicap

In the 1977 International Classification of Impairment, Disability and Handicap (ICIDH), the World Health Organization defined "handicap" as "a societal disadvantage for a given individual that limits or prevents the performance of a social role or participation." In recent years, use of this term has dropped steadily, "out of deference to those who feel that handicap is a denigrating term when used to describe a person" (Pope & Tarlov, 1991). In 2001, the WHO joined a long list of organizations, including the federal government and its various agencies, in ending its use of the term.

Chronic Care

Chronic care encompasses a broad range of health, medical, and supportive services to treat and manage a chronic condition. It includes but also entails moving beyond episodic, symptomatic acute care services that treat the patient's medical problems. The full range of services that constitute chronic illness care includes:

- Primary prevention. Services to prevent the initial onset of a chronic condition include immunizations and education programs to help individuals modify their behavior (e.g., smoking) to reduce their risk

- Screening programs to identify people at higher risk for a chronic condition

- Tests and procedures to diagnose a chronic condition

- Medical and/or surgical interventions to treat a chronic condition to reverse, stop, or slow the progression of the condition

- Medical and/or surgical interventions to treat acute exacerbations of a chronic condition (e.g., acute asthma attack)

- Medical and/or surgical interventions to treat an unrelated acute condition in a patient with a chronic condition, such as a respiratory tract infection in a patient with diabetes

- Complementary and alternative medicine, such as acupuncture, naturopathic medicine, aromatherapy, and other practices and products that are not presently considered to be part of conventional Western medicine

• Supportive services, including counseling; physical, speech, and occupational therapy; rehabilitation; assistance with diet, exercise, and other lifestyle issues; self-care skills; and patient education about and support for managing their illness

• "Indirect" services such as case management, care coordination, assessment, and geriatric evaluation and management (GEM)

• Long-term care, such as:

Informal (i.e., unpaid) support and care from family and friends
Formal (i.e., paid) care, including personal care, meals, homemaking, and other home care or community-based supportive (custodial) services
Supportive services in nursing homes and assisted living settings
Technologies such as assistive devices and environmental adaptations in housing

In this book we use the terms "chronic care" and "chronic illness care" interchangeably. (We do not use "chronic disease care.") Both terms are meant to capture the full spectrum of health and supportive services needed to appropriately respond to the ways in which a chronic condition affects a person's life and health.

Long-term Care

Chronic care and long-term care are closely intertwined and overlap. However, there are important differences. In contrast to chronic care, long-term care is a narrower concept and is defined as "personal care and assistance that an individual might receive on a long-term basis because of a disability or chronic illness that limits his or her ability to function" (Kane & Kane, 1987). Long-term care includes medical, social, personal care, and supportive services that help those in need perform what are called the Activities of Daily Living (ADL) and Instrumental Activities of Daily Living (IADL). ADLs refer to six basic personal activities required for daily life: bathing, dressing, grooming, feeding, toileting and transfer (getting around inside the home). More complex tasks such as cooking, light and heavy housework, grocery shopping, using the telephone, managing money and paying bills, are examples of IADLs. Most people who need long-term care have underlying chronic illnesses. Thus, good long-term care must be actively tied to chronic care. Unfortunately, these two worlds are often represented as reflecting conflicting social and medical models. In truth, it should not be necessary to forgo one to achieve the other.

Summary

Acute conditions and chronic conditions differ on a variety of important dimensions. So, too, does the appropriate response to these two categories of ailments. Treating and managing chronic conditions entails moving beyond episodic, symptomatic acute care services and addressing the myriad ways in which these conditions affect patients' functioning, their lives, and the lives of those who care for them. Individuals with chronic conditions receive care from the same health care system as people with acute conditions. But the same system that works well for discrete acute events does not work well for continuous chronic conditions. To provide optimal chronic care, a new approach, indeed a new philosophy of care, is needed. The new approach must differ from the old in terms of goals, timelines, and the roles of clinicians and patients. Whereas acute care aims to cure, managing a degenerative condition to mitigate functional limitations and maximize quality of life is the central aim of chronic illness care. Because chronic care is long-term, patient/clinician encounters are best viewed as part of an ongoing planning and review process and what occurs away from health care settings is at least as important as what takes place while patients are in the hospital, clinic, or clinicians' office. Effective chronic illness care will require an inversion or, at a minimum, an adjustment in the balance of power between clinician and patient.

2. The Dimensions of Chronic Illness

♣ When I awoke one morning at age 12, with pain in my ankles, knees, hips, and wrists, I did not realize that my life would be changed forever. I was diagnosed with juvenile rheumatoid arthritis (JRA). The prognosis was grim. I was told I would never go to college, never get married, never have children, never lead a normal life. Instead, I would need to live my life in bed, with others caring for me day and night.

Arthritis affects every joint in my body. I now take 23 different medications, over 50 pills every day. I have had over 60 surgical procedures. I have only five original large joints remaining in my body—two ankles, two elbows, and one wrist. My family and friends call me the bionic woman.

Life with a chronic illness is complicated—certainly more so than it should be. Simple things become difficult. For instance, because I can't raise my arms high enough, caring for my hair is a challenge. I rest my arm on one of the grab bars in our shower and with shampoo in hand, bend my head down and wash my hair. To apply hair spray, and not spray it all over the wall and mirror, I put the spray can on a towel rack, stabilize the can and use two fingers to press the spray button, rotating my head in the spray.

Shoes, socks, buttons, and earrings present unique obstacles. I have a long, flexible shoe horn to get shoes on. To tie them I need to put my foot on a stool and lean against a wall for balance. When I can't manage alone, I do what anyone else would do—go to my local pharmacy (with which I had a wonderful, caring relationship for over 30 years) and ask the pharmacist to help button the buttons, tie the shoes, put my earrings in my ears, and whatever else I need help with.

There was a time I bought all my prescription medications through this pharmacy. They treated me like I was family. Because I have difficulty with the caps used for medicine bottles, they kept a supply of the easy-open containers in a box labeled "Gay's bottles." The pharmacists knew all the medications I took, what I'd tried previously, and the results. When there was a question, I would always receive a call for clarification. Or they would follow-up with the doctor's office.

Now I'm "forced" to buy my prescriptions through the mail. Insurers say it's more cost-effective. The "one-size-fits-all" mentality of these companies costs a very heavy price. For example, I cannot be approved for certain medications until it's been proven that I've already tried at least two other drugs in the same family and that neither helped. Many times deliveries of my medications are delayed. Decisions are made about me without ever consulting either me or the doctor who prescribed the medication. Generic drugs are substituted for brand-name drugs or prescriptions are not filled and no one notifies me. To them, I'm just an account number.

Today, HMOs have forced doctors to reduce the time spent with each patient. Doctors no longer take a personal interest in their patients' personal lives. Granted, I am an HMO's worst nightmare, but I still deserve to be treated as a person. I feel as if I'm penalized even more for having a chronic illness. Companies such as these choose not to care about patient needs because it might cost them a little more.

It took me 15 years after my original diagnosis to finally find a rheumatologist who could help. He and I developed a partnership for my health care. I'm alive and thriving today, largely because of that partnership. He encouraged me to learn more about my illness, become my own advocate, and communicate effectively with the medical community. He was far more than just my doctor; he was my coach and cheerleader, too. He convinced me that no one can walk in my shoes, and that no one knows my body better than I do.

I now average one to two doctors' appointments every week, sometimes more. Through the years, I've learned a number of things. Among them are that I don't have to take "no" for an answer and I can say "I don't understand," and wait for them to explain until I do. Because managing my care requires a partnership between my doctor and me, information has to flow in both directions. If my doctors and staff cannot communicate with me, or I cannot communicate with them, they won't be part of my care team. And if I don't obtain the proper knowledge, I cannot take care of myself. The medical professionals who care for me become an integral part of my life and well-being.

I try to live my life in a positive way and look at it as an adventure. Life will not adapt to me, so I have to find a way to make my journey easier. I've always believed that it's mind over matter. If you don't mind, it doesn't matter.

Gay Bloom, Minneapolis

CAREGIVER VIGNETTE

♣ Like everyone else, I vividly recall September 11, 2001. But for me the day also signifies something more personal. My oldest brother died that day (for reasons unrelated to 9/11) and his death seemed to coincide with profound changes in my mother's and father's health.

I first helped my parents, both now 88 years old, deal with the grief of losing their oldest son. For my mom, however, the difficulties lay deeper. It seems almost as if my brother's death triggered a rapid decline in my mother's physical and mental health. She suffered a series of small strokes and also had a variety of serious medical complications that truly threatened her life at that time. As a result, she now has multiple health and supportive care needs.

Up until this time, it was my mother who mostly was managing the care-taking of my father, who has Alzheimer disease. My dad's needs are also many, although they are quite different from my mom's because he was and still is in robust physical health. Before my mom's strokes, she was able to do a good job of tending to my father's confusion. After 9/11, however, she no longer could manage this alone. These changes for both my parents were dramatic, because they were each thriving well into their eighties, living in-dependently in their own home in a suburb of St. Paul.

I am 54 years old, married, and a mother of two teen-aged sons. I am also a full-time psychologist with a private practice in Minneapolis. I am my parent's only daughter, the youngest of their three children. I am also now their primary caregiver and feel as if I am responsible for almost everything in their lives. My other brother is in on many of the decisions (regarding my parent's finances, housing, health care, and so on), but because he lives in Massachusetts, he can only provide indirect support, not the direct care.

My father has always been a dignified man exuding pride, authority, and control. He rarely, if ever, needed to rely on others; and certainly not on me—his daughter! I am not supposed to know more about his life than he does or be the one to manage legal, financial, health, and daily living issues for him. But neither he nor my mother can make these decisions any more. So they fall to me (and my brother). As a result, my relationship with my par-ents has flipped. Formerly, I enjoyed a peer relationship as an adult daugh-ter with a fondness for aging parents who were totally independent in their lives. Now I am responsible for them and they depend on me, frequently without knowing about it. So in one sense, my dad and mom are no longer my parents and I no longer expect anything from them. Our roles are dra-matically changed and, in the classic sense, reversed.

To make decisions, and get my father to accept them, requires a creative and well-thought-out strategy and the perseverance and emotional strength to see it through. Most of the time these plans require the help of others so that my dad does not know that I am the one who is managing them. I do this to avoid his intense anger born out of his own sense of pride, helpless-ness, and anxiety from an oblique understanding that he is no longer able to be in charge of his life and his decisions. For example, for his own safety and that of others, he needed to stop driving. Only by devising a complex, lengthy strategy, involving at various points his clinician, a private competency-testing agency, several very good friends, the local police, and the traffic court (after he drove on a revoked license), were we able to get the car and the car keys from him. Selling my parents' home and getting them to move to an assisted living facility (where they now live) required a similar, roundabout strategy, with me managing it from behind the scenes. These were ultimately successful strategies but also time consuming, anxiety producing, and exhausting. There are few resources to learn about doing such things and most families come to these situations without preparation.

I am always tired. Besides managing all their mail and paying their bills I also drive and participate in all my parent's many health care appointments. At a minimum, each trip takes 3 hours. I do this so that my parents' get the best health care possible, as they are no longer good reporters or collaborators regarding their health needs. I maintain my private practice, though at a reduced level, by scheduling my clients' appointments around these trips. Clearly, I couldn't do this if I were not self-employed and did not have a caring and supportive spouse who shares roles with me at home and also enjoys doing all the cooking.

When I visit my parents it seems I always have a list of secondary tasks as well—following up with them about any current living or health complaints, helping my mom schedule her hair and nail appointments (I have known since I was a small girl that these are essential ways she feels good about herself), making sure my parents have the right clothes available for the right season and that the clothes fit, trying to assess whether my dad is taking showers, checking the cabinets for supplies and shopping for essentials, making certain the phone is hung up and the clocks are working, watering the plants, and on and on. Too rarely do we merely gather as a family, wherein I visit them as just their daughter with my family along. I am their caregiver first now, their daughter second. I work hard to relax and just let myself be with them, to enjoy my dad's articulate, passionate, and interesting stories from his past (though they are mostly all repeats for me now), to share news with both of them, and to have the conversations I know my mom enjoys having with me.

My discretionary time has mostly slipped away. I miss time with my friends. I work to maintain my sense of humor, to relax, to play, to travel. Personal decisions that are hard to make get pushed to the bottom and sometimes are delayed too long. My own medical appointments do not get scheduled. Though the assisted living facility provides many services, there are still gaps that I must fill. What I can't do for my parent's myself, I arrange for others to do. I look forward to natural breaks in the caretaking for my mom and dad that come along the way, just as I am aware of worrying about what the newest serious medical situation will be.

For all the hardship and exhaustion, there is also much satisfaction. I am delighted that I still have both of my parents alive at this time in my and my children's lives. I would not change what I am doing or my level of involvement with my mom and dad. In circumstances such as mine, the amount of care and support provided can distract from the ever-increasing sense of loss. There has also been an amazing gift for me related to the last remaining psychological resolution within both of these important relationships in my life. And I truly experience the caregiving as a wonderful and concrete way to love each of them. Taking care of my mom's and dad's health, happiness, well-being, and daily comforts is what I want to do. At this particular time in their lives, this is my own way of loving these two dear people who each are so important to me. I can only hope that when the time comes, someone will love me in these ways as well.

Katherine Kegan, Ph.D., Minneapolis

The burdens of chronic illness fall most squarely on chronically ill people themselves but also affect their families and friends, their communities, and society as a whole. The effects are multiple and varied. Chronic conditions extract a physical, emotional, and financial toll from family members who provide care; they tax the expertise and fortitude of clinicians faced with patients whose inexorable decline challenges their roles as healers; they reduce productivity for employers due to time off (for both those who have chronic conditions and those who care for them); and they fuel rapidly escalating health care expenditures that are ultimately shared by all payers.

The overall burden of chronic illness in America is staggering:

- 125 million Americans report having at least one chronic condition and 60 million of them have more than one chronic condition (Wolff, Starfield, & Anderson, 2002)

- Chronic conditions account for more than 75% of total national health care expenditures

- Chronic conditions claim the lives of more than 1.7 million Americans each year, representing more than 7 of every 10 deaths

- Chronic conditions represent the top 4—and 7 of the top 10—leading causes of death among Americans of all ages (table 2.1)

Projections call for these burdens to increase:

- By 2020, a projected 157 million Americans will have at least one chronic

TABLE 2.1.
Ten Leading Causes of Death in the United States, 2000

Condition	Number of Deaths
Heart disease	710,760
Cancer	533,091
Stroke	167,661
Chronic lower respiratory tract disease	122,009
Accidents	97,900
Diabetes	69,301
Pneumonia/influenza	65,313
Alzheimer disease	49,558
Nephritis, nephritic syndrome, and nephrosis	37,251
Septicemia (blood poisoning)	31,224

Source: Data from Centers for Disease Control and Prevention, National Center for Health Statistics, www.cdc.gov/nchs/fastats/lcod.htm (accessed July 28, 2003).
Note: Chronic conditions in italics. Pneumonia and septicemia are often secondary to a chronic condition.

condition, an estimated 81 million (25% of the population) will have multiple chronic conditions (Wolff, Starfield, & Anderson, 2002)

• By 2020, more than 80% of all health care expenditures will be spent for people with chronic conditions (Wu & Green, 2000)

Moreover, the burden is not unique to the United States; every country faces similar problems. Chronic conditions are accelerating globally.

• Chronic conditions were responsible for 46% of the "global disease burden" in 2000; this disease burden will increase to 60% by the year 2020[1]

• Chronic conditions account for 70% of the world's deaths (World Health Organization, 2002)

In the United States, the prevalence of chronic conditions, that is, the proportion of Americans with a chronic condition at a particular time, is also increasing. That means the number of Americans with chronic conditions is rising faster than the population itself. The percent of the population with a chronic condition increased from 44.7 in 1995 to an estimated 45.4 in 2000 and is projected to rise to 48.3 in 2020, as shown in figure 2.1 (Partnership for Solutions, 2002a).

Although the reasons for the increase in the percentage of the population with a chronic condition are vigorously debated, among those typically seen as the most probable explanations are the many medical advancements that have enabled people to live longer; changes in Americans' diet, behavior, and lifestyle; and the aging of the population. Medical advancements such as new drugs and health care devices have transformed what were once

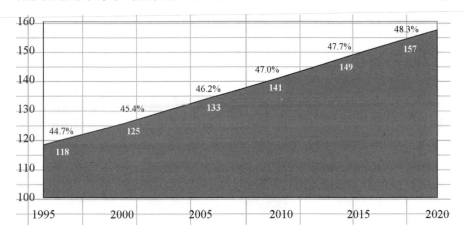

FIGURE 2.1.

U.S. population with a chronic condition, 1995–2020: Total number
(in millions) and percentage of population.

Partnership for Solutions, 2002a.

fatal, acute diseases into chronic conditions. For example, only a few years
ago, a diagnosis of HIV/AIDS invariably proved to be fatal for the patient
within a relatively short time. With the development of new treatments, such
as the so-called antiretroviral "drug cocktail," many patients with HIV/AIDS
now live 10 years or longer after their initial diagnosis. Changes in dietary
patterns, level of physical activity, and stress are among the behavior and
lifestyle factors that likewise affect the prevalence of chronic conditions. A
dramatic example of the influence of such risk factors is the rapid rise since
1980 in the number of Americans with type 2 diabetes mellitus, which has
been linked to changes in the American diet (Mokdad et al., 2001).

The aging population is also a factor because older adults are more
likely than younger people to have a chronic condition, especially since
chronic conditions accumulate with age. As Americans live longer, with a life
expectancy today of 76.9 years compared with 49.2 years in 1900, they are
more likely to develop and die of a chronic condition than an acute condition. However, the ultimate impact of the aging of the population on future
needs and costs of chronic care is a topic of much debate. Under one assumption, people will live longer but still get sick or become disabled at the
same age as now, lengthening the time spent sick or disabled. Under an alternative, "compressed morbidity" assumption people who take active preventive steps would live longer without disability or disease and compress
the time of sickness to the very end of their lives. A decline in the rate of dis-

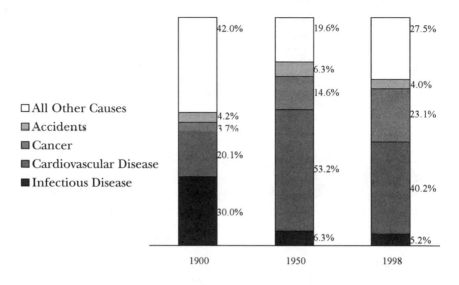

FIGURE 2.2.

Changes in the leading causes of death in the U.S. population, 1900–1998.

Data from U.S. Bureau of the Census, Statistical Abstract of the United States: 2000;
Robert Wood Johnson Foundation, 1996.

ability among older persons is now well documented (Cutler, 2001; Spill-man, 2004). Between 1984 and 1999, the number of older Americans who reported having a chronic disability declined from 22.1% to 19.7%. Most of this decline, however, is concentrated at lower levels of disability, a result of the decreasing rate of older persons who need assistance with activities such as shopping and financial management. During the same 15–year period there was almost no change in the rate of older persons with more severe disabilities, commonly due to chronic conditions (Spillman, 2004). Some people fear that the current pandemic of obesity, with all its negative health consequences, will offset this trend of declining disability (Flegal et al., 2002; Surgeon General, 2001).

At the same time that medical advances, behavior and lifestyle changes, and (possibly) the aging population have raised the prevalence of chronic conditions, a variety of public health initiatives and the large-scale introduction of vaccines and antibiotics have reduced the prevalence of many acute health conditions. Combined, these developments have led to a major shift in the pattern of diseases. As seen in figure 2.2, the morbidity and mortality profile of the American population has dramatically shifted over the past century from one heavily weighted toward acute conditions to a profile dominated by chronic conditions. Compared with previous decades, far fewer Americans today have or die of infectious diseases and other acute conditions.

Who Are the Chronically Ill?

"No one is immune to chronic conditions" (Summer, 1999). Anyone can have or develop a chronic condition and almost everyone will have a chronic condition at some point during his or her lifetime. Even though no one is immune, not everyone has the same odds of having or developing a chronic condition. Chronic conditions are not evenly or randomly distributed throughout a population. Instead, multiple interacting factors, including age, gender, socioeconomic factors such as poverty, cultural factors such as diet, environmental exposure, and genetic predispositions for certain types of chronic conditions, affect the rates of chronic conditions.

The chance of having a chronic condition increases steadily with age (fig. 2.3). This is no surprise, since chronic conditions are by definition long term, often life long, and thus accumulate as a person ages. In 2000, 84% of Americans aged 65 years and older reported having one or more chronic conditions. Among people aged 20–44 years 38% reported having at least one chronic condition. The prevalence of a chronic condition for the population as a whole was 45%. Older Americans are also more likely to have chronic conditions that are more disabling, such as arthritis and heart disease. Nonetheless, although the prevalence of chronic conditions is higher

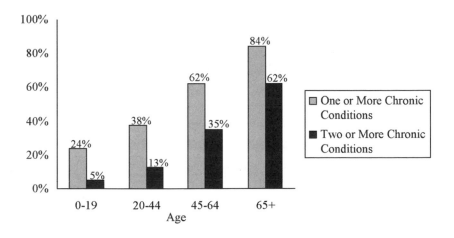

FIGURE 2.3.

Percentage of U.S. population with chronic conditions, by age.

Partnership for Solutions, 2002a.

among older persons, it is important to note that the absolute number of persons with chronic conditions is greater among the working-age population. In 2000, about 29 million Americans aged 65 years and older had one or more chronic condition, compared with more than 75 million Americans aged 20–64 years.

For the population as a whole, women are more likely than men to have a chronic condition. Among all ages, the five most common chronic conditions are, in order, hypertension, mental conditions, respiratory diseases, arthritis, and heart disease (fig. 2.4). Among specific age cohorts, however, the makeup and ranking of the five most common conditions differ. For example, among males, heart disease is one of the five most common chronic conditions for those aged 45 years and older; among females it is in the top five only for the 75 years and older age group. The prevalence of some chronic conditions also varies according to race. Overall, the proportion of blacks that have one or multiple chronic conditions is higher than the proportion of whites.

Chronic conditions disproportionately affect the poor, who are more likely to lack access to necessary health care services, may lack the resources needed to protect themselves from disease, and are more likely to have risk factors (e.g., tobacco use, overweight) associated with chronic conditions (Bach et al., 2004). Among Americans aged 50 years and older, for example, those with higher incomes are less likely to have multiple chronic conditions than those with lower incomes. The pernicious link between chronic conditions and poverty fuels a vicious cycle: chronic conditions can lead to poor health, which in turn can reduce the ability to participate in the work

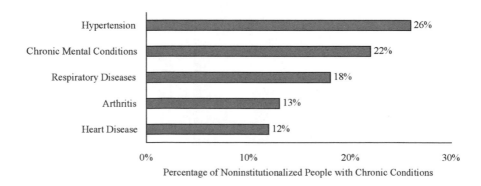

Percentage of Noninstitutionalized People with Chronic Conditions

FIGURE 2.4.

Five most common chronic conditions in the United States, 1998.

Partnership for Solutions, 2002a.

force, which can reduce the income available to pay for health care services, which (to complete and restart the cycle) can exacerbate the chronic condition and so on (World Health Organization, 2002). America's reliance on a job-based health insurance system only adds to the disparities in access to chronic care services and care quality among socioeconomic groups.

Multiple Chronic Conditions

Comorbidity is defined as having more than one medical condition at a time. For people with chronic conditions, comorbidity can be the direct result of the initial condition, as when a person's diabetes leads to blindness. It can also stem from the same risk factor, as when a person's smoking leads to both lung cancer and heart disease. Finally, comorbidity can be completely unrelated as, for example, in a person with hypertension and Alzheimer disease. Of course, people with chronic conditions may also have acute health problems that are unrelated to their chronic conditions.

Of the people who have at least one chronic condition, about 55% have only one and 45% have two or more chronic conditions. The number of chronically ill Americans in 2000 with more than one chronic condition was estimated at 60 million, about 21% of the total population (fig. 2.5). This number is projected to rise to 81 million by 2020 (Partnership for Solutions, 2002a). Not only are people more likely to have a chronic condition as they get older, they are then also more likely to have multiple chronic conditions. About 70% of people aged 65 years and older have two or more chronic con-

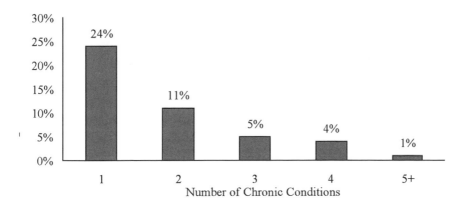

FIGURE 2.5.

Percentage of U.S. population with one or multiple chronic conditions, 2000.

Partnership for Solutions, 2002a.

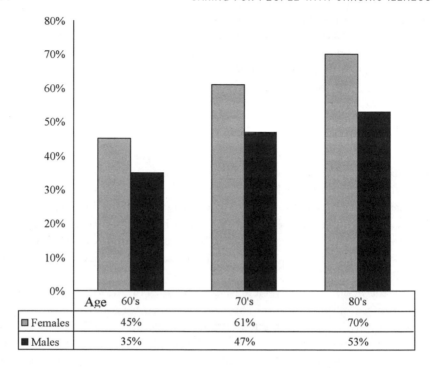

Age	60's	70's	80's
▣ Females	45%	61%	70%
■ Males	35%	47%	53%

FIGURE 2.6.

Percentage of elderly U.S. population with multiple chronic conditions,
by age and gender.

Robert Wood Johnson Foundation, 1996.

ditions, compared with only 13% of adults aged 20–44 years. Also, women
are more likely to have comorbidities than men; for example, among people in their sixties who are chronically ill, 45% of women have a comorbidity, compared with 35% of men (fig. 2.6).

Impact of Chronic Conditions

Some chronic conditions severely limit daily activities and change the way
people live, whereas others are less disruptive. Most people with chronic conditions live in their community and most of them lead active, productive
lives. Only a minority reside in a nursing home, hospital, or other institution. Nonetheless, the burden on people with chronic conditions—even for
those who seem to be doing well—can be overwhelming. The impact often
extends far beyond a person's physical and mental health. Chronic condi-

tions can disrupt a person's relationships with his or her spouse, children, or other family members; challenge their friendships and social life; interfere with their ability to earn a living; and impose substantial financial hardship (Pearlin et al., 1990; Zarit, 1996). People with chronic conditions have said that their illness changes almost every aspect of their lives.

Impact on Peoples' Health

The overall health status of people who report having a chronic condition is worse than the general population. About 56% of all Americans say their overall health is excellent or very good, compared with only 25% of those who report having a chronic condition. Similarly, about 33% of those with one or more chronic conditions describe their health as fair or poor, compared with only 13% of the total population (fig. 2.7). People with certain chronic conditions are even more likely to identify their health status as fair or poor, including those with coronary artery disease (42%), diabetes (40%), and arthritis (34%) (Robert Wood Johnson Foundation, 2002).

People with chronic conditions are about twice as likely to have a "bad health day" as other Americans (Robert Wood Johnson Foundation, 2002). Although12% of the general population report having at least 7 bad physical health days in the past 30, over 40% of people with arthritis and coronary artery disease report having at least that many. About 14% of people with chronic conditions report having a bad physical health day *every day,* confirming their extremely poor physical health (Robert Wood Johnson Foundation, 2002).

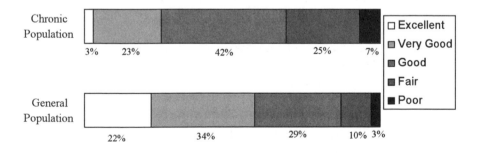

FIGURE 2.7.

Self-reported health status of general adult and chronic adult populations, 2001.

Reprinted with the permission of the Robert Wood Johnson Foundation in Princeton, New Jersey.

The impact of chronic conditions has also been measured by the degree to which a person's daily activities are limited. A person's activity limitation can be defined as "a long-term reduction in a person's capacity to perform" the major activity usually associated with their particular age group (Robert Wood Johnson Foundation, 1996). The "major activity" associated with particular age groups are, for example, "attending school" for children ages 5–17 years, and "working and keeping house" for working-age adults. With these definitions, people with chronic conditions can then be classified into one of four categories with regard to their activity limitation:

- 58% are not limited in any way

- 12% are not limited in a major activity but are limited in the kind and amount of other activities

- 17% are able to perform the major activity but limited in the kind and amount of this activity

- 12% are unable to perform the major activity (Robert Wood Johnson Foundation, 1996)

In general, people with multiple chronic conditions are more likely to have activity limitations, with the extent of limitation directly related to the number of conditions.

Impact on Use of Health Care Services

People with chronic conditions are heavy users of health care services (fig. 2.8). They account for nearly 76% of hospital admissions, 80% of total hospital days, 55% of emergency room visits, 88% of prescriptions, 96% of home care visits, and 72% of physician visits (Partnership for Solutions, 2002a; Robert Wood Johnson Foundation, 1996). On average, people with chronic conditions see a doctor more often—7.4 visits per year, compared with 1.7 visits for people with no chronic conditions (Partnership for Solutions, 2002a).

The use of most types of health care services increases with each additional chronic condition. While people with 1 chronic condition on average have 3.5 physician visits annually, people with 3 chronic conditions have 7.7 annual visits; for people with 5 or more chronic conditions, the number of visits rises to 14.8. Similarly, people with 3 chronic conditions are more than twice as likely to be hospitalized than those with only 1 chronic condition (Partnership for Solutions, 2002a).

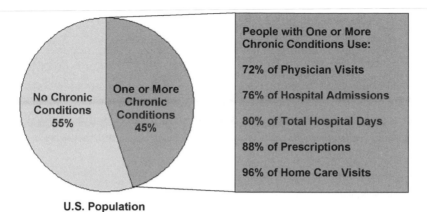

U.S. Population

FIGURE 2.8.

Use of health care services by people with chronic conditions.

Data from Partnership for Solutions, 2002a, and Robert Wood Johns Foundation, 1996.

Impact on Access to Health Care

People with chronic conditions are in special need of frequent and prompt access to health care. Although the vast majority of chronically ill people have a regular doctor, many do not get timely access to the services they need or do not receive those services at all. Nearly one in five report not getting a timely appointment when they needed care and 12% could not get the care as soon as they needed it (Robert Wood Johnson Foundation, 2002). Some needs go unmet altogether: about two-thirds of chronically ill persons who say they need home health or personal care services say they do not receive them (Robert Wood Johnson Foundation, 2002).

Among the barriers to getting needed chronic illness care are the cost of care and the lack of assistance with coordinating needed services. Although people with chronic conditions are more likely to have health care coverage (about 7% are uninsured, compared with 15% of the overall population) paying for care is still difficult for them. More than 2 of every 5 say the financial burden associated with their chronic condition is a problem and an additional 17% say it is a "major problem." Nine of ten people with chronic conditions report difficulties in obtaining insurance. Among those who obtain insurance, 22% report that it does not cover all the types of care they need (Harris Interactive Inc., 2001).

The high cost of care is an even greater barrier to care for persons with certain chronic conditions. For example, 32% of people with depression were not able to get medical care sometime in the past year because they could not afford it, compared with 23% of the overall population (Robert Wood Johnson Foundation, 2002). Problems in accessing needed medical care are typically more severe for people with chronic conditions who are from households with low income, without insurance coverage, and among African Americans and Hispanics, groups that already have higher than average rates of chronic conditions (Robert Wood Johnson Foundation, 2002). As would also be expected, access difficulties are compounded for people with multiple chronic conditions.

Impact on Families

Family members and friends are the "first line of support" for many people with chronic conditions. An estimated 52 million spouses, children, siblings, other relatives, and friends serve as informal (that is, unpaid) caregivers. Typically, one family member—most often a spouse or adult daughter— serves as the primary caregiver, sometimes with assistance from other family members and friends. Women are nearly twice as likely to be caregivers as men. Over one third (38%) of caregivers are age 55 years and older, with the likelihood of being a caregiver greatest for individuals between ages 55 and 64 (Partnership for Solutions, 2002a).

The type and amount of care provided by informal caregivers varies and includes assisting with physical tasks such as cooking and shopping, managing financial and legal issues, coordinating health care, and providing assistance with personal care such as bathing and eating. What caregivers provide most often, however, is emotional support and companionship to the care recipient. Caregivers who live in the same household as the care recipient provide more types of assistance and are far more likely to provide personal care assistance. They also provide more hours of care per week, 36.6 hours per week compared with 13 hours if the recipient lives outside the household. The number of caregiving hours increases with the age of the caregiver, from less than 15 hours per week for caregivers aged 15–24 years to more than 34 hours per week for caregivers older than 74 years. The number of hours devoted to caregiving is also affected by the competing demands caregivers face. Those who are employed full-time, for example, provide about 19 hours of care per week, compared with nearly 30 hours for caregivers who are not employed. On average, caregivers provide assistance to a family member or friend for 5 years. Although spouses provide care for more hours per week on average than other caregivers, adult children provide care for the longest periods of time, 9.6 years (Alcecxih, Zeruld, & Olearczyk, 2001).

Many informal caregivers report no or minimal untoward effects of their helping role and describe caregiving in positive terms (Kramer, 1997). Some caregivers "simply survive," whereas still others suffer severe consequences (Montgomery & Kosloski, 2001). The overall physical, emotional, and financial hardships of caregiving are collectively referred to as "caregiver burden."

Studies of caregiver burden have documented a wide range of negative consequences. Some of these stem from the physical demands of caregiving. For example, caregivers report difficulty in lifting or moving their care recipient or in performing personal care tasks. Far more common are psychological and emotional burdens, including feelings of isolation, family conflict, and the loss of friends and activities as a result of caregiving. The time-consuming responsibilities of caregiving inflict various limitations on the caregiver's life, including restrictions on one's personal and social life. How to balance the competing demands of the care recipient, other family obligations, and employment responsibilities is a major challenge. Full-time employees, for instance, find that caregiving responsibilities can affect their careers in many ways. In one survey nearly 40% reported that caregiving affected their ability to advance in their job (for example, 29% passed up a job promotion, training, or assignment). Caregiving obligations can also reduce a worker's income (e.g., through reduced hours worked).

Caregiving spouses often worry about their own health and what would happen if they became ill, and experience some form of generalized anxiety about the future. The emotional and physical strains of caregiving can also lead to deterioration in the caregiver's own health. Almost one in five caregivers suffer from depression, nearly twice the rate in the general population (Robert Wood Johnson Foundation, 2002). Caregivers must also often adjust to a new role since being a caregiver may change the former relationship between the caregiver and the care recipient.

The degree of caregiver stress increases as the care recipient's level of functional impairment becomes more severe. In general, caregiver burdens are usually more pronounced when the care recipient has Alzheimer disease or another form of dementia. Disruptive behavior and improper social functioning, such as aggressiveness, forgetfulness, repetitive behaviors, embarrassing behaviors, wandering, and sleep cycle disturbances, are key factors in explaining why dementia caregiving is so difficult for most informal caregivers.

Caregiver burden may be a particular concern for the growing number of people in the so-called "sandwich generation," primarily adults in their fifties. Nearly 75% of people aged 50 to 54 years have at least one living child and one living parent. As family size continues to decrease among American families and family support networks get smaller, the number of family

TABLE 2.2.
Out-of-Pocket Spending per Person, by Age and Number of Chronic
Conditions, 1996

Age	Spending per Person				
	All	Healthy	1 disease	2 diseases	≥3 diseases
Total population	$427	$249	$433	$733	$1,134
0–19 years old	219	170	288	502	441
20–44 years old	337	258	380	616	814
45–64 years old	593	356	553	186	1,055
65–79 years old	777	421	610	815	1,130
80 years or older	1,162	617	540	1,074	1,828

Source: Adapted from Hwang et al., 2001.

members who simultaneously care for their children and for their own parents or elderly relatives will likely increase.

Impact on Personal Health Care Spending

On average, people with chronic conditions pay more for health care out of their own pocket than other Americans. Out-of-pocket expenditures include coinsurance, deductibles, and payments for health care services, drugs, and supplies that are not covered by the person's health insurance.[2] Among all Americans who used health care services in 1996, the average out-of- pocket expenditure was $427 per person (table 2.2). As would be expected, out-of-pocket spending across all ages was lowest for people with no chronic condition ($297), higher for people with one chronic condition ($433), and increased for each additional chronic condition, up to $1,134 for people with three or more chronic conditions (Hwang et al., 2001). It is not unusual for a family with one member who has multiple chronic conditions to spend more than 10% of their total income on health care.

A positive, linear relationship between out-of-pocket expenditures and the number of chronic conditions existed across all age groups. Such expenditures were highest for people older than 80 years of age with three or more chronic conditions ($1,828). High out-of-pocket spending for people with chronic conditions is likely to persist over multiple years, since such conditions are by definition long-term and the clinical course for most chronic conditions is toward progressively worse health and lower levels of functioning (Hwang et al., 2001).

Impact on National Health Care Expenditures

Direct health care expenditures for chronic conditions (which include expenditures for physician, hospital, and all other health care services) were estimated at $1 trillion in 2000, or 78% of all health care expenditures. Annual per person spending for persons with a chronic condition was about $6,000, or more than six times higher than for a healthy person ($800). Among persons with chronic conditions, average per capita health care expenditures go up rapidly with the number of chronic conditions, from $1,900 for people with one chronic condition to $11,500 for people with five or more such conditions. Overall, more than half of the nation's health care spending is for care for people with multiple chronic conditions (fig. 2.9).

Medicare expenditures are similarly concentrated among the program's enrollees who have multiple chronic conditions (fig. 2.10). In 1999, average per beneficiary spending for Medicare enrollees with one chronic condition was $1,154, $2,394 for those with two chronic conditions, and more than $13,973 for those with four or more chronic conditions. In contrast, per capita expenditures were only $211 for Medicare enrollees with no chronic conditions. Beneficiaries with two or more chronic conditions represent 65% of the Medicare population but are responsible for nearly 95% of total Medicare expenditures (Wolff, Starfield, & Anderson, 2002).

In addition to direct health care costs, chronic conditions create substantial indirect costs that affect all of society. These indirect costs include (1) "morbidity costs" such as the cost of goods and services not produced by

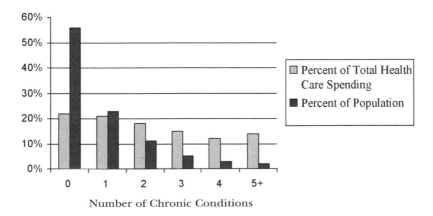

FIGURE 2.9.

Health care spending and chronic conditions.

Partnership for Solutions, 2002a.

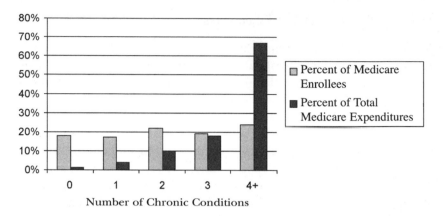

FIGURE 2.10.

Percent of Medicare spending by number of chronic conditions.

Partnership for Solutions, 2002a.

persons with chronic conditions because they are unable to work and the cost of housekeeping services that they are unable to perform themselves; (2) "mortality costs," defined as "the value of the goods and services that would have been produced over the remaining lives by persons [with chronic conditions] who died prematurely"; and (3) the costs to employers when employees are absent from work to provide care (usually to a family member) and the cost of such care (Hoffman, Rice, & Sung, 1996). Though difficult to measure, indirect costs of chronic conditions have been estimated to equal nearly half the direct health care costs. Indirect costs are much higher for some chronic conditions; annual direct health care expenditures for patients with heart disease, for example, were estimated at $478 per person in 1995, compared with indirect costs of $3,013 per person (Hodgson & Cohen, 1999). Researchers estimated that in 1990 total costs for people with chronic conditions were $659 billion, of which $425 billion was for direct health care costs and $234 billion was for indirect costs (Hoffman, Rice, & Sung, 1996). Using the same ratio, total expenditures for chronic care in 2000 would be an estimated $1.5 trillion: $1 trillion for direct health care costs, and $500 billion for indirect costs.

Summary

Chronic illnesses affect everyone, in one way or another. Nearly half of all Americans have one or more chronic conditions and thus experience daily the many ways these conditions affect their health and lives. In addition, millions of Americans—including many who are chronically ill themselves—provide assistance to a family member or friend who has a chronic condition. Even the small minority of Americans who neither has a chronic condition nor is caring for someone who does is indirectly affected, even if only by helping to finance a health care system that devotes three-fourths of its resources to the care of people with chronic conditions. The health, psychological, emotional, financial, and other burdens of chronic illness will grow as the number of people with a chronic condition continues to rise and the cost of their care continues to increase.

3. How the Current System Fails People with Chronic Illnesses

PATIENT CARE VIGNETTE

♣ Mrs. Fernandez is a 75-year-old Hispanic female with obesity, diabetes mellitus, congestive heart failure, atrial fibrillation, and degenerative joint disease. She lives alone in Milwaukee on a limited fixed income and takes care of her three grandchildren at her house several days per week. Mrs. Fernandez quit driving five years ago and now uses the city bus for transportation.

Mrs. Fernandez has three scheduled visits per year with her primary care physician, who works at a multispecialty clinic. Several years ago he referred her to a diabetes education program at a clinic not far from her house. Though she attended the program, Mrs. Fernandez has failed to follow through with the recommendations. She consistently tells her primary care physician that she will "do better" with the suggested changes in diet and exercise. Her diabetes and hypertension are poorly controlled, as they have been for years. Mrs. Fernandez is reluctant to change or increase medications in her regimen. Her physician has never discussed with her the cost of her medications, and Mrs. Fernandez has never mentioned to him that at times their costs exceed her budget.

During the past several years Mrs. Fernandez has been seen multiple times with complaints of fatigue, joint pain, and shortness of breath at the urgent care (UC) center where her primary care physician works. At the UC she sees a different clinician each time—never her primary care physician. Although the UC staff always has a chart with her medical information, Mrs. Fernandez believes it may be incomplete. For example, at the last visit the UC clinician did not know of her visit with her primary care physician two weeks earlier. And they don't seem to know about all her medications, sometimes prescribing drugs she is already taking.

Four times in the past two years Mrs. Fernandez has been hospitalized for congestive heart failure. She has been told to "weigh herself" every day and call her physician if she gains "too much" weight, but she isn't sure what that means. She does not own a scale and no health care professional has ever asked if she owned one.

Mrs. Fernandez is treated with coumadin (a blood-thinning drug) to prevent strokes. She recently saw her orthopedic surgeon (who works at a

44

different clinic across town) about persistent knee pain caused by arthritis. The surgeon, apparently unaware she was taking coumadin, gave her samples of a nonsteroidal anti-inflammatory drug (NSAID) pain medication that caused her to have a significant gastrointestinal bleed requiring hospitalization and transfusion of three units of blood.

During this most recent hospitalization, the staff performed a comprehensive "geriatric evaluation" of Mrs. Fernandez. The evaluation revealed that:

1. Mrs. Fernandez is only sporadically taking her diabetes and blood pressure medications due to the overwhelming monthly cost.

2. She snores very loudly and has low oxygen levels during the night. Subsequent work-up revealed a significant sleep disorder that is contributing to her hypertension and congestive heart failure.

3. Mrs. Fernandez has yet to follow up with a cardiologist, as she was strongly urged to do after her last hospital admission for heart failure. Indeed, because that admission was at a different hospital in the city, with which her clinic is not affiliated, her primary care physician was not even aware that she had been hospitalized.

4. Mrs. Fernandez is very depressed regarding her poor health status, limited financial resources, and family stressors (such as her grandchildren's disjointed day care). She feels she has "no energy" to address her multiple medical problems and relies on her primary care physician to "tell her what to do" when she is sick.

5. Mrs. Fernandez has prescriptions for 11 different medications for her medical conditions. She is not actively treated for her depression.

When she was discharged from the hospital she was given prescriptions for heart medications, diabetes medications, and antidepressants that cost $562 at the pharmacy. She did not keep an appointment for an overnight sleep test because she was unable to get a ride across the city to the sleep center and the bus trip would have been more than two hours each way. At her next visit with her primary care physician the geriatric evaluation from the hospital had not yet been forwarded to the clinic. She was found to have an elevated blood pressure and high blood sugar. Mrs. Fernandez again told her doctor she would work harder on modifying her diet and increasing her exercise. She was scheduled for a return appointment in four months.

(This case is hypothetical. Any resemblance to persons living or dead is purely coincidental.)

Teresa McCarthy, M.D., University of Minnesota

In its influential 2001 report, *Crossing the Quality Chasm: A New Health System for the 21st Century*, the Institute of Medicine's Committee on the Quality of Health Care in America found serious deficiencies in our health care system and concluded that "between the health care we have and the care we could have lies not just a gap, but a chasm" (Institute of Medicine, 2001). Although the IOM committee focused only on the quality of health care, the chasm the committee identified is in fact much broader. In addition to quality concerns, the lack of access to care for millions of Americans, the financial barriers to care, the high cost of care, inadequately trained and too few health care professionals, and other dimensions of our health care system further expose the gap or chasm between "what is" and "what should be."

The deficiencies in the health care system are particularly troubling for people with chronic conditions. On average, people with chronic conditions rely more heavily on the health care system; they use the system more frequently, consume more health care resources, and are more likely to see multiple health care professionals and have long-term relationships with them. When the health care system fails, chronically ill patients are often harmed the most. Regarding chronic illness care, the deficiencies of our health care system can be grouped into three categories: structure and function, payment, and personnel.

In this chapter, we explore some, but by no means all, of the deficiencies in each of these categories and briefly examine how they hinder the provision of optimal chronic illness care. We return to many of these issues, in more detail and with an eye toward solutions, in the second section of the book.

Structure and Function

The structure and function of the health care system refers to the way in which hospitals, physician practices, clinics, rehabilitation centers, long-term care facilities, health plans, and the other components of the system are configured, both as independent entities and as parts of a larger whole. It also refers to how those components relate to and interact with one another. The "structure and function" of the health care system thus encompasses both how the components of the system are put together and how they, and the system as a whole, perform or do their jobs. Deficiencies in the structure and function of the health care system that hinder optimal chronic illness care include fragmented and poorly coordinated care, restricted roles for patients and families, failure to practice evidence-based medicine, and inadequate use of information technology. But the fundamental failure of our health care system relative to chronic care is that the conceptual model of care that lies at the system's foundation does not support optimal chronic illness care.

Wrong Model of Care

At its core, the structure and function of our health care system rests on a conceptual model. Conceptual models are designed to make sense out of complex events in the world and to help organize our responses. Microeconomics, for example, uses Adam Smith's conceptual model of a perfectly competitive market to both understand economic transactions and shape policies to achieve desirable economic goals. In a similar fashion, the conceptual model that underlies our health care system constitutes the reference framework we use to understand and treat health problems. The model helps, for example, determine what counts as a "disease," set the proper boundaries of health care professionals' responsibilities, establish the appropriate response of the health care system to those who are "sick," and shape societal attitudes toward patients.

The conceptual model at the foundation of America's health care system is the acute care model. As a result, this system is structured first and foremost to prevent, diagnose, and treat acute medical conditions. The acute care model adopts a disease orientation, is firmly grounded in science (or so we like to believe), and is principally focused on the pathology and pathophysiology of body functions and structure.[1] In this model, diseases are narrowly defined as abnormalities or deviations from what is normal. The language of science (primarily the biological sciences) is used to establish both what is "normal" and which deviations from the norm are sufficient to warrant the label "disease." Thus, the model helps determine, for example, whether a child who is markedly shorter than his peers can be said to have a disease, rather than being merely short. Short stature due to a deficiency in human growth hormone is recognized as a disease, whereas short stature due to no known natural causes (idiopathic short stature) typically is not. The model also influences the response: treatment for a child with growth hormone deficiency is accepted medical practice, whereas medical interventions to increase the height of a short child without a recognized disease are seen as inappropriate. Health insurers typically pay for the former but not the latter.

The acute care model has been enormously successful for understanding and treating many medical conditions, resulting in remarkable achievements in identifying the causes and mechanisms of disease and in developing effective treatments. This has vastly reduced the incidence of infectious diseases and ameliorated many other medical problems. Whereas it is important to acknowledge the successes of this model in improving treatment for acute conditions, the acute care model nonetheless is not a sound framework for responding to chronic conditions. The acute care model leaves little if any room for the social, psychosocial, and behavioral dimensions of chronic illness (Tinetti & Fried, 2004). It does not provide for the commitment to continuing care. It is also not broad enough to account for and aid understanding of the types of human distress experienced by people with chronic conditions. These include challenges to the "person's self-image and sense of meaning and purpose in life" (Jennings, Callahan, & Caplan, 1988) and the suffering that occurs due to disruptions in the patient's "extended system," including their family, friends, work associates, and community (Cassell, 1991). Furthermore, the acute care model undervalues the importance of a variety of other key facets of chronic illness care, including the influence of lifestyle factors such as nutrition and exercise in preventing or managing a chronic condition, the likelihood of depression or other mental health issues accompanying a chronic condition, the vital role of families in supporting and caring for a chronically ill family member, and the influence of the environment in understanding the causes of and developing appropriate responses to chronic conditions.

To paraphrase the IOM Committee on Quality, between the care encompassed by the acute care model and the care needed by people with chronic conditions lies not just a gap, but a chasm. Health care based on the acute care model focuses on treating immediate presenting symptoms and often discounts the sustained impairments that threaten the health status and diminish the functioning of people with chronic conditions. Similarly, acute care's emphasis on cure seems misplaced when directed to chronic conditions, most of which can never be resolved. The episodic nature of acute care is also at odds with the long-term monitoring and continuous support and care needed by people with chronic conditions to prevent exacerbations and maintain their functional abilities.

Because America's health care system is structured principally to respond to acute conditions it fails to effectively meet the needs of people with chronic conditions (Tinetti & Fried, 2004). The predictable consequence of a system built on the acute care model is the current chasm between the reality of having to respond to chronic illness in our society and the way our health care system actually deals with chronic illness. The system does not ignore chronic conditions themselves, but it continues to respond to them as if they were acute and episodic, treating symptoms as they occur. The care for persons with chronic conditions is often a "poorly connected string" of clinician-patient encounters (Rothman & Wagner, 2003). Consequently, the system ignores the fundamentally different approach that is needed to care for people with chronic conditions, that is, managing the conditions long term and responding to the myriad ways they affect peoples' lives. The problem is not that people with chronic conditions do not receive care in our health care system; rather, the problem is that their care is provided in a system principally designed to treat a wholly different type of condition and thus is ill equipped to adequately respond to chronic conditions.

In sum, the distance between "what is" and "what should be" for chronic illness care persists as the health care system continues to emphasize acute care—in the provision of services, the education of health care professionals, the research and development of new technologies, and the system's financing. The foremost reason America's current health care system cannot optimally provide the full complement of services needed by people with chronic conditions is that the system remains based on an episodic, acute care medical model.

Fragmented, Poorly Coordinated Care

In the current system, care for people is often fragmented and poorly coordinated. Although this may jeopardize health care quality and efficiency for any patient, it is particularly troublesome for those with more than one chronic condition, such as Mrs. Fernandez in this chapter's vignette. To meet their complex needs, patients such as Mrs. Fernandez often receive care from multiple clinicians, who may work independently from each other. Each of the clinicians may provide one or more of the services that constitute the full spectrum of care the patient needs, such as medical, mental health, rehabilitation, prevention, and supportive services. Yet the clinicians rarely communicate with each other about the patient's care. By functioning in separate "silos," the clinicians (and the clinics and health care organizations where they practice) often do not have complete information about the patient's condition or treatment history, a major source of medical errors. For example, Mrs. Fernandez's latest hospitalization, for a gastrointestinal bleed, was a direct result of her orthopedic surgeon not being aware of all the drugs her other physicians had prescribed for her.

This "silo-based" approach to care is a hallmark of our fragmented system, hampering the "coordinated, seamless care across settings and clinicians and over time" that is needed to effectively meet the needs of people with chronic conditions (Institute of Medicine, 2001). It also results in inefficiencies because discrete health care providers will often duplicate laboratory and radiological investigations and other diagnostic services, especially if medical records and other patient care information are not shared. Compounding the complexity and inefficiency, each of these segments of care may have its own distinct management information system, payment structure, financial incentives, and quality oversight. Patients find this complicated, uncoordinated "system" extremely confusing and a "nightmare to navigate" (Picker Institute, 1996).

The fragmented system hampers the follow-through and coordination of care across the entire spectrum of care processes. Information about a patient's health and treatments is rarely centralized, well organized, or easily retrievable, "making it nearly impossible to manage many forms of chronic illness that require frequent monitoring and ongoing patient support" (Institute of Medicine, 2001). The important findings from Mrs. Fernandez's geriatric evaluation, for example, were not available to her physician at her latest visit, leaving him with incomplete information on which to base decisions. Coordination of care for a chronically ill patient is particularly important when many different individuals—including various health care professionals and the patient, family members, and other informal caregivers—are involved in managing the patient's conditions. The discrete, yet interconnected tasks performed by these individuals, often in disparate areas of the health care system as well as in the patient's home, must be linked and coordinated to ensure that desired outcomes are achieved efficiently.

But the coordination of care for chronically ill patients, including the integration of medical with nonmedical services, is often overlooked. Rarely in a fragmented, poorly coordinated health care system is a single health care professional or entity responsible for a patient's overall care. Instead, clinicians and other health care professionals may feel responsible only for the care and services they themselves provide, and they neglect or overlook integrating and coordinating all the care their individual patients receive. Even when a clinician strives to stay abreast of their patient's overall care, the system's fragmentation may thwart such efforts, as when Mrs. Fernandez was hospitalized without her primary care physician's knowledge at a hospital with which he had no affiliation. Imprecise clinician responsibility increases the chance that some services may conflict with others (e.g., medications prescribed by different clinicians may interact and harm a patient) and that still other needed services may not be provided at all. Among people with chronic conditions 71% report having no help in coordinating their care (i.e., making appointments, arranging and getting needed services, assisting with insurance issues) and 17% say they have received contradictory medical information from health care professionals (Partnership for Solutions, 2002c).

Patients with chronic conditions suffer from fragmented services in another sense—when they are treated not as persons but instead are segmented or compartmentalized into discrete organs or body systems. If health care professionals treat a malfunctioning system of the body rather than the person as a whole (i.e., treat disease in the patient rather than treat the patient with disease), treatment can become a series of medical interventions that target only the disease and ignore the ill person. Such a disease-centered—as opposed to a person-centered—approach risks providing care that the person may not want. By treating a patient's diabetes, for example, rather than treating the patient who has diabetes, a clinician may focus narrowly on using intensive monitoring, aggressive follow-up, and systematic assessments to control blood sugar levels and other aspects of the disease, thereby reducing the risks of future complications. Even if the patient shares the goal of reducing the chance of blindness or other complications of diabetes, a singular focus on such narrow medical goals may ignore the patient's interest in keeping the management of the disease from overwhelming other aspects of his or her life (Wolpert & Anderson, 2001).

Restricted Roles for Patients and Families

For chronically ill patients, the condition and its consequences "interact to create illness patterns requiring continuous and complex management" (Holman & Lorig, 2000). Effectively managing chronic conditions requires intimate understanding of these illness patterns. Patients, not their clinicians, are in the best position to accurately detect and characterize such patterns. Only they can provide the personal information regarding the impact of the condition on their health and well-being that is necessary for effective management. Effective chronic illness care must therefore allow and encourage patients to be more engaged in their own care. "Self-management" refers to a variety of activities individuals undertake with the intention of limiting the effects of their illness. These include participating in decisions about treatment and sharing responsibility for them by, for example, monitoring their health status, reporting changes or unexpected events, and adhering to agreed-upon treatment. "Unlike much acute care, effective care of the chronically ill is a collaborative process, involving the definition of clinical problems in terms that both patients and providers understand; joint development of a care plan with goals, targets, and implementation strategies; provision of self-management training and support services; and active, sustained follow-up" (Von Korff et al., 1997).

In general, people with chronic conditions have better health outcomes and are more satisfied with their care if they participate actively in the management of their health and health care (Leveille et al., 1998; Lorig et al., 1999). Yet many patients do not have the skills and competencies needed for this role. Some patients desire a more passive approach to their health and health care or may be uncomfortable managing their own care and thus may not seek to acquire such skills and competencies. For patients who want to become more actively engaged, however, health care providers and health plans often fail to prescribe, provide, or reimburse the necessary educational materials and empowerment tools to build self-efficacy and self-management skills or to support their efforts to manage their own care.[2] Although Mrs. Fernandez, for example, expressed some desire to better manage her own health, she was not given the necessary tools, with some clinicians failing even to make sure she understood their instructions. Even when patient education services are provided, they are often sporadic, unplanned, and superficial, given the lack of coordination among providers (Institute of Medicine, 2001). In addition, the current system often fails to acknowledge and address the impact of a person's chronic illness on other family members, both as caregivers and as family members. (The roles of patients and families are discussed in greater detail in chapter 6.)

Failure to Practice Evidence-based Medicine

Evidence-based medicine (EBM) is defined as "the conscientious, explicit, and judicious use of current best evidence in making clinical decisions about the care of individual patients" (Sackett et al., 1996). In a nutshell, EBM is designed to take the best available scientific information and help clinicians apply the results in clinical practice. All too often, innovations in clinical practice have had little effect beyond a few leading medical groups and institutions.

In theory, evidence-based medicine will improve the quality of care by closing the gap between the treatment recommended on the basis of clinical evidence and the treatment actually provided—between knowing and doing. Examples of this so-called treatment gap, that is, the differences between the treatment recommended on the basis of clinical evidence and the treatment actually provided, include the failure to prescribe the most effective medications, inadequate follow-up and monitoring, and many examples where the care provided failed to follow widely accepted practice guidelines, resulting in the underuse, overuse, and misuse of services in the care of patients.[3] Such problems have been well documented for patients with chronic conditions throughout the health care system (Institute of Medicine, 2001; McGlynn et al., 2003). For example:

- The Diabetes Quality Improvement Project recommends annual retinal eye examinations for diabetics. In 1995–96, only 45.3% of the 3.1 million Medicare enrollees who were diagnosed with diabetes received one or more eye examinations.[4]

- The Diabetes Quality Improvement Project also recommends routine monitoring of HgbAlc protein, a marker for glucose. Only 29% of diabetic patients reported having this test during the previous year (Saadine et al., 2002).

- Twenty-four percent of patients with unstable angina who were "ideal" candidates for treatment with aspirin during hospitalizations did not receive aspirin during their hospital stay (Simpson et al., 1997).

- The United States Task Force on Preventive Disease guidelines recommend mammograms at least once every two years for female Medicare enrollees aged 65–69 years. In 1995–96, only 28.3% of women in this age group received at least one mammogram.[5]

- Less than 25% of Americans with major depressive disorders are receiving adequate treatment (Kessler et al., 2003).

- Overall, even when evidence-based guidelines exist, a chronically ill patient has just a 56% chance of receiving the recommended care (McGlynn et al., 2003).[6]

Efforts to promote EBM include the identification and dissemination of research findings about effective clinical practice, the development of innumerable (sometimes competing) practice guidelines, and assessments of the safety and effectiveness of existing and emerging health care technologies. The common aim of these activities is to find out what works in health care and what does not, and to promote the appropriate use of those interventions that work and minimize the use of those that do not.

However, evidence-based medicine has several limitations. The base of evidence about the safety, effectiveness, and cost-effectiveness of health care interventions is not as great as some believe, certainly not evidence derived from well-executed scientific studies. When such evidence does exist, it may be restricted to carefully defined instances that do not directly relate to actual practice, especially when patients' chronic conditions are made more complex by the interactions of other diseases. In many instances, scientific evidence to support EBM has had to be supplemented by professional consensus. Still, even where good scientific evidence does exist, clinicians unfortunately may not use it.

Failure to Optimize Information Technology

Information technology (IT) is critical for delivering good chronic care. In the context of health care, IT encompasses all forms of technology used to create, store, exchange, and use information to support the delivery and processes of health care. IT includes single-task systems, such as computerized patient health records, as well as complex, integrated systems that can meld together multiple tasks such as ordering medications and lab tests, billing, and patient records. The IT toolbox in health care includes discrete devices, such as PCs and handheld computers, and e-mail and Web-based technologies that allow health care providers to communicate with patients and monitor patient care remotely.

Health information technology can play several crucial roles, including:

1. Providing clinical decision support

2. Collecting and sharing clinical information

3. Reducing medical errors

4. Enhancing patient-clinician interactions

5. Educating and informing patients

Many believe that IT has significant untapped potential for improving chronic illness care. IT is expected to improve the flow of information and improve the quality of decisions by getting the right data to the right people at the right time—when decisions need to be made—and thereby producing better care and providing care more efficiently. Nevertheless, the rate of adoption of IT in health care has been slow, relative to many other industries. The health care sector spends 3% to 5% of its operating budget on IT, whereas industries such as banking and financial services spend over 10%. Despite its promise, there has been great reluctance within health care to invest heavily in IT, outside of financial accounting and billing. As a result, "the U.S. health care system remains mired in a morass of paper records and bills, fax transmittals and unreturned phone calls" (Goldsmith, Blumenthal, & Rishel, 2003). (Different types of information technologies and their potential to improve chronic illness care are discussed in chapter 7.)

Personnel

Workforce Shortages

Patients with chronic conditions will continue to receive care from a wide range of health care practitioners. Although projecting the future demand and supply of health care professionals in chronic illness care is imprecise at best, the consensus is that without significant changes in health care professional education, too few practitioners will be trained to deal with the manifold needs of patients with chronic conditions. One concern is the decline in the number of primary care clinicians. Because primary care is the foundation for most chronic illness care, this decline is troubling, especially in light of the projected increase in demand for chronic care services.

Another concern is the number of clinicians who care for particular subpopulations of chronically ill patients, such as elderly patients with multiple chronic conditions. Because of their special training in aging and age-related disease, maintaining and improving functional status, and managing chronic conditions, geriatricians are often the most qualified to treat such patients. There are, however, relatively few practicing geriatricians and their number is expected to decline in the near future as practicing geriatricians retire at a faster rate than new trainees enter practice. Beyond the shortage of geriatricians is the inadequate training for medical students who do not specialize in geriatrics. Although most physicians will see elderly patients at some point in their practice regardless of their specialty, few receive much formal training in the specific needs of this population.

Though the projected supply and demand for physicians caring for chronically ill patients is hotly debated, the shortage of nurses is well-documented and unquestioned. As with physicians, the shortage of nurses with special training to care for older persons is a particular concern. The demand for advanced practice nurses (registered nurses with advanced education and clinical training in fields such as adult or pediatric health) has increased in recent years and the number of such clinicians has risen as well. However, there are relatively few advanced practice nurses with specific geriatric training to respond to the unique needs of elderly patients.

Inadequate Training in Chronic Illness Care

Managing chronic conditions demands skills and knowledge that extend beyond traditional biomedical training for preventing, diagnosing, and treating acute conditions. Care coordination abilities, behavior modification techniques, and patient education are among the broader set of skills health care professionals will need to provide optimal chronic care. Health education curricula, however, have not kept pace with changes in the health needs of the population, such as the rise in chronic conditions. Specifically, the current curricula for many health care professionals, but particularly for physicians, do not provide adequate training in the principles of good chronic illness care, such as promoting patient-centered care, using information technology and information systems, practicing evidence-based medicine, and working in interdisciplinary teams.

In addition to less-than-adequate training in these key chronic care competencies, health care professional students do not receive enough of their training in the settings in which they will provide the vast majority of care to patients with chronic conditions. Most medical and clinical training continues to transpire in hospital settings, even though the system is rapidly moving more care into ambulatory practice. Moreover, because a hospital admission for a chronically ill patient typically results from an exacerbation of the illness, a breakdown of normal caregiving systems, or further deterioration in function, health profession trainees see such patients at their worst, rather than in less crisis-oriented ambulatory settings. (Health care workforce issues are discussed further in chapter 5.)

Payment

Misaligned Financial Incentives

Financial incentives can serve as primary motivators or reinforcers for behavior change among providers, patients, and other stakeholders. Yet few incentives in the current health care system promote effective chronic care. Instead, the predominant payment schemes represent major barriers. However motivated some health care stakeholders may be to implement changes to improve chronic illness care, few will operate counter to their economic interests (Leatherman et al., 2003). A core element for reform will thus be to develop and adopt payment approaches that include appropriate financial incentives.

Payment methods in America's health care system are varied and complex, linking health plans, providers, patients, and other stakeholders through various financial transactions. Current methods often do not align financial incentives with the goal of optimal care for patients with chronic conditions. For example, the primary methods of clinician reimbursement (that is, the methods for paying clinicians for the services they provide) include fee-for-service, capitation, and salary. Each creates perverse incentives for patient care. The incentive under fee-for-service (FFS) reimbursement is to provide as many reimbursable services as possible, creating the potential for overuse of services, and not to provide uncovered services that may ultimately be cost-effective, such as active patient monitoring by phone or computer. An example of just how this perverse payment system can undermine good chronic care is shown in the exhibit. On the other hand, FFS minimizes incentives for avoiding patients who are difficult to treat, such as patients with multiple chronic conditions.

Capitation arrangements, which pay clinicians based on the number of people they care for and not the quantity of services they actually provide, have the opposite economic incentives. Clinicians paid by capitation bear the financial risk, creating the potential for underuse of services. Under capitation, clinicians have the incentive to sign up more consumers (patients)

EXHIBIT 3.1

Payment Barriers to Good Chronic Care

An article in the *New York Times* (August 11, 2004) illustrates how the fee-for-service (FFS) payment approach is directly opposed to good chronic care. Whatcom County in the State of Washington has introduced a special program to better address the needs of persons with diabetes and congestive heart failure. The program uses specially trained nurses who stay in close contact with targeted patients. Physicians who opted to participate were required to purchase an electronic medical record subsystem with which they could track patients' courses and communicate with the patients by e-mail. But these activities were not billable; moreover, they displaced billable office visits. The county's physicians now face a dilemma. They can readily appreciate the impact of this new program and its benefits for patients and for health care financing overall, but they are individually losing money as a result. Some doctors have altruistically opted to stay with the program despite its financial implications, but many have withdrawn. (Kolata, 2004)

and do less for each, as well as to avoid high users of care, such as patients with multiple chronic conditions. Salary methods may be the most neutral form of clinician reimbursement; however, they have "the potential for reduced productivity if sufficient rewards are not built in" (Stoline & Weiner, 1993). FFS is the dominant payment method for physicians, the popularity of capitation methods waxes and wanes, and though an increasing number of physicians now earn at least part of their income as salary, fully salaried doctors remain the exception to the norm. In contrast, most other clinicians, such as advanced practice nurses, are salaried employees.

Our health care system may create perverse financial incentives at the health plan level as well. Most of the discussions about creating suitable incentives for health plans focus on the problem of selecting enrollees. Capitated health plans, such as health maintenance organizations (HMOs) and other managed care plans that receive a predetermined per-capita fee, should theoretically have incentives to provide to their enrollees preventive and other services designed to keep them healthy, slow the progression of disease, or otherwise reduce enrollees' future use of health care services. However, the financial reward of such efforts sometimes isn't captured until 10 or 20 years in the future, particularly for efforts targeting slow-developing and long-term chronic conditions (e.g., diet and exercise programs to reduce risks for diabetes). A health plan would thus reap a reward only if enrollees who participate in the plan's health promotion and risk reduction programs remain with the plan long-term. However, annual open enrollment and other features of our health care system facilitate and encourage consumers to switch among health plans. This undercuts incentives to provide such programs because the health plan that incurs the programs' costs is not necessarily the same plan that captures the financial pay-off. The same arguments also apply to hospitals, integrated health systems, and other provider organizations. While diabetes management programs and other quality improvement initiatives, for instance, improve health outcomes and may save health care dollars over the long run, current payment policies do not offer provider organizations financial incentives to develop and implement such initiatives. The prospect for a positive return on investment within a reasonable time for the parties that invest in these initiatives, that is, the "business case," is weak or nonexistent (Leatherman et al., 2003).

Another feature of the health care-financing system provides a second disincentive for health plans to improve chronic illness care. Insurance spreads the financial risk of unexpected events. The essential logic of health insurance is to spread this risk across "a very broad pool in which the currently well subsidize the currently ill" (Kuttner, 1998). The structure of the U.S. health insurance market of competing health plans, voluntary participation, choice among health plans, and payments that generally do not take into account individuals' health status means that the market currently rewards those health plans that enroll more of the "currently well" and avoid the "currently ill." When health plans pursue these rewards, the burden falls most heavily on people with chronic conditions, who constitute the majority of the "currently ill" and are, on average, the most costly enrollees for a health plan. Furthermore, health plans that achieve good outcomes for such enrollees would not want that information publicized if it leads to increased enrollment of more people with chronic conditions. Being identified as a health plan that is good for people with chronic conditions could be financially harmful to the plan.

Health plans have begun to aggressively pursue strategies for turning the unexpected events that trigger utilization of health care services into predictable occurrences. One such strategy, "predictive modeling," uses sophisticated software to attempt to accurately predict who will develop a chronic condition that may require expensive services (McCain, 2001). While such strategies would theoretically allow a health plan to target timely health care interventions to prevent or at least ameliorate the predicted condition, under the current financing system the plan would also have a financial incentive to identify and then remove such patients from their enrolled population.

Coverage Gaps

Many private health insurance plans as well as public programs such as Medicare do not cover or inadequately cover some of the most important services that people with chronic conditions need. In general, health insurance plans give priority to acute, provider-directed medical care over the clinical and nonclinical supportive services needed by people with chronic conditions. The coverage and benefits policies of public and private health plans also often encourage costly, institutionally based care in favor of less costly supportive home- or community-based services. Specific coverage problems for patients with chronic conditions include inadequate coverage for preventive services, patient assessments, and the coordination and management of care. Similarly, few health plans reimburse physicians for teaching patients how to better manage their own chronic condition. The most pernicious coverage gap, of course, concerns the 40 million and counting uninsured Americans, many of whom have a chronic condition, who consequently suffer the greatest hardship in our patchwork health care system. (Payment issues are further discussed in chapter 9.)

Summary

Improving chronic illness care will require more than minor adjustments and accommodations to a health care system based on the acute care model. Optimal care for people with chronic conditions requires a different type of health care system. The solution, however, does not require discarding the infrastructure in place for acute care, which will need to continue to treat acute medical conditions. Rather, a new system is needed that overlays the current system that can only respond in a fragmented and disjointed way to the needs of patients with chronic conditions. A conceptual model of care is needed that would then serve as the foundation for the chronic care component of the system by encompassing the health as well as the social, psychosocial, and behavioral dimensions of illnesses. The contrast between the current care arrangement and such an ideal chronic care model can be seen in table 3.1, which identifies the distinct processes of care needed by a person with a chronic condition and contrasts how these are handled in the current acute care-dominated system with how they would be addressed in a more ideal system that prioritizes chronic illness care.

In reviewing table 3.1 it is possible to imagine that even if the current acute care system meets the needs of a relatively healthy person with one chronic condition, it breaks down quickly when confronted with a patient with multiple chronic conditions (comorbidity). The reactive, crisis-oriented

TABLE 3.1.
Comparison of Care Processes in Current and Ideal Health Care Systems

Care Process	Current Health Care System, Based on Acute Care Model	Ideal Health Care System, Prioritizing Chronic Care
Assessment	Disease-centered	Person-centered
	Focus on clinical considerations	Focus on implications for function and quality of life
Treatment/intervention	Provider initiates; patient expected to comply	Patient and provider jointly involved in decision, risks, benefits, and costs considered
	Disjointed, little coordination	Coordination among multiple providers
	Primarily medical or pharmacological	Includes behavior change and adaptation
	Care often planned on an ad hoc basis	Clinical pathways used whereve feasible to inform both providers and patients
Monitoring/adjustment	Intermittent	Continuous
	Encounters triggered by problems or arbitrary time period	Encounters triggered by change in clinical course
	Interventions frequently initiated after decline	Early intervention at first sign of change or deviation from expected course
	Reporting tied to encounters	Ongoing, frequent, and possibly remote reporting of signs and symptoms
Acute care—exacerbation of chronic condition	Focus on stabilization/return to steady state	Focus on stabilization then identifying and rectifying the case of exacerbation
	Event perceived as a somewhat inevitable part of disease course	Event perceived as a system failure or breakdown in care management
Acute care—other diagnosis: chronic condition is a comorbidity	Chronic condition viewed as problem or ignored	Addressing chronic condition integral to the treatment
	Resolution of principal problem defined as success	Functional status part of definition of success
Post-acute care	Driven by efforts to reduce hospital stay	Most important outcomes identified. Decisions based on balancing benefits, risks, and costs
	Minimal patient/family support; little time for careful decision making	Maximal patient/family involvement in decision making. Efforts made to separate stages of decision into choice of venue and vendor
	Sporadic monitoring	Continuous monitoring
	Limited information transfer	Patient-centered record goes with patient as patient moves to another source of care

acute care model focuses on treating a patient's immediate needs or symptoms and views each patient interaction with the health care system as an isolated encounter. It typically ignores the interdependent nature of multiple conditions; thus failing, for example, to connect a diabetic person's depression with the resultant loss of appetite, which can lead to malnutrition, which can exacerbate their diabetes, and so on. Treating and managing multiple conditions highlights the fact that effective chronic care entails moving beyond a series of encounters to monitoring patients over the long term and providing "longitudinal care." Such care must be consistent over time and coordinated, so that the various services reinforce each other toward achieving common goals. The care provided over the long term varies primarily in intensity, responding to changes in the patient's health status. An ideal health care system should also follow a patient with chronic conditions through successive acute care episodes and facilitate the transitions prior to and after intensive treatment such as surgeries or hospitalizations.

In the next section, we revisit many of the deficiencies reviewed above, but we shift our focus to what is needed to turn a system that fails people with chronic illnesses into one that can provide optimal chronic illness care.

PART II

Opportunities for Change

4. Reorganizing Care in the Face of Chronic Illness

Major changes are needed to reorient our health care system so that it responds more appropriately to the needs of people with chronic conditions. Minor changes at the margins will not be enough. What is required is nothing short of shifting the health care system from its current emphasis on acute health conditions to a system that gives chronic conditions top priority. But recognizing the need for major change is one thing; bringing it about is quite another.

The current health care system has a great deal invested in the status quo. Health care is one of the nation's largest industries. In 2001, national health care expenditures were $1.424 trillion, or 14.1% of the gross domestic product (GDP). Projections are for health care expenditures to reach $3.0 trillion in 2012, or 17% of total GDP. Although some bemoan the relentless increases in health care expenditures, others point out that in health care, as in any other industry, what is expenditure from one perspective is income from another. And in an industry as large as health care, millions of people share in that income. About 12 million Americans work in the health care sector, many of who are in some of the most highly compensated and revered professions. Millions more invest in the health care sector, which includes some of the country's most profitable companies. Health care is an important component of local economies as well. In many locales, and especially in rural areas, hospitals and other health care organizations (along with schools) are often the largest employers. Our health care system, which already accounts for one of every seven dollars in the nation's economy and employs one of every eleven workers, is rife with powerful vested interests that may understandably resist change. The very size of this economic investment in the status quo makes it more difficult to achieve the needed infrastructure reforms.

Not only is health care one of our country's major industries, many Americans strongly believe that ours is the best health care system in the world, despite the frequently cited international statistics to the contrary (Anderson, 1997). We revel in the knowledge that we possess the technology that promises to undo years of unhealthy behaviors or lifestyles. We celebrate those who intervene to bring people back from the point of death.

We willingly pay for costly, heroic saves—even if preventing the need for them would have been more efficient.

Barriers to reforming this vast and highly valued health care system to one that is more attuned and responsive to chronic illness are numerous and profound. A brief look at one major component of the existing system, the Medicare program, is illustrative. Medicare, the federal social health insurance program for the elderly, was designed with more of an eye toward paying providers than paying for the care that Medicare beneficiaries need. When it was enacted in 1965, the program sought to extend the then traditional insurance coverage to a distinct vulnerable population (i.e., adults aged 65 years and older) and deliberately minimized any potential impact on the manner in which health care services were delivered. As a result, the program was weighted toward hospital and institutional care.

Medicare, according to most observers, does poorly for people with chronic conditions. The program does not cover (or covers poorly) some of the health care services, such as many long-term care services, which are important for the care of beneficiaries with chronic conditions. Medicare's reliance on unmanaged fee-for-service reimbursement fails to promote continuity and coordination of care. This form of reimbursement is also event driven, providing no incentive for the long-term management of chronic conditions. Reimbursements are not adjusted adequately for the added complexity of chronic conditions. And the program continues to pay clinicians more for using technologies and performing procedures than for spending time talking with patients.

Although some savings are possible by reducing the program's waste and fraud and increasing its efficiency, changing Medicare to better meet the needs of its enrollees with chronic conditions will require either an infusion of more money into the program or a major redistribution of existing resources. Both of these options face major challenges. Despite (or perhaps because of) the recent enactment of the prescription drug benefit (scheduled to go into effect in 2006), increasing the Medicare budget is unrealistic in the current economic and political climate, and a major rearrangement of Medicare's priorities is difficult in light of our political system's bias against any kind of major reform—in health care or elsewhere.

There was a flirtation with managed care as a vehicle to shift incentives but the managed care organizations seemed more interested in marketing to lucrative clients than to changing the fundamental approach to care (Kane, 1998). The upshot of the experience with Medicare managed care was it provided about the same quality of service at a slightly higher price (because of favorable selection) (Brown et al., 1993; S. Retchin, Clement, & Brown, 1994; S. M. Retchin & Brown, 1990, 1991; S. M. Retchin et al., 1992, 1997).

Redistributing Medicare dollars to improve chronic illness care would mean that some stakeholders within health care would have to reduce or give up certain revenue streams. It may also require Medicare beneficiaries to give up some high-cost, high-tech health care or to forgo some of the services that benefit only a few in favor of services that benefit many. A prerequisite to these changes is a new social ethic, one that differs significantly from today's dominant individualistic ethic. Yet there are few calls for such a new social ethic.

For the moment the attention to Medicare is focused on controlling its costs, not on changing the care infrastructure. A rapid reorientation of the Medicare program in the near term is unlikely; instead, only limited changes can be expected. Although the Medicare program has historically relied on contracting with managed care as a means to control its costs, recent developments suggest that it is now considering other strategies that will allow it to exert more direct influence by creating cost-saving incentives that can actually transfer savings back to the Medicare program.[1]

Similarly, for the health care system as a whole, revolutionary changes implemented in one swoop are not likely; instead, a series of small, incremental changes that will improve chronic illness care in selected areas or for certain conditions or specific populations is the more likely scenario.

Shifting the health care system's primary focus to chronic illness care is akin to turning around a ship the size of the Titanic. Ultimately we will have a radically different system from the one we have today; but instead of a single major, abrupt transformation from the system we have to the system we should have, improving chronic illness care will be a step-wise process. It will require an effort that is:

- Incremental; increasing gradually by regular additions until it involves all stakeholders and all segments of the health care system, as well as individuals and organizations providing long-term supportive services to patients with chronic conditions

- Integrated; linking, to the extent possible, changes throughout the health care system to each other and identifying and minimizing the negative consequences of changes in one area of the system on another area

- Sustained; creating and implementing a wide variety of changes and maintaining the momentum for additional change over the long term

A blueprint for a solution may not yet exist, but a fast-growing body of knowledge points us in the right direction. Indeed, we know more than we think we do. A long list of publications points to needed changes (Institute of Medicine, 2001; Kohn, Corrigan, & Donaldson, 2000; Lawrence, 2002;

Wagner, 2001; Wagner, Austin, & Von Korff, 1996b; Lynn, 2004). A number of pieces of the puzzle have been shown to be meritorious, but no one has yet put it all together to create a new system of care. This chapter reviews what is known about a range of interventions and strategies for improving chronic illness care. This review is deliberately selective and will focus only on changes in the structure and process of care. It will not cover clinical interventions, such as new drugs or surgical procedures; these are beyond the scope of this book. Unlike clinical interventions, the interventions and strategies reviewed here are generic, addressing issues that cut across chronic conditions. Furthermore, this review is not meant to be exhaustive of all structure and process changes; rather, it is limited to selected interventions and strategies that have been shown, in well-designed studies, to improve the quality and/or reduce the cost of chronic illness care. The ones reviewed in the following sections—self-management, interdisciplinary team care, group visits, disease management, case management, and geriatric evaluation and management—have been used both in isolation and in various combinations. Some of them overlap: self-management, for example, is both a component of disease management and a stand-alone strategy. Although the optimal configuration of these interventions and strategies has yet to be determined, there is growing consensus that these are among the building blocks needed to reorganize the health care system to more effectively respond to chronic conditions.

Self-management

The term "self-management" represents the idea of patients' active involvement in their own care. In the context of chronic illness care, self-management refers to a variety of activities individuals can undertake with the intention of limiting the effects of their illness. The key premise underlying self-management is that since patients live with their conditions 24 hours a day, they develop a level of expertise that is different from but at least as, if not more important than that held by their clinicians. By living with their chronic conditions, patients are in the best position to notice subtle changes in their health or well-being as a result of the disease's course or treatment modifications and to quickly respond to such changes.

However, the term may be misleading. Self-management does not imply complete independence from clinicians. Rather, it connotes collaboration and establishing partnerships between clinicians and informed, empowered, and motivated patients.

Creating and sustaining effective partnerships, with decision-making responsibility shared between patients and clinicians, requires that clinicians be taught how to communicate effectively with their patients and that they understand better the aspects of care for which patients are willing and able to take responsibility. At the same time, patients need to become more active participants, for example, by organizing their ideas and observations in advance of clinic visits and communicating them to their clinicians in a coherent manner (Greenfield et al., 1988) and by assuming greater responsibility for the day-to-day monitoring and management of their chronic conditions. Sustaining these partnerships requires clinicians to nurture and support their patients' active participation in the care process.

Self-management programs for patients with chronic conditions are designed to achieve two closely related goals. First, they seek to help patients acquire and improve skills needed for assuming a major role in managing their chronic conditions. This entails not just educating them about the medical and related dimensions of their conditions but also providing them with problem-solving skills and other tools needed to monitor and change their behaviors. Second, self-management programs aim to enhance patients' self-efficacy, defined as people's belief in their own ability to succeed at something they want to do. Increasing patients' self-efficacy in the context of chronic care contributes to their confidence that they can assume more responsibility in their own care, strengthens their motivation, and promotes perseverance. But just as self-management does not mean patients are on their own, promoting self-efficacy should not be interpreted as creating a competition for control between patients and clinicians. The goal is patient-clinician collaboration.

The role of patients as collaborators in managing their own chronic conditions is best viewed on a continuum. Some patients may be more actively involved in managing one aspect of their condition and more passive about other aspects. Also, self-management may not be the answer for every patient. Some patients are physically or mentally incapable of self-management. Others do not want to take part in shared decision making or are not comfortable with taking responsibility for their own health. In many respects, self-management represents a middle-class approach, which works best with proactive personalities. It may not be as effective with other cultural or socioeconomic groups. Indeed, younger adults are more drawn to this active role than are elders, although some dismiss this as simply a generational artifact.

Compared with standard care, self-management programs can provide important benefits for patients with any of a variety of chronic conditions. Self-management programs have been found to reduce the use of health care resources, improve health outcomes, and increase patient involvement in medical decision making. Specific reductions in the utilization of health care services have been found for physician visits (Lewin et al., 1992), hospitalizations (Lorig, Mazonson, & Holman, 1993), readmissions to hospitals (Leveille et al., 1998; Lewin et al., 1992), total hospital days (Leveille et al., 1998; Lorig, Mazonson, & Holman, 1993), and use of psychoactive medications (Leveille et al., 1998). Documented positive health outcomes of self-management programs include:

- Improved emotional well being

- Improved physical functioning

- Fewer and less severe symptoms

- Slower progress of disease and fewer complications

- Improved health behaviors such as exercise and diet

- Improved patient satisfaction

Evidence also supports the cost-effectiveness of self-management programs. Although only a few studies have formally evaluated the programs' cost-effectiveness, studies that address costs consistently note the relatively low cost per patient of self-management programs. Several studies that compared the costs of self-management programs and standard care found that the programs saved costs; that is, on a per-patient basis, the cost of the program is less than the amount of money saved due to reduced use of health care services (DeBusk et al., 1994; Leveille et al., 1998; Lorig et al., 1999). Studies of self-management programs have not been sufficiently detailed, however, to permit teasing out within a specific program the precise factor or factors that reduce costs or lead to improved health outcomes.

Unlike other strategies for improving chronic illness care, most of which have been designed, implemented, and tested with reference only to patients with a specific chronic condition, self-management programs have now been developed for use with heterogeneous groups of chronically ill patients. One successful model is the Chronic Disease Self-Management Program (CDSMP) developed by Kate Lorig and her colleagues at Stanford University. Initially developed for patients with arthritis, the CDSMP has since been adapted for use by patients with different chronic conditions. The CDSMP, which is based on self-efficacy theory and emphasizes problem solving, decision making, and confidence building, is based on the following assumptions:

1. Patients with different chronic diseases have similar self-management problems and disease-related tasks,

2. Patients can learn to take responsibility for the day-to-day management of their disease(s), and

3. Confident, knowledgeable patients practicing self-management will experience improved health status and will utilize fewer health care resources (Lorig et al., 1999).

The six-week CDSMP program is typically conducted by trained lay people, usually in community settings such as senior centers or churches. When conducted with patients with a mixture of chronic conditions, CDSMP participants improved control of their symptoms and were less restricted in their activities (Lorig et al., 1999). More recent studies confirm that the CDSMP leads to positive results in "real-world" clinical practices and not only in controlled research settings (Lorig et al., 2001b).

Based on this success, large-scale dissemination of CDSMP programs has begun. The most notable may be the plan by the National Health Service (NHS) in England to introduce lay-led, self-management training programs, modeled on the CDSMP, for patients with chronic disease. After conducting an initial pilot phase and evaluation, the NHS plans to mainstream the programs within all NHS service areas between 2004 and 2007.[2]

Interdisciplinary Team Care

Team care, first proposed in the 1940s as a way to deliver primary care services, has since been used in a variety of inpatient and outpatient settings. Interdisciplinary team care is the model commonly proposed for improving chronic illness care. In this model, team members come from different professions and each member contributes his or her expertise as needed, maintaining distinct professional responsibilities and individual assignments. In contrast to the multidisciplinary model—in which members, frequently with diverse goals, work in parallel to each other—members of interdisciplinary teams work interdependently toward jointly developed outcomes and goals that are regularly reevaluated.

Many patients with chronic conditions need a range of medical and support services. Those with a single chronic condition, such as sinusitis or other conditions that have a relatively minor impact on health and functioning, may need only limited medical services. Patients with multiple chronic conditions, however, typically need a broader set of health care and supportive services from a variety of practitioners. To respond appropriately and to treat the "whole" person, rather than focusing only on the physiological dimensions of a specific medical problem, care for these patients often requires a team approach. Their complex health and psychosocial problems may require skills and knowledge that go beyond what one practitioner, or even one discipline, can provide. These patients may be best served by an integrated group of professionals who can coordinate care across a variety of disciplines—including, for example, various combinations of physicians, nurses, pharmacists, social workers, therapists, dieticians, and counselors. Unlike individual providers, an interdisciplinary team can use their collective insight to integrate ideas about patient needs and intervention strategies to address the disparate aspects of a patient's chronic conditions.

For interdisciplinary teams to effectively and efficiently meet the needs of chronically ill patients, members should be skilled not only in their own disciplines but also in communication and conflict resolution and understand and respect the roles and expectations of other team members. Open and continuous communication among and between team members is crucial. Furthermore, active involvement of the patient and family with the team is seen as important. Team members should join with the patient and family to establish common goals and objectives and to create a management plan that integrates and addresses the various aspects of the patient's health and supportive care needs. Achieving this level of effective team function requires a substantial investment in building and maintaining team skills (Drinka & Clark, 2000).

One controversial and unresolved issue for interdisciplinary teams concerns the locus of responsibility for a patient's care. From one perspective, interdisciplinary teams work best using a collaborative rather than a delegative model. In a delegative model, one team member (traditionally the highest ranking member) leads the team and retains overall responsibility for patient care. In a collaborative model, members of the team share both leadership functions and responsibility for patient care and are willing to sacrifice some professional autonomy in working together for common goals. However, this model for team care may not only be difficult to implement in the traditionally hierarchical health care system, it may be anathema to some practitioners. Physicians are "used to calling the plays, are trained to so do, expect to do so, and can be highly resistant to sharing that power and authority" (Cooper & Fishman, 2003). Even among those who extol the benefits of patient care teams, some note that "most successful interventions in chronic disease management entail the *delegation* of responsibility by the primary care doctor to team members for ensuring that patients receive proved clinical and self management support services" (Wagner, 2000, emphasis added).

Potential benefits of interdisciplinary team care include increases in efficiency, team member satisfaction, patient satisfaction, patient compliance with treatment regimens, and the use of health care providers other than physicians. The efficiency of team care depends heavily on the ability of team members to communicate effectively without the need for frequent face-to-face meetings. Such communication relies on trust of each other's observations and judgments and an information system that allows information to be shared easily. The expected benefits of interdisciplinary team care from the patients' perspective include reduced fragmentation, greater integration of care for the health and related services they need, and support for their active involvement in their own care. For health care providers, team care is expected to enable them to focus on their individual areas of expertise while learning new skills and approaches to care from team members from other disciplines. Moreover, "a greater sense of completeness of care, a more stimulating practice, and the shared management of very complex patients all add to a more effective clinical environment" (Grant & Finocchio, 1995). Interdisciplinary team care has also reduced the number of missed or broken appointments, decreased hospitalizations, decreased the use of physicians, and reduced costs (Baldwin, 1994). A 1996 Institute of Medicine report strongly endorsed interdisciplinary team care and "asserted its belief that the quality, efficiency, and responsiveness of primary care are enhanced by the use of interdisciplinary teams and recommends the adoption of the team concept of primary care wherever feasible" (Donaldson et al., 1996).

Nonetheless, despite the enthusiasm for interdisciplinary team care and its conceptual advantages, a strong empirical base does not yet exist to show that it consistently results in better chronic care. There is limited direct evidence of the effectiveness of team care itself. Instead, studies that show improved outcomes and costs as a result of chronic care interventions that use interdisciplinary teams as an integral component, such as geriatric evaluation and management, have typically focused on the primary strategy, not on the team care. Rarely is the interdisciplinary team itself the object of the study (Cooper & Fishman, 2003). A review of published studies of interdisciplinary teams in health care and human services settings found the "literature repeatedly endorsed the team model, with little empirical evidence of efficacy" (Schofield & Amodeo, 1999). Accordingly, there is only limited hard evidence concerning the impact of interdisciplinary team care on the outcome and costs of chronic illness care.

It is important to note that this does not mean that interdisciplinary teams do not improve outcomes or reduce costs of chronic illness care; rather, it means only that the available evidence does not yet support those conclusions. Furthermore, several successful programs that have interdisciplinary teams at the "heart of their operations"—including the Program for All-Inclusive Care for the Elderly (PACE), a program of comprehensive services for frail elderly patients that integrates Medicare and Medicaid financing for dually eligible enrollees and hospice programs for terminally ill patients—provide indirect evidence of the value of interdisciplinary teams (Cooper & Fishman, 2003).

Three studies of interdisciplinary home care (IHC) for functionally disabled older people found that, compared with traditional home care, IHC was associated with consistent trends toward lower use of inpatient and outpatient services. In each of the IHC programs, a team—including nurses, occupational and physical therapists, and home health aides but under the leadership of a physician—provided an integrated set of medical and supportive services.[3] The IHC teams met regularly to discuss the cases under their care. Although IHC was also associated with significantly greater use of in-home services, overall, it resulted in lower use of total resources and thus, "unlike traditional forms of home care, IHC may be cost-effective" (Boult, Boult, & Pacala, 1998).

Group Visits

Group visits offer a way to reorganize outpatient care for patients with chronic conditions (Beck et al., 1997). As the term suggests, a group visit entails getting together a small group of patients (usually no more than 15–20 patients) with their principal clinicians for a block of time (usually two to three hours) to facilitate the delivery of health care and other services in a group setting. A group of health care professionals, including, for example, a physician, nurse, social worker or therapist, and pharmacist, typically conducts the group visits. Although these health care professionals provide different services to group-visit participants, they do not necessarily function as an interdisciplinary team.

Group visits, usually conducted on a monthly or bimonthly basis, are designed to facilitate interactions with health care professionals, allow patient monitoring and follow-up, and foster patients' informal discussion about shared health care issues. The group visits usually include a brief social time followed by an educational session or structured group discussion about a specific topic—usually selected by the group—such as lifestyle changes or problems the patients encounter due to their chronic conditions. The meetings also provide time for one-on-one interactions between patients and their clinician. See sample agenda in Table 4.1.

Participants in a group visit may all share certain characteristics, such as the same chronic condition or level of function and impairment. Disease-specific groups are particularly useful for patients with conditions that require extensive patient education or for patients such as newly diagnosed diabetics who have never completed a formal diabetes education program. More frequently, however, group-visit participants are more heterogeneous,

TABLE 4.1.
Group Visit: Standard 2-Hour Model

15 minutes	Greeting and warm-up exercise*
10 minutes	What questions need to be addressed today?
30 minutes	Presentation of topic chosen at last meeting or outside presenter
20 minutes	Break†
15 minutes	Questions and answers
	Wrap-up of discussion
10 minutes	Topic brainstorm for next date
	Confirm next date
20 minutes	Closing
	One-on-one time with physician

*Group process techniques are imperative and not to be underestimated.
†It is important to allow ample unstructured time for one-on-one questioning with physician, blood-pressure check, snack, rest room, etc. (Wellington, 2001).

including patients who do not all have the same medical conditions but may still share certain characteristics (e.g., high utilization of health care services). To form these groups, a clinician may simply invite a number of patients from his or her practice, say 25 elderly patients who have at least one chronic condition.

Group visits aren't for everyone. Clinicians who have experience with group visits estimate that about half of the patients they invite will attend. About 40% of patients dismiss the idea immediately, and another 20% may agree to attend but fail to appear. However, satisfaction with group visits among the patients who do attend is high.

Group visits represent an attempt to move away from the brief office visits that are best suited for identifying and solving a discrete problem, toward a structure that is more appropriate for chronic illness care. These visits are designed to address issues for which there is insufficient time in the normal 18–minute office visit. For example, they may allow clinicians more time to address the preventive, psychological, and social needs of patients with chronic conditions. The structure also allows the clinicians to establish a rapport with the patients and encourage better communication (Wellington, 2001). Another goal is to facilitate patient self-management, promoted through enhanced patient education and expanded opportunities for professional and, even more important, peer support. The encouragement and support patients receive from the other patients is cited as a key advantage of group visits over normal office visits. This is particularly true for chronically ill patients, who often have a greater need for support and reassurance from others.

Studies of group visits have documented a variety of benefits. Group visits for chronically ill older adults in a health maintenance organization (HMO) have been shown to reduce the use of emergency departments

(Coleman et al., 2001). Emergency department use has been associated with subsequent functional decline, increased use of health care services, and increased nursing home admissions; it may also be "an important sentinel event signifying a breakdown in care coordination" (Coleman et al., 2001). Another study of chronically ill older adults in an HMO found that group visits reduced repeat hospital admissions and emergency care use, delivered flu shots and other preventive services more effectively, increased patient and physician satisfaction, and reduced the overall cost of care (Beck et al., 1997).

Disease Management

Disease management (DM) is perhaps the most well known and widely adopted strategy designed to promote cost-effective, quality care for patients with chronic conditions. This strategy is not only popular in the United States, but also "commands wide international support as the optimal approach to planning and delivering" chronic illness care (Hunter, 2000). In its relatively short history since the early 1990s as a structured systems response to chronic conditions, DM has given rise to a national trade association of organizations providing DM programs, several professional journals, a new $1 billion industry, and, most recently, efforts by national health care organizations to establish accreditation standards for DM programs.[4] Although some view disease management as a novel and innovative strategy, others maintain that DM "is as old as medicine itself" and is little more than a sophisticated packaging of fundamental precepts of providing good medical care for a population or group of patients (Bodenheimer, 1999).

There are multiple competing definitions for disease management. The Disease Management Association of America (DMAA), for example, defines disease management as "a system of coordinated healthcare interventions and communications for populations with conditions in which patient self-care efforts are significant."[5] A recent literature review defined the term as "an intervention designed to manage or prevent a chronic condition using a systematic approach to care and potentially employing multiple treatment modalities" (Weingarten et al., 2002). Choosing among these definitions may be less helpful than identifying the common components included in all definitions of disease management. These components include:

- Strategies, such as patient surveys or claims data, to identify patients who have or are at high risk for developing the targeted condition (In some cases high utilization may be the identifying factor.)

- Patient assessment and enrollment

- Supporting adherence to state-of-the-art, evidence-based practice guidelines

- Services designed to enhance patient self-management and adherence to the patient's care plan

- Monitoring patients' status between visits and intervening where appropriate, either by means of advice to the patient or communication to the clinician concerning the patient's condition

- Collaboration among providers and between the patient and providers

- Collection and analysis of process and outcome measures

Despite this common thread across the definitions of disease management, not all DM programs include all these components. The specific components included vary across different health care settings and disease states. According to the DMAA, programs that provide less than the full complement of services listed above are more appropriately termed "disease management support services."

The philosophy underlying disease management is that health care "resources can be used more effectively if the patient becomes the pivot around which health care is organized" (Hunter, 2000). By focusing on patients as "entities experiencing the clinical course" of their chronic conditions, disease management brings a coordinated and sustained approach to patient care over the long term and avoids viewing care as a series of discrete encounters (Hunter, 2000). Thus, in theory, DM is an approach that is particularly well suited for the care and management of patients with chronic conditions.

Two Models

There are two basic models for disease management programs: a contracted "carve-out" model and a primary care-based model (Bodenheimer, 1999). In the carve-out model, an independent organization contracts with a managed care organization, health plan, or employer to provide disease management services to a selected group of patients (e.g., enrollees in a health plan who have a specific chronic condition such as diabetes). This approach is often used by insurance companies and health plans because few of their contracted physicians have enough patients covered by a single insurer or health plan to warrant changing their practice styles. This model is thus run in parallel with primary care. Among the organizations that offer commercial DM programs are pharmaceutical benefits management firms and dedicated DM organizations (see exhibit 4.1).

EXHIBIT 4.1

Medicare's Chronic Care Improvement Program

The Medicare Prescription Drug, Improvement, and Modernization Act of 2003 (MMA) includes several provisions designed to enhance chronic illness care. Among the most important is the Voluntary Chronic Care Improvement under Traditional Fee-for-Service Medicare program, or CCI. Phase I of the CCI, the pilot phase, calls for the phased-in development, testing, evaluation, and implementation of chronic care improvement projects for selected subgroups of Medicare beneficiaries. This project is especially noteworthy because it represents an example of Medicare acting as an HMO, developing programs that can potentially save money for the program by investing in better near-term care.

In Phase I, the Centers for Medicare and Medicaid Services (CMS) will contract with private organizations, such as health insurers and disease management organizations, to establish approximately 10 regional CCI projects, collectively serving approximately 150,000–300,000 chronically ill beneficiaries in Medicare's fee-for-service plan. The Phase I projects will operate for three years and be evaluated through randomized controlled trials. The principal objectives are to develop and test new strategies that can cost-effectively improve quality of care and beneficiary and provider satisfaction for chronically ill patients. Successful elements of Phase I projects could be expanded after the pilot phase to reach more Medicare beneficiaries with chronic health conditions. CMS solicited proposals from interested organizations for Phase I on April 23, 2004. CCI projects are scheduled to begin in 2005.

Initially, the CCI projects will focus on beneficiaries who have congestive heart failure (CHF), complex diabetes, or chronic obstructive pulmonary disease (COPD). Beneficiaries with these conditions account for a disproportionate share of Medicare expenditures (for example, the 18% of Medicare beneficiaries with diabetes account for 32% of Medicare spending). Their health care experience is also modifiable in the short term, increasing the potential to document changes in the three-year timeframe for evaluating results.

The CCI initiative is based on but goes beyond existing chronic care strategies such as disease management and case management programs. Thus, for example, each CCI project will offer self-care guidance and support to chronically ill beneficiaries to help them manage their health, adhere to their physicians' plans of care, and ensure that they seek (or obtain) medical care that they need to reduce their health risks. The projects will also include collaboration with participants' providers to enhance communication of relevant clinical information. The projects are intended to help increase adherence to evidence-based care, reduce unnecessary hospital stays and emergency room visits, and help participants avoid costly and debilitating complications.

CCI organizations will be required to develop a care management plan with each participating beneficiary and, in carrying out these plans, the organization must:

- Guide the participant in managing the participants' health,
- Use decision-support tools such as evidence-based practice guidelines, and
- Develop a clinical information database to track and monitor each participant across settings and to evaluate outcomes.

The CCI initiative is designed to foster innovation. It therefore does not identify which approach (e.g., disease management or case management) best suits Medicare's needs. Although CMS anticipates that CCI projects will have some elements in common with existing private-sector disease or case management programs, it also anticipates that these will need to be adapted to suit the unique needs of Medicare's FFS beneficiaries and that new elements will need to be developed. Accordingly, CCI projects are given flexibility in tailoring support services to participants' needs and will be held accountable only for meeting broad performance improvement goals, including population-based measures of clinical quality, costs, and satisfaction (Foote, 2004), not for adhering to rigid protocols.

For Medicare beneficiaries, participation in CCI will be strictly voluntary. Eligible beneficiaries do not have to change plans or providers or pay extra to participate, leaving intact Medicare beneficiaries' freedom of choice of provider. They will be able to stop participating at any time.

Ideally, the CCI initiative will not only improve chronic illness care for Medicare beneficiaries, it will "create a financially sustainable means of catalyzing private sector efforts" and thus contribute to a broader reorientation of the health care system to improve chronic care (Foote, 2004).

Source: Information about the CCI program is at www.cms.hhs.gov/medicarereform/ccip/

In the primary care-based model, health care organizations, such as integrated health systems or managed care organizations, develop their own in-house disease management programs designed for selected groups of patients with certain chronic conditions. To date, nearly all disease management programs in both models have targeted patients with a single, relatively well-defined chronic condition, such as diabetes or asthma. The programs then apply standardized approaches to the similar needs of their enrollees with this condition.

A major point of controversy with regard to disease management programs is the extent to which the services they provide are integrated with the patients' other medical care. Principles of chronic care management would suggest that a high degree of integration is important in establishing effective clinician-patient partnerships. The two models for DM programs differ significantly on the level of integration. In the "carve-out" model, health plans that contract with many clinicians and have relatively little control over those clinicians (or health plans with insufficient resources to develop their own in-house DM programs) may contract with disease management companies to provide DM programs for some of their enrollees.[6] Some commercial disease management programs augment traditional medical care by adding services such as patient education, preventive services, or transportation but do not include actual treatment of the patient's condition. Other commercial DM programs, however, take the added step and assume primary responsibility for managing the patient's chronic condition. In so doing, they typically separate management for the chronic condition from the care provided by the patient's personal clinicians.

In essence, these latter arrangements carve out the management of the patient's chronic condition and essentially establish a treatment program that is parallel to the patient's primary clinicians and customary care. Commercial DM programs are not responsible for the patient's general well-being or problems related to diagnoses other than those they have been contracted to manage. "Carving out" the management of one condition and assigning it to someone other than the patient's personal clinicians could therefore result in more fragmentation as well as missed opportunities to treat important comorbidities. For example, the DM program may not know the full range of drugs the patient is taking. Although it is in the health plan's interests to establish linkages and promote communication between the disease management program and the patient's clinicians, as an add-on approach this model of DM will nonetheless pose difficulties for efficiently and effectively managing the patient's overall care.

In contrast, DM programs based on the primary care-based model are developed and implemented by health care organizations as in-house programs. They typically use the organizations' own health care providers and other resources. For such DM programs a health care organization may, for example, reorganize some of its staff into interdisciplinary teams to address all aspects of care for selected groups of enrollees. Even if the teams' responsibility is limited to the care of the enrollees' chronic condition, the team nevertheless works within the organization, uses the same communication and information systems as the organization's other personnel, and shares the organization's goals, values, and patient care responsibilities. It should therefore be easier to integrate such an in-house DM program with the care provided by the enrollees' primary caregivers. Because the primary care-based model builds on the enrollees' existing care system (Bodenheimer,

1999), it should reduce fragmentation and reinforce rather than undermine continuity and coordination of care.

Beyond the criticisms of the "carve-out" model, other concerns regarding disease management programs include:

- Most DM programs target a single chronic condition, only a few manage care for patients with more than one chronic condition. Separate DM programs for different chronic conditions merely add more stovepipes to an already fragmented health care system. The trend, however, is away from a "disease-centric" approach to a more "patient-centric" one, allowing for multidisease management programs (Villagra, 2004).

- The need of commercial DM companies to make a profit may encourage them to attract healthier patients, pull out of markets that are less profitable, or chose not to offer programs for particularly difficult or expensive chronic conditions (Bodenheimer, 2000).

- The growth of commercial programs and the separation of DM from the primary care site could lead to fragmentation of care rather than the cost savings and improvements in quality hoped for by the programs' purchasers.

Despite these concerns, the private sector has enthusiastically embraced disease management as an approach that could compensate for some of the deficiencies in how the current health care system provides care for people with chronic conditions. States have also implemented disease management programs in their efforts to control costs in their Medicaid programs while improving the quality of care. They have used both models of DM programs, with some states developing in-house programs whereas others contract with commercial vendors. Medicare has now also embraced DM, making the strategy a core component of the chronic care improvement initiative included in the Medicare Modernization Act of 2003 (see exhibit 4.1).

Still, the effectiveness of DM programs in improving health care outcomes or mitigating health care costs is largely unknown (Villagra, 2004). Evaluating DM programs has been difficult in part because only the individual components have been studied, not the combined package of services that constitute a typical disease management program. Moreover, current research has not addressed whether some components or combinations are more effective than others (Weingarten et al., 2002). A recent review of published reports on disease management programs for patients with chronic conditions evaluated the following program components: provider education, provider feedback, provider reminders, patient education, patient reminders, and patient financial incentives. The review concluded that all these components were associated with improvements in provider adherence to practice guidelines and disease control. However, because only a few studies have compared the effectiveness of the various components of DM programs, there is little information on the components' relative effectiveness. It is not clear which disease management strategy, or combination of strategies, can achieve the greatest benefits (Weingarten et al., 2002).

Uncertainty surrounds disease management's potential for cost savings as well. The recent growth in DM may be attributable in part to the program's focus on the small subset of patients who account for the vast majority of medical expenditures. Typically, about 10% of a population accounts for nearly 70% of total medical expenditures, and people with chronic conditions make up a disproportionately large share of this top 10%. By targeting selected subsets of patients with high-cost chronic conditions for close day-to-day monitoring and rapidly reacting to any trouble signs as they appear, disease management programs seek to avoid costly hospitalizations and emergency room visits. Although focusing narrowly on a few high users may indeed reduce costs, this approach does not advance the stated population health goals of DM programs.

It is unclear whether more broadly targeted DM programs actually save money. Fewer than half of HMOs reported that DM programs for patients with diabetes had saved money and only about 1 in 4 reported savings from DM programs for asthma (Bodenheimer, 2000). Bodenheimer notes that the lack of cost savings to HMOs for asthma treatment "is surprising since proper management of asthma would be expected rapidly to reduce the number of days spent in hospital and visits to the emergency rooms." Savings with diabetes may be even harder to demonstrate because the benefits of preventing complications may not become apparent for years. In the context of managed care, these benefits may arise after the patient has disenrolled from the plan that made the initial investments in such care. Preliminary data from a comprehensive DM program addressing 17 specific chronic conditions show substantial cost savings and a return on investment of at least 2 to 1 (exhibit 4.2).

Case Management

Interest in case management[7] has surged since the early 1980s and it has been implemented in all patient care settings, including acute, ambulatory, long-term, and community-based settings. However, there is still little consensus regarding what case management is and this absence of agreement on its definition and component activities fuels the ongoing dispute regarding its impact and its appropriate role in chronic illness care.

EXHIBIT 4.2

BCBSM / American Healthways Initiative

In 2002, Blue Cross and Blue Shield of Minnesota (BCBSM) embarked on a 10-year initiative with American Healthways to better meet the needs of BCBSM enrollees with 17 specific chronic conditions. BCBSM is the largest health insurer in Minnesota; American Healthways promotes itself as "the nation's leading provider of specialized, comprehensive care enhancement and disease management services." The 10-year "strategic alliance" marked a significant step for both companies. For BCBSM it replaced two 5-year-old internal disease management programs that targeted only patients with diabetes and /or heart disease and vastly expanded their population-based approach to disease management. For American Healthways, the contract represented the first opportunity to implement its "total care enhancement" program.

The Blueprint for Health care support program targets a total of 17 conditions in two categories: (1) high-volume chronic conditions (e.g., diabetes, coronary artery disease, congestive heart failure, COPD, asthma, and end-stage renal disease) and (2) selected "impact conditions" (e.g., low-back pain, atrial fibrillation, osteoporosis, fibromyalgia, arthritis, and six others).

These conditions were chosen based on evidence showing that more aggressive monitoring and disease management can have a positive impact on outcomes and patient satisfaction. However, the sponsoring organizations acknowledge that convincing data may not yet exist for all of the 17 conditions.

An estimated 12–15% of BCBSM enrollees have one or more of these 17 conditions, accounting for about 45% of BCBSM's annual health care expenditures. About 100,000 BCBSM enrollees were enrolled in the first year of the program. Compared with BCBSM's previous efforts, the new model provides more frequent and intensive communication (between clinicians and patients), patient monitoring, and follow-up. Specific elements of the new model include:

- A "neural-net" predictive model to identify enrollees who have or are at risk for the targeted conditions
- Enhanced risk stratification of program enrollees (based on severity) to allow more effective matching of clinical interventions with patient needs
- Monitoring patient enrollees via telephone calls from a nurse (minimum four to five calls per year, on average)

Nurses are American Healthways employees working only on the BCBSM contract and are based in a Minnesota call center built specifically for this project.

Nurses use computer-driven protocols to guide patient care and management of disease.

Nurses are empowered to make home visits to patients, particularly for certain conditions where biomedical device monitoring is used.

"On the ground" nurses (Provider Support Managers) interface with and support physicians who have patients in these programs.

- Concerted efforts to support and reinforce existing clinician-patient relationships and to avoid "carving out" care for the chronic condition from the patient's ongoing (primary) care.
- Intensive patient education and heavy reliance on patient self-management

BCBSM and American Healthways have identified five measures ot success for the new model:

1. Higher patient satisfaction
2. Higher physician satisfaction
3. Greater adherence to recommended practice guidelines
4. Improved clinical outcomes
5. Cost savings

The final measure of success may be the most important. The services included in this new initiative represent new expenditures. Though BCBSM acknowledged there was no track record for the new model itself, the organization expects to save money in the long run, based on its experience with its older disease management programs.

Outcomes: In October 2003, BCBSM reported that:

- More than 100,000 members were enrolled in the care support program during the first year.
- Preliminary results at six months into the program showed high patient satisfaction and a decrease in days lost from work for employed enrollees.
- There were demonstrable decreases in emergency room utilization and hospitalizations and decreases in per-member, per-month costs for both the core chronic diseases and the impact conditions.
- Savings at six months were estimated at a 1.9:1 return on investment.
- Results at one year have shown a statistically significant decrease in mean HgbA1c levels for diabetic members enrolled in the program and persistent decreases in emergency room use (11%) and hospital admissions (14%).
- Costs for the population enrolled in the program increased 6%, compared with an increase of slightly higher than 20% for those who did not have access to the program.
- The estimated return on investment at one year was between 2.9 and 3.9:1, and the savings were in the range of $36–49 million.

Source: Based on conversations with Steven Eisenberg, M.D., Medical Director, Blue Cross and Blue Shield of Minnesota, January 2002 and October 2003.

Case management has been variously identified as a set of specified activities, a patient care delivery system, a practice model, or a process of care delivery. As defined by the Case Management Society of America, case management is a collaborative process that assesses, plans, implements, coordinates, monitors, and evaluates the options and services required to meet an individual's health needs. This "process" thus includes patient screening and case finding, advocating for the patient and family, ongoing reassessment of patients needs, evaluation of patient care services, and referral for community-based services. Combined, these activities seek to manage the clinical services needed by patients, assure appropriate resource utilization, enhance the quality of care, and facilitate cost-effective patient care outcomes.[8] Case management is proactive, focusing on the present to prevent adverse outcomes and hospitalizations in the future, and continuous over an extended time.

Case management comes in many forms, only some of which offer advantages to chronic diseases. Broadly, a case manager's role is twofold. One role is associated with the patient and family, and its aims are to improve the patient's health status, functional abilities, and accessibility to health care. Case management is designed to achieve positive health outcomes through patient education, information, advocacy, and patient empowerment. The second role, associated with the health care organization, aims at cost containment and the appropriate use and allocation of resources. Case management may save money by avoiding care associated with medical complications that can be prevented, eliminating inappropriate care, and by reducing duplication, overbilling, or system inefficiencies. Table 4.2 illustrates the variation in case management roles.

Though it shares many features, case management can be differentiated from disease management. In contrast to disease management, which is by definition disease-specific and thus targets people with a discrete (usually chronic) condition, case management programs are non-disease-specific, targeting persons who are at high risk for adverse outcomes and expensive care because of their complex medical (usually chronic) conditions. Accordingly, case management generally adopts a more individualized approach to address the unique needs of "at-risk" patients than the more standardized approach of disease management programs for a group of patients who share the same condition and thus similar needs.

Continuity and consistency of care are keys to successful case management and are assured by linking each patient to a case manager (also called a "care manager" or "health coordinator"). The case manager is someone other than the provider of direct care and is responsible for managing, facilitating, and coordinating the care of a caseload of patients across the continuum of care. Case managers work with each patient, and family and

TABLE 4.2.
Variations in Case Management

Type of Case Management	Case Manager	Components
Eligibility management	Social worker or nurse	• Assessment to see if client reaches threshold for eligibility • Care plan • Implementations • Cursory monitoring for change in status that would affect eligibility
Care coordination	Social worker or nurse	• Structured assessment to identify needs • Care plan addressing each need • Arrangement of services to meet each need • Follow-up to ensure services are delivered • Periodic reassessment to adjust care plan
Utilization management	Usually a nurse	• Identification of high-volume/high-cost cases • Work with high users to change clinical course • Intensive monitoring • Counseling to encourage compliance • Preventive problem solving • Flagged charts to alert clinicians
Disease management	Usually a nurse, possibly M.D.	• Focus on a single disease • Provision of reminders • Counseling • Monitoring • Usually not coordinated with primary care
Chronic care management	Nurse or nurse practitioner	• Expected clinical course established • Monitoring of salient parameters for each condition treated • Patients responsible for most of the monitoring • Communication with clinicians by phone, Web • Intervention when actual course differs from expected course • Indication for active intervention • Clients seen primarily when their condition changes significantly • Many conditions monitored simultaneously • Both function and disease addressed

health care team, over the long term—both when the patient is feeling well and when the patient has immediate health care needs. By establishing an individualized and personalized relationship with the patient and family, the case manager can help ensure that all needed health and social services are obtained. The case manager is expected to work closely with the patient and health care team to create a plan that meets the patient's needs and is acceptable to all involved.

The case manager role can be performed by professionals with varying backgrounds. Some groups, such as the American Nurses Association, have developed specific definitions of case management practice for use within their profession. The vast majority of case managers are nurses with at least a bachelor's degree, a minority are advanced practice nurses, and some are social workers. Who assumes the case manager's role may influence the component activities. The core competencies for case managers include communication (with patients and families as well as with other health care professionals), collaboration, delegation, and knowledge of health care resources, community resources and support, and insurance and reimbursement issues.

Evaluations of case management have examined the impact on utilization (e.g., length of stay), clinical outcomes, patient satisfaction, and cost-effectiveness. As with case management programs themselves, most evaluations also focus on patients with chronic illnesses. There are problems with the quality of these studies, however. Most are of a single case management program, using a pre-post design where the outcomes are compared before and after the introduction of the program. This type of study does not control for other variables that may also affect the outcome. The published studies also do not clarify which elements of a case management program lead to which outcomes.

A nurse case management program with diabetes education guidelines, diet and exercise reinforcement, and systematic treatment adjustments was found to significantly improve glycemic control and other health indicators (Aubert et al., 1998). A study of patients discharged from hospital with congestive heart failure found that case management can significantly reduce the rate of readmission, improve the quality of life, and decrease the overall cost of medical care (Rich et al., 1995). In a study of patients with at least one chronic illness who received case management services in their own homes (in person or by telephone), the number of hospital admissions and emergency department visits were significantly reduced (Boyd et al., 1996). Case management works best with significant patient input and cooperation. As discussed previously, patients who are actively involved in their treatment often obtain better outcomes. Patients are also more willing to share information with a case managers with whom they have good rapport; this in turn helps the case manager in coaching and guiding patients toward desired outcomes.

Other studies are more equivocal. For example, a Canadian study of frail older people over age 70 found that nursing case management had no impact on the number of hospital admissions or the length of hospital stay (Gagnon et al., 1999). Moreover, not everyone agrees with the reported financial outcomes. One review of the literature concluded that, despite the cost savings reported by some studies of case management programs, "a technically correct and rigorous cost-effectiveness analysis has not been performed in any assessment of case management" (Institute for Clinical Systems Improvement, 1998). Regardless of these concerns, however, evidence suggests that case management has promise in improving care, outcomes, and costs for persons with selected chronic conditions.

Geriatric Evaluation and Management

Geriatric evaluation and management (GEM) is perhaps the most thoroughly studied care coordination strategy for improving the care of a specific subset of chronically ill elderly persons. GEM, which has been used both in inpatient and outpatient settings, combines comprehensive geriatric assessment with sustained treatment and care management for high-risk older people. The assessment is a diagnostic process, using standardized instruments and procedures, to determine an older person's physical and mental health, functional capabilities and limitations, and level of social supports (including informal caregivers' capabilities). This evaluation then forms the basis for the development of an overall plan for treatment and follow-up, tailored to the person's identified needs. Typically, an interdisciplinary team (including, for example, a geriatric nurse practitioner, physician, and social worker) conducts both the evaluation and care management components of GEM.

Inpatient GEM units are typically separate hospital wards that have been redesigned specifically for geriatric patients. Interdisciplinary team rounds and patient-centered team conferences are hallmarks of care on these specialized units, which, in contrast to less structured geriatric consultations, have direct control over the implementation of team recommendations (Agostini, Baker, & Bogardus, 2001). Early studies of inpatient GEM found dramatic improvements in patients' survival and functional status (Stuck et al., 1993). Over the past two decades "usual [geriatric] care has become progressively more like the programs of geriatric evaluation and management in earlier studies" (Cohen et al., 2002). As a result, "there may be relatively little additional improvement *in mortality* that can be gained with the use of geriatric evaluation and management in the population of frail patients" (Cohen et al., 2002, emphasis added). A recent multicenter study of GEM in both inpatient and outpatient settings found no significant effects on survival or on subsequent function. However, inpatient GEM had a significant positive effect on "health-related quality of life" at the time of discharge, reflecting its usefulness for "improving functional status and management of pain while patients are in the hospital." In the same study, outpatient GEM significantly improved patients' mental health status at one year after discharge (Cohen et al., 2002).

The cost of inpatient GEM programs has remained high, prompting more efforts to deliver GEM in outpatient settings. One study at an outpatient clinic at a community hospital found that GEM preserved functional ability, reduced restriction in daily activities, decreased symptoms of depression, increased patient satisfaction, and reduced the burden felt by family caregivers. The program was estimated to cost about $1,350 per person for the screening, the tests, and all professional services (Boult et al., 2001). The study's authors conclude that it will be up to patients, consumers, and third-party payers to decide if these "valuable, but not free" benefits are worth the investment. A recent review of 13 randomized controlled studies of GEM in outpatient settings reported that 6 of the 13 found improved maintenance of physical functioning. None of the 13 studies demonstrated a reduction in hospital admissions (though one showed a reduction in nursing home utilization) and none demonstrated a reduction in mortality (Cooper & Fishman, 2003). In a large randomized trial of GEM programs in the United Kingdom, patient management by a hospital outpatient geriatric team versus the primary care team resulted in significant improvements in quality of life, in terms of mobility, social interaction, and morale (Fletcher et al, 2004).

The benefits of geriatric evaluation and management, in both inpatient and outpatient settings, have thus shifted from reducing mortality (where additional improvement may no longer be possible) to improvements in patients' physical and mental health status and functioning. The challenge is to integrate these programs into other inpatient and outpatient services for frail elderly patients.

Summary

Though the interventions and strategies reviewed in this chapter are not necessarily unique to chronic illness care (interdisciplinary team care, for example, has a long history in the acute care system), each responds to characteristics that differentiate chronic from acute conditions. Among the targeted differences are that chronic conditions are enduring and thus require ongoing management; that the majority of such management will take place not in hospitals and physician's offices but elsewhere; that patients themselves are often in the best position to monitor and manage chronic conditions; that the skills and competencies needed to effectively manage chronic conditions are dispersed across different health care disciplines; and that persons with chronic conditions may need more information and support than clinicians can provide in traditional office visits.

These interventions and strategies are among the most promising elements of modern chronic care management. They can increase the likelihood that optimal chronic care will be rendered, health outcomes and patient satisfaction improved, and costs moderated or reduced. A few organizations at the cutting edge of reform (some of which are outlined in chapter 11) have comprehensive programs that put all or most of these elements of chronic care management into practice. Many more organizations have adopted only a single element, most often disease management. A positive impact on patients, however, is more likely with a more comprehensive approach (Renders et al., 2001). These interventions and strategies should be included in any multidimensional effort for improving chronic illness care, although which combinations are most likely to achieve best possible outcomes have yet to be determined.

5. The Right Health Care Workers with the Right Skills

Providing optimal care for people with chronic conditions will put new pressures on a health care professional workforce already buffeted by major changes in the health care system. The projected growth in the number of people with such conditions, in particular, those with multiple chronic conditions and thus more complex needs, will increase the demand for most types of health care professionals.[1] These projections, calling for a larger workforce and a different mix of health care professionals to care for patients with chronic conditions, come at a time when the supply of some health care professionals, such as nurses and primary care physicians, is shrinking. Pressure from inside and outside the health care system for greater accountability, improved quality, and greater efficiency will prompt new staff configurations, a reshuffling of health care professionals' roles and responsibilities, and changes in their interactions with each other. Interdisciplinary team practice, for example, will become more common and clinicians such as advanced practice nurses will increasingly perform tasks previously performed by physicians. This will expedite the shift from a physician monopoly to a sharing of clinical authority among health care disciplines.

Caring for chronically ill patients and managing their conditions requires skills and competencies that extend beyond traditional biomedical training for preventing, diagnosing, and treating acute conditions. Health care professionals who care for chronically ill patients will need to:

- Communicate effectively (both listening and explaining) with patients and with colleagues

- Relate to patients, including being comfortable sharing power

- Employ behavior modification techniques and motivate lifestyle and behavior changes

- Coordinate patient care with health care professionals from other disciplines and settings

- Use electronic communications, including becoming proficient with structured data systems

To competently provide care and avoid burnout, health care professionals must also be able to derive satisfaction from helping people delay the course of their chronic conditions without curing them. Likewise, a health care system designed for optimal chronic illness care will place new demands on informal (or unpaid) caregivers and on patients themselves.

Demographic and workforce projections forecast a shortage of clinicians to care for people with chronic conditions, whereas economic projections indicate that current cost trends in health care are unsustainable. New ways must therefore be found to train and use health care professionals more efficiently and in clinically appropriate ways. Redoubling past efforts to increase the supply of clinicians who care for patients with chronic conditions will not be enough. New options include:

- Expanding training in chronic illness care, both for a distinct cadre of chronic care clinicians and for all clinicians, by focusing on the skills and competencies that are central to good chronic care. Ensuring that clinicians have the right skills and competencies requires changes in both training and practice environments (one without the other will not change clinician behavior).

- Reconfiguring the roles and responsibilities of clinicians who care for patients with chronic conditions

- Using information technology to substitute for some in-person contacts

- Using information technology to allow more care to be delegated to personnel with less training

This chapter concentrates on changes for the health care professional workforce. Proposed new and expanded roles and responsibilities for patients in caring for their own chronic conditions are discussed in chapter 6, as are the roles and responsibilities of family members and other informal caregivers.

Workforce Supply and Demand

Patients with chronic conditions will continue to be cared for by a wide range of health care professionals, including general internists, family practitioners, and other physicians; advanced practice nurses, nurses, and nursing aides; and social workers, occupational and physical therapists, and other practitioners. Projecting the future supply of and demand for these professionals is imprecise at best, especially in light of anticipated role changes. Long-term supply projections are notoriously difficult because of the long timeframe for health professional education (four to five years after medical school for geriatricians, for example), the uncertain impact of current worker shortages and declining job appeal for some health careers on future recruitment efforts and enrollment in training programs, and the expanding range of opportunities for health care professionals to pursue their careers in administrative and other non-patient-care jobs.

Projecting future demand is similarly inexact. Simple demographic projections are typically given as a range. For example, the projected total population for the Unites States in 2020 will fall somewhere between 303 million and 354 million, of whom about 50%, or 152 million to 177 million, will have at least one chronic condition. To maintain the current (1996) ratio of 180 active physicians per 100,000 population means that demand in 2020 will be for 545,000 to 673,000 physicians, a nearly 20% range. Compounding the difficulty is the complex relationships among aging, chronic illness, and disability. Some researchers suggest, for example, that a decline in disability rates among the elderly may partially offset demographic factors such as the aging population and thus lead to a healthier population overall (Cutler, 2001; Spillman, 2004) and a corresponding decrease in demand for health care professionals. Most believe, however, that future advances in medicine will continue to transform previously fatal events into lengthy chronic conditions and, when these trends are combined with the sheer volume of people reaching age 65 (who are more likely than younger people to have or develop a chronic condition), they will overwhelm any social and demographic changes in the next few decades that would suggest a possible plateau or decline in the demand for chronic care services. The real debate, according to them, is over the size of the increase in demand. Regardless how the controversy over the magnitude of the future demand for chronic care services is resolved, the consensus is that, without significant changes in health care professional education, there will be too few practitioners trained to deal with the often complex and wide-ranging needs of people with chronic conditions.

Concerns regarding the health care professional workforce for chronic care mirror those raised for the primary care workforce (Grumbach & Bodenheimer, 2002), because so much of chronic care is fundamentally primary care.[2] The core functions of primary care—comprehensiveness, accessibility (or first-contact care), continuity, and coordination—are also central to chronic illness care (Rothman & Wagner, 2003). Although chronic care overlaps with primary care, the two are not equivalent. Nonetheless, given their similarity, chronic care practitioners suffer many of the same problems faced by those in primary care disciplines, including financial inequities and diminished reputation. In an increasingly specialized health care system, primary care clinicians are, on average, paid less and, on balance, valued less, than their specialist colleagues. Interest in primary care careers is declining (R.A. Cooper, Laud, & Dietrich, 1998; Grumbach & Bodenheimer, 2002). Overall, the same factors that curtail health care students' and practitioners' interest in primary care also apply to chronic care.

Three types of health care professionals—physicians, advanced practice nurses (and physician assistants), and nurses—provide the vast majority of formal (as opposed to informal or unpaid) health care services to patients with chronic conditions. Practitioners from these three disciplines, the focus of this chapter, are typically also the lead health care professionals in managing and coordinating chronic illness care. These practitioners are supported by a wide range of health care professionals from other disciplines, including social workers, pharmacists, and rehabilitation and other therapists, who offer narrower and more targeted health and supportive services.

Physicians

Physician supply and demand is endlessly debated, with little agreement on whether we currently face a physician surplus or deficit and on future projections. The overall trend, though, is toward a workforce with more specialists and fewer primary care physicians. For the types of physicians who care for certain subpopulations of chronically ill patients, however, there is no debate about surpluses or deficits. For instance, geriatricians, that is, physicians with expertise in aging-related health issues or gerontology, will be particularly important in any effort to improve chronic illness care because so much chronic illness is concentrated in the elderly population. Regarding geriatricians, the clear consensus is that we face a shortage, both now and in the future.

Geriatricians are most often primary care-oriented physicians who have completed at least one additional year of training in geriatrics after their initial training in family practice, internal medicine, or psychiatry. Geriatrics integrates many aspects of medicine and emphasizes problems that are more common in older adults, such as chronic pain management, dementia, and sensory impairments.

Many experts agree that a "large core of geriatricians will be needed to provide care for the 15 to 20 percent of the elderly who are the oldest and most frail" (Firshein, 1999). Geriatricians may also be needed to advise and train the other health care professionals who see elderly patients but who have had little or no geriatric training. But the supply of geriatricians and forecasts for growth fall far short of what would be needed to make even a dent in the needs.

Concerted efforts over the past 25 years have led to significant growth in geriatric training programs in U.S. medical schools and residency programs. In 2001, nearly 9 of every 10 U.S. medical schools had a distinct geriatric medicine program. The number of first-year positions in geriatric medicine fellowship programs has also risen dramatically, but many of these training slots remain unfilled (Warshaw & Bragg, 2003). Other challenges remain. Most geriatric medicine programs are a part of other medical school departments; only 6 of the 126 accredited medical schools have a distinct geriatrics department. And there are still relatively few practicing geriatricians. A total of 10,207 physicians were certified as geriatricians from 1998 through 2002. The number of geriatricians is expected to decline in the near future—a projected 26% reduction, from 9,256 in 1998 to 6,806 in 2004—as practicing geriatricians retire at a faster rate than new trainees enter practice (Warshaw & Bragg, 2003). The field is thus shrinking just as the number of people needing this type of special care is rapidly increasing.

Beyond the shortage of geriatricians is the deficiency in geriatric training for medical students who do not specialize in geriatrics. Although most physicians will see elderly patients at some point in their practice regardless of their specialty, few receive any formal training in the specific needs of this population. In 1995, only 10% of all U.S. medical schools required their students to complete a separate course in geriatrics. In medical schools where geriatrics is offered as an elective, only 3% of students take the course (Firshein, 1999).

This lack of training may help explain why many physicians find it so hard to care for elderly patients. A recent survey revealed that, although primary care physicians, on the whole, enjoyed interactions with their elderly patients, "the high prevalence of multiple medical problems and declining physical and cognitive function among these patients gave rise to interacting medical, interpersonal, and administrative difficulty" (Adams et al., 2002). Many physicians felt they lacked confidence in dealing with the special needs of elderly patients, particularly those with chronic conditions. Common concerns expressed included the physicians' "frustration at their perceived inability to help with older patient's chronic conditions." Indeed, research in other areas has in fact shown that people who must deal with strangers they feel unable to help may actually develop negative feelings toward them (Lerner & Simmons, 1966). Physicians who perceive themselves as unable to effectively assist geriatric patients may then become negatively disposed to these very persons who need their help most. With increased geriatrics training, such as mandatory geriatrics rotations during medical school, primary care physicians "could become more skilled and comfortable with the special needs of elderly patients" (Adams et al., 2002).

Advanced Practice Nurses

The problem of attracting the right types of people into primary care physician careers has been discussed for many years. At one point, creating separate tracks in medical school was suggested as a means of recruiting people who have better interpersonal skills and who are also particularly interested in fields of practice that offer extensive and sustained patient contact. The idea of creating such a distinct physician corps was abandoned, but it may be resurrected in another form. The new corps of primary care providers may be clinicians trained in disciplines other than medicine.

The past decade has been marked by rapid growth in the number of such clinicians, who can be grouped into 10 disciplines "that most strongly overlap the scope of medical services provided by physicians"[3] (Cooper, 2001). The professionals trained in these disciplines are authorized to assume "principal responsibility for patients, under at least some circumstances" (Cooper, 2001). The combined number of graduates from programs in these 10 disciplines doubled from 8,850 in 1992 to 18,500 in 1997 (Cooper, Laud, & Dietrich, 1998). Advanced practice nurses (including nurse practitioners, clinical nurse specialists, certified nurse midwives, and nurse anesthetists) are by far the largest group, accounting for 42% of the 18,500 graduates in 1997. For some of these disciplines that provide primary care the rate of growth is projected to accelerate.

Nurse practitioners (NPs) are registered nurses who have advanced education (at a minimum, a master's degree) and clinical training in fields such as adult, family, pediatric, psychiatric, or geriatric health.[4] The supply of nurse practitioners has increased sharply in recent years, partly driven by the rapid expansion among managed care organizations, which use proportionately more NPs than non-managed care settings. Between 1990 and 1995, the number of active NPs doubled to 58,000. By 2005 the number of NPs (115,000) is projected to be similar to the number of family physicians. If enrollment plateaus at current levels, 175,000 NPs will be in clinical practice by 2015 (Cooper, 2001). Although most nurse practitioners now train in primary care, a growing number are training in specialty disciplines (Cooper, Laud, & Dietrich, 1998). NPs have been shown to be effective substitutes for physicians in primary care settings. (Mundinger et al., 2000)

Clinical nurse specialists (CNSs), like nurse practitioners, are registered nurses who have graduate preparation. Unlike NPs, however, CNSs have by definition an area of clinical specialization, such as community health, psychiatric-mental health, or gerontology. The number of clinically active CNSs is projected to double from 15,500 in 1995 to an estimated 31,000 in 2015 (Cooper, Laud, & Dietrich, 1998).

As with geriatricians, advanced practice nurses specializing in care for elderly patients are particularly important to chronic care. Geriatrics is a relatively new field in nursing, identified as a distinct practice with advanced training requirements only during the last three decades. Whereas most training programs for adult and family nurse practitioners include a geriatric component, geriatric nurse practitioner (GNP) programs provide a more in-depth curriculum to prepare students to respond to the unique needs of elderly patients. The United States now has 55 programs that train geriatric nurse practitioners, but they graduate only a mean of five students annually, that is, 275 total GNPs per year (Mezey & Ebersole, 2001). Moreover, of the estimated 4,200 certified GNPs nationwide, approximately 60% work in institutional long-term care settings and thus provide care for only a small segment of the elderly population. Gerontology is also one of the specialty options for CNS training but is offered by only 20% of CNS programs (Walker et al., 2003).

Registered Nurses

Though the projected supply and demand for physicians caring for chronically ill patients is hotly debated, the shortage of registered nurses (RNs) is well documented and unquestioned.[5] Today, the number of unfilled nursing positions is at an historic high.[6] The problem is likely to get worse before it gets better. In contrast to the increasing enrollment in nurse practitioner programs, the number of students in generic nursing programs is declining. Enrollment in baccalaureate RN programs, for example, declined each year between 1995 and 2000. Despite increases in enrollment in nursing schools in 2001 and 2002, there are still 10,000 fewer nursing students today than there were in 1995. The reduced number of new entrants into nursing has also contributed to the aging of the nursing labor force. The average age of working RNs increased by 5 years between 1983 and 2000, from 37.4 to 42.4 years, and is projected to increase another 3 years to 45.4 years by 2010 (Buerhaus, Staiger, & Auerbach, 2000).

Unless the decreased interest in nursing as a career and the corresponding decline in enrollment in nursing training programs are reversed, by the year 2020 the total number of RNs nationwide will be about the same as in the year 2000, although the nation's total population will have increased by a projected 50 million people. Phrased another way, the demand for nurses in 2020 will outstrip supply by more than 400,000 RNs. Even if the number of students entering nursing significantly increases in the next few years, the short-term impact on RN supply would be nominal because "the size of the RN workforce during the next 20 years is largely determined by

the size of the cohorts that have already entered the labor market" (Buerhaus, Staiger, & Auerbach, 2000).

Like other female-dominated professions, nursing has lost much of its
allure as a wide range of career opportunities have opened to women. To
restore its social role, nursing must redefine itself and develop new role models. It must once again become an attractive career path for those who want
to serve others. Thus far, nursing has not yet attracted an adequate complement of men to remove its genderized association. The shortage of nurses
has, however, increased the pay rates, which should facilitate recruitment of
new students and increase supply. And some new approaches have begun.
Post-baccalaureate programs (especially nurse practitioner programs), for
example, have increased their enrollment by streamlining training for persons who have completed college in another field. Similar initiatives are
needed to renew student interest in nursing at the undergraduate level.

Chronic Care Skills and Competencies

Health care professional education, in general, has not kept pace with recent changes in the health care system, such as the growth of managed care,
or with changes in the health care needs of the population, particularly the
increased prevalence of chronic conditions. But this varies across the disciplines. For practitioners in some disciplines the skills, competencies, and
perspective needed to improve chronic illness care already form the foundation or are key elements of their training. For example, core principles of
a chronic care model have been part of academic training for decades in
the rehabilitative fields, including rehabilitative nursing, occupational therapy, and physical therapy. Client-centered practice, interprofessional care
planning, ongoing therapeutic relationships, wellness models, and intervention goals based on patients' abilities and maximizing their quality of life
have held precedence over a curative approach. The rehabilitative disciplines support a holistic model of care in which restoring, remediating, or
compensating for loss of function form the core philosophy of practice
(Moyers, 1999).

For practitioners in other health care disciplines, however, the learning
curve will be steep. This is particularly true for physicians and others whose
training focuses on acute care. As one physician educator notes, "despite its
prevalence, chronic illness has not been adequately treated as a subject for
medical education at either the medical school or the residency training
level" (Cohen, 1998).[7] Contemporary medical education (that is, the training of physicians in medical school and during residencies) is still dominated
by an acute care model that is more concerned with disease than with pa-

TABLE 5.1.
Top 12 Topics That Medical School Deans Believe Should Be Required in Medical Students' Learning Experiences

1. Effective patient-provider relationships/communication
2. Outpatient/ambulatory care
3. Health promotion / disease prevention
4. Primary care
5. Professional values
6. Use of electronic information systems
7. Biomedical / health care ethics
8. Care for the elderly
9. Interdisciplinary teamwork
10. Psychosocial care
11. Community social problems
12. Patients as partners in health care

Source: Adapted from Graber et al., 1997.

tients and more concerned with treatment and cure than with care management. It is thus not compatible with the totality of needs of patients with chronic conditions. As a result, most physicians entering practice in today's health care system are unprepared to provide optimal chronic illness care. Without changes in their training, they will be even less prepared in the future as the burdens of chronic conditions across the population intensify.

Physicians and physician-educators agree with the perception that medical education in chronic illness care is deficient (Partnership for Solutions, 2002b). The deans of U.S. medical schools included among the top 12 topics that they feel need more emphasis in an "ideal" medical curriculum many that are central to optimal chronic illness care (Graber et al., 1997). The skills and competencies that require more emphasis, according to the deans, are not in the hard sciences or clinical knowledge (in which American medical students receive exemplary training); rather, they are linked to the methods of doctoring (table 5.1). Virtually all of these skills and knowledge would improve care for chronically ill persons. Assuring that physicians have the skills and competencies to adequately respond to the medical and non-medical needs of people with chronic conditions may thus require medical schools to recalibrate the balance between training in basic science and clinical knowledge, on the one hand, and seeking to improve physicians' patient relationship skills and molding their character and values, on the other (Graber et al., 1997).

In contrast to the limited movement toward such a rebalancing of physician education at the undergraduate level, graduate medical education (i.e., residency training) has taken a major step in this direction. As part of its broad initiative to ensure that physicians are "adequately prepared to practice medicine in the changing health care delivery system," in 1999, the Accreditation Council on Graduate Medical Education (ACGME), the accreditation body for residency training programs, identified six core competencies for all such programs. The ACGME's core competencies are:

1. Patient care that is compassionate, appropriate, and effective for the treatment of health problems and the promotion of health

2. Medical knowledge about established and evolving biomedical, clinical, and cognate (e.g., epidemiological and social-behavioral) sciences and the application of this knowledge to patient care

3. Practice-based learning and improvement that involves investigation and evaluation of their own patient care, appraisal and assimilation of scientific evidence, and improvements in patient care

4. Interpersonal and communication skills that result in effective information exchange and teaming with patients, their families, and other health professionals

5. Professionalism, as manifested through a commitment to carrying out professional responsibilities, adherence to ethical principles, and sensitivity to a diverse patient population

6. Systems-based practice, as manifested by actions that demonstrate an awareness of and responsiveness to the larger context and system of health care and the ability to effectively call on system resources to provide care that is of optimal value[8]

Medical education has traditionally emphasized the first two competencies, which focus on medical science and clinical knowledge. The remaining four focus more on the methods of doctoring, crucial for the effective long-term clinician-patient relationships that are hallmarks of good chronic care. Combined, these six competencies, according to the ACGME, form the required building blocks for assessing physicians' educational and professional development in all residency training programs nationwide.

Both the medical school deans' list of curriculum topics and the ACGME's core competencies represent ideals. Health care education for physicians, and for some other health care professionals as well, does not yet provide adequate training in the skills and competencies required for effective chronic illness care. Current medical education is particularly deficient in providing physicians with training in promoting patient-centered care, using information technology and information systems, and working in interprofessional teams. These three skills and competencies, capturing the dominant themes of the recommendations of ACGME and the medical school deans, are essential for optimal chronic illness care.

Reorganizing chronic illness care will require instilling in health care professionals these new skills and competencies. A major challenge for medical education will be to go beyond mere instruction. Students should not only be exposed to the principles of good care, they should have the opportunity to witness the differences that good care makes in the lives of their patients. Such an educational experience may motivate them to adopt such practices in their own careers. But physicians must also be taught how to use these skills and competencies within the parameters of actual practice. The medical education community has not traditionally undertaken the responsibility of making the transition from training into practice. It has been content to establish standards for good care and leave it to others to determine how real world constraints, such as limited time and resources, can be overcome. Such an attitude will no longer suffice.

Promoting Patient-centered Care

Chronically ill patients have significantly different relationships with their clinicians than acutely ill patients. Because chronic conditions are enduring, their management requires ongoing clinician-patient partnerships, often lasting years. Clinicians need to be skilled not only in the physical aspects of disease but also in interviewing, communicating, negotiating, and other skills crucial to creating and sustaining relationships with their chronically ill patients.

At the core of the long-term partnerships for effective chronic illness care are (1) a philosophy or orientation to care that encourages sharing control with the patient of decisions about health care interventions and overall management of the patient's health problems and (2) a focus on the patient as a whole person, acknowledging his or her individual preferences and values as well as resources and situational limitations (in contrast to a focus on a body part or disease) (Lewin et al., 2002). Health care that incorporates these two elements is termed patient-centered care. Yet the term "patient-centered" may not be specific enough. Physicians have long been happy to put patients at the center of attention, but they also have been accustomed to making decisions for and about patients. In one survey, more than 90% of medical students and residents believed that physicians should have more say in decisions about medical treatment than their patients; moreover, the longer the trainees were beyond medical school, the stronger was the belief in physician-only decision making (Beisecker et al., 1996).

Care that is truly patient-centered individualizes treatment recommendations and decision making in response to the patient's own preferences
and beliefs. Such care is possible only with full and open communication between clinician and patient (McNutt, 2004). Communicating with patients
who are full partners in the management of their chronic illness is different
from informing patients about relatively discrete topics, such as the benefits
and risks of a short-term antibiotic treatment. Effective management of
chronic conditions through the long-term associations between clinicians
and their patients requires a "deliberate discussion about the patient's principal health concerns and priorities and designing strategies to address
them" (Safran, 2003). It demands ongoing communication and many small
and large negotiations regarding diagnostic tests, treatment strategies, monitoring and responding to symptoms, and adjusting to physical and psychological changes (Cohen, 1998).

These types of patient-clinician interactions demand more highly developed and nuanced communication skills than simply imparting health care
information to the patient. Many techniques to improve communication between clinician and patient are relatively straightforward and almost second
nature for some clinicians, but for most they are difficult to master, despite
their seeming simplicity (see exhibit 5.1).

Although good clinician-patient communication and a respectful attitude toward patients are essential for patient-centered care, this type of care,
which emphasizes the patients' needs and perspectives, requires even more
of both clinicians and patients. It requires physicians (and other clinicians,
where appropriate) to be willing both to share decision making with patients
and to have patients assume greater responsibility for their own care. It also
means maximizing "the effectiveness of patients to manage their chronic illness themselves" (Von Korff, Glasgow, & Sharpe, 2002). To achieve this
broader goal, patients must have not only the required knowledge and understanding but also the skills, confidence, and motivation to assume a larger
role in their own care. For clinicians, this requires not only that they know
their patients' preferences, values, beliefs, and their attitude toward self-management, but also that these clinicians have the skills to help their patients
achieve greater self-management. This means clinicians must understand
theories of behavior modification and be able to use those techniques to in-
still patient confidence. Yet clinicians state that they are ill prepared to offer behavioral interventions to improve patients' self-management abilities
(World Health Organization, 2002). (Self-management is discussed further
in chapter 6.)

Although these requirements of patient-centered care fit with the medical profession's traditional stated commitment to the primacy of the pa-

tient's welfare and interests, many believe this commitment has eroded and needs to be restored. For instance, in response to the perceived deterioration of medicine's traditional service commitments, the American Board of Internal Medicine Foundation, in cooperation with other U.S. and European physician organizations, issued a new Charter on Medical Professionalism in 2002. The Charter's three patient-centered "Fundamental Principles"—(1) the principle of the primacy of patient welfare; (2) the principle of patient autonomy; and (3) the principle of social justice—are designed to restore medicine's professionalism and its "dedication to serving the interests of patients" (ABIM Foundation, 2002). By clarifying the professional commitment to the patient, the Charter is intended to make patient-centered care a reality, not just a slogan.

EXHIBIT 5.1

Effective Clinician-Patient Communication

Effective communication techniques derived from studies of the clinician-patient relationship include:

- Attend to the patient (signaled by cues such as making eye contact, sitting rather than standing when conversing with the patient, moving closer to the patient, and leaning slightly forward to attend to the discussion).

- Elicit the patient's underlying concerns about the condition.

- Construct reassuring messages that alleviate fears (reducing fear as a distraction enables the patient to focus on what you are saying).

- Address any immediate concerns that the family expresses (enabling patients to refocus their attention toward the information being provided).

- Engage the patient in interactive conversation through use of open-ended questions, simple language, and analogies to teach important concepts (dialogue that is interactive produces richer information).

- Tailor the treatment regimen by eliciting and addressing potential problems in the timing, dose, or side effects of the drugs recommended.

- Use appropriate nonverbal encouragement (such as a pat on the shoulder, nodding in agreement) and verbal praise when the patient reports using correct disease management strategies.

- Elicit the patient's immediate objective related to controlling the disease and reach agreement with the family on a short-term goal (that is, a short-term objective both provider and patient will strive to reach that is important to the patient).

- Review the long-term plan for the patient's treatment so the patient knows what to expect over time, the situations under which the physician will modify treatment, and the criteria for judging the success of the treatment plan.

- Help the patient plan in advance for decision making about the chronic condition (such as using diary information or guidelines for handling potential problems and exploring contingencies in managing the disease) (Clark & Gong, 2000).

Training in Patient-Centered Care

A few training programs have successfully promoted patient-centered care in clinical practice and increased patients' satisfaction with the care they receive (Dickstein, 2001; Lewin et al., 2002). There is ample evidence supporting a positive impact of patient-centered care on a variety of outcome measures (Lorig et al., 1999). Patients can be taught to be more effective communicators with their physicians (Greenfield, Kaplan, & Ware, 1985; Greenfield et al., 1988; Levin, 1975). As the social distance between doctors and patients narrows (Starr, 1983), such communication should become easier, and patients should be more willing to demand a bigger role in their own care.

Nevertheless, it remains unclear whether the programs designed to help providers promote patient-centered care themselves ultimately change patients' health behavior or improve their health status. In other words, we can teach clinicians to provide patient-centered care and we now know that patient-centered care improves patient satisfaction, but what is still unclear is the impact of interventions to promote patient-centered care on the ultimate goal, that is, on patients' health (Lewin et al., 2002). At present, the new wave of enthusiasm for programs promoting patient-centered care is based only on assumptions of their effectiveness in achieving this goal. Accordingly, two strategies—one targeting clinicians, the other targeting patients—are needed to maximize the potential of "patient-centered care." The first strategy is to expand effective methods to train health care professionals to be more patient centered. The second is to document that such methods not only boost patient self-management but also increase patient satisfaction and, most important, improve health outcomes.

Using Information Technology

In health care, "information technology" encompasses all forms of electronic technology used to create, store, exchange, and use information to support the delivery and processes of health care. It includes handheld computers and other discrete devices as well as complex technology systems that combine multiple components to perform complex integrated tasks. Information technology is best seen as a tool, whose appropriate use and application can enable more patient-centered care and promote other components of effective chronic illness care.

There are many reasons why clinicians need to become more proficient in the use of information technology. Clinical knowledge is expanding rapidly, driven by greater investments in biomedical research; the development of new medical technologies, drugs, surgical techniques, and approaches to care; and increased numbers of clinical trials conducted and published. As a result, it is now virtually impossible for clinicians to keep abreast of advances in health care across all areas of specialty. Even keeping up with the rapid expansion of knowledge within their own field of expertise poses significant challenges.

To ensure that clinicians use the most up-to-date clinical knowledge in caring for their patients, health care professional education may need to shift from information acquisition to information management. That is, instead of seeking to expand clinicians' base of clinical knowledge (increasingly difficult, given the exponential growth in such knowledge), health care professional education should pay more attention to ensuring that clinicians have the skills needed to obtain, manage, and correctly use such knowledge. This means that instead of attempting to add more knowledge to the already overloaded clinical curricula of health care professional students, training programs should provide trainees with the skills needed to quickly find and apply such information in a clinical setting.

The current level of interest in expanding training for health care professionals in the use of information technology may outstrip the documented usefulness of such training. The training's effectiveness in preparing clinicians to use information technology skills in practice remains in doubt. Still, we are fast becoming a technological, information-based society. An irrefutable trend in health care and many other aspects of society is the continued development of technologies to create, store, manage, and provide ready access to information. Research has also shown that such information technology can enhance clinical performance and improve patient care (see chapter 7). The appropriate response, therefore, to the unknown impact of information technology training on health care practice and outcomes is to conduct research designed to clarify its impact and then expand the types of training shown to be effective.

Expanded training in the use of information technology may also change the nature and attraction of chronic illness care for health care professionals by minimizing aspects of such care that are unappealing. Computerized information systems in which patient's medical records and treatment plans can be updated electronically can save clinicians significant time by reducing paperwork. Communication technologies such as telemedicine can cut travel time by reducing the number of in-person visits. They also facilitate remote consultation among practitioners, increasing opportunities for interaction with peers with whom they would have been otherwise unlikely to communicate.

Perhaps more important, training in information technology can enhance for clinicians the positive aspects of chronic illness care, such as demonstrating improved health outcomes. Health care professionals frequently see their patients with chronic conditions deteriorate despite their best efforts and care. When they see themselves unable to affect the prognosis of the people they serve, it is easy to understand why these practitioners become discouraged. Without information that allows a comparison of the actual outcomes of care with those expected if such care were not rendered, practitioners are unable to appreciate the difference their care makes. However, information that is collected to monitor patients' health can also be used to provide feedback to health care professionals on the effectiveness of their actions. Health care professionals can use information technologies to present these data in a way that lets them see the impact of their efforts. By harnessing the power of information about the clinical outcomes of health care interventions and their effect on patients' quality of life, information technology could transform the way health care professionals view their accomplishments. It can provide them with positive reinforcements regarding the impact of the care and services they provide.

Working on Interdisciplinary Teams

Members of an interdisciplinary team supply different kinds of relevant data and can provide insight into different aspects of the patient's chronic conditions. (See the discussion of interdisciplinary team care in chapter 4.) Ideally, interdisciplinary teams set common goals, consistently share relevant information (both among team members and with the patient), coordinate complete care, solve problems too complex for one discipline, and work interdependently, reaching joint decisions with the patient. Among the specific skills needed to work effectively on interdisciplinary teams are:

- Understanding and respect for other professions

- Group problem solving, critical thinking

- Conflict management

- Communication

- Trust building

- Group dynamics and facilitation

- Knowledge of health care and organizational systems

Conveying teamwork skills to health care professional students only in classroom sessions will not be enough. For students to internalize the skills of interdisciplinary care, they must be exposed to these skills during the daily care of patients throughout their clinical training as well. Frequent and consistent exposure of health care professional students to models of efficient interdisciplinary collaboration is essential for preparing them for a world where cross-disciplinary teamwork is increasingly common. Such exposure will prepare them to successfully work as health care professionals in teams that address the psychosocial and the biomedical aspects of a patient's chronic condition. To the extent possible, trainees should be exposed to faculty and practitioners from the other professions, not just trainees; for example, they should see faculty role models participate in interdisciplinary care of patients.

Yet only a minority of health care professional training programs have interdisciplinary instruction. "We train health care professionals, in the classroom and at the bedside, with an almost exclusive emphasis on honing their individual knowledge and technique so that they can perform their clinical role with excellence. We are superb at teaching clinicians to be soloists in the ballet of medicine" (Safran, 2003). Health care profession students are typically trained without sufficient exposure to other health care professional disciplines for them to "appreciate each other's strengths or recognize weaknesses except in crisis," leaving them unprepared to work in settings using a team approach to provide health care (Institute of Medicine, 2001).

The timing of interdisciplinary education for health care professionals is still debated, even among proponents. Many suggest that, to maintain the integrity and enhance the excellence of the core disciplines, interdisciplinary education in the classroom should begin only after trainees have become sufficiently familiar with the basic precepts and philosophy of their own profession, but before they are socialized into professionally segmented approaches. In other words, competence in one's own discipline is a prerequisite for interdisciplinary competence. If other disciplines are to appreciate the contributions of another discipline they must observe that practitioner working in a way that demonstrates added benefit. Novice trainees are not likely to provide such positive interdisciplinary experiences.

Expanding interdisciplinary team care must overcome barriers to both interdisciplinary education and practice. To be useful in practice, team care must be shown to be efficient. As with some other innovations in chronic illness care, however, the benefits of interdisciplinary team care have not yet been well documented. A Cochrane Library evaluation of the effectiveness of interdisciplinary education was abandoned because of the lack of any rigorous studies on the topic.[9] However, there is some evidence to show that interdisciplinary training improves the interdisciplinary nature of practice and that it improves patient care (Headrick, Wilcock, & Batalden, 1998).

To ensure that health care professionals will in fact be able to provide more chronic illness care through interdisciplinary teams, changes will also be needed in "scope of practice" legislation, professional certification and licensure, and the boards that regulate health care professional practice. A central goal of these regulatory initiatives is to ensure patient safety. The mechanisms they use, however, such as minimum competency standards in licensure laws, may inhibit the use of interdisciplinary teams and other flexible approaches to care delivery. Inadequate payment for interdisciplinary care presents an additional barrier.

Settings for Health Care Professional Education

In addition to less-than-adequate training in the key competencies reviewed above, many health care profession trainees, particularly medical students and residents, still do not receive enough of their training in the settings in which they will provide the vast majority of care to patients with chronic conditions. Recognizing the shift toward ambulatory care, many medical schools and academic health centers have begun to move a greater percentage of clinical instruction to ambulatory settings. Yet most clinical training continues to occur in hospitals.

Even if inpatient settings are best for acute care training and the most efficient training sites, they are less than ideal for training in chronic illness care. Because hospital admissions for chronically ill patients typically result from an exacerbation of the illness, a breakdown of normal caregiving systems, or further deterioration in patients' function, health care profession trainees who see such patients in the hospital rather than in less crisis-oriented ambulatory settings would see them at their worst. Seeing patients only in the hospital provides a "crisis snap shot" that does not allow the provider-in-training to observe the course of the illness, including the patients' recovery and return to baseline, deterioration, or other consequences that follow a hospitalization.

Environmental Changes to Support Training

A goal of expanded training in the three areas reviewed—providing patient-centered care, using health information technologies, and working on interdisciplinary teams—is to help provide clinicians with the skills, competencies, and perspective they need to provide optimal chronic illness care. However, assuring that the health care professional workforce is able to provide such care will entail more than just reconfiguring the training for health care professionals. The practice environment may have as much or more to do with successfully developing the right workforce for chronic care than the training itself.

Practice environments must be realigned to be more consistent with the needs of people with chronic conditions. New models of care are needed, because the dominant acute, episodic model, where patients come into brief contact with health care professionals and the health care system, no longer meets the needs of most patients. Indeed, improving chronic illness care may need to begin with a change in clinical practice environments. Furthermore, health care professional students currently have relatively few opportunities during their clinical training in chronic illness care to obtain exposure to positive models of such care in clinics and other nonhospital settings. A critical first step in creating the training grounds for future practitioners may thus be to establish models for effective chronic care (see chapter 11 for a discussion of selected models).

Changing Roles

The projected changes in the supply of and the demand for clinicians with new chronic care skills and competencies will affect their future patient care roles and responsibilities. Although the precise impact remains unclear, a significant trend in the care of patients with chronic conditions is likely to be a reduced and more circumscribed role for physicians and a broader and more expansive role for other clinicians, especially for advanced practice nurses (APNs). This trend is supported by a growing body of evidence showing that the care provided by advanced practice nurses is of high quality, is cost-effective, and leads to a high level of patient satisfaction (Brown & Grimes, 1995; Mundinger et al., 2000). In addition, changes in APNs' professional autonomy, prescriptive authority, and reimbursement will further broaden their roles and responsibilities in providing care for patients with chronic conditions.

All 50 states license nurse practitioners and clinical nurse specialists as nurses, which gives them the right to practice. Other state laws and regulations, such as state practice acts, and (in some states) certification by a recognized professional body, then define more precisely the scope of practice for these clinicians, their level of authority, as well as the degree, if any, of physician oversight required. Although these provisions vary considerably among the states, the clear trend is toward granting APNs greater autonomy as clinicians, more authority in prescribing medications, and authorization to provide a broader set of health care services. Advanced practice nurses have some authority to prescribe medications in all 50 states. In about half the states, they can write prescriptions, including ones for controlled substances, without any physician involvement.

How APNs are paid is also critical to determining their future role and responsibilities in chronic illness care. In general, direct reimbursement is a clinician's ticket to practice autonomy. Historically, APNs who worked in clinics and other ambulatory settings were reimbursed only through payments made to their employer, typically a physician. (APNs working in institutional settings are almost always employees of the institution and do not bill for their services.) As a result of changes to the Medicare and Medicaid programs and in state laws regulating private health plans, in many situations nurse practitioners and clinical nurse specialists can now be directly reimbursed for their services. Changes made in 1997 to the Medicare program, for example, permit APNs to receive direct Medicare reimbursement regardless of the setting or place of service. Although other reimbursement policies still vary among the states and among private programs, a growing number of APNs are allowed to bill directly for the services they provide, in a manner similar to physicians and sometimes at the same rates.

These trends will allow APNs to assume greater responsibility at all stages of chronic illness care, including diagnosis, coordinating and managing care, monitoring and controlling symptoms, preventing and responding to exacerbations, and following the progression of the illness. It also suggests that the services APNs are allowed to provide will increasingly overlap with services that physicians have traditionally provided. A key question in delineating future roles and responsibilities in chronic illness care for physicians and advanced practice nurses is to what extent these clinicians will deliver the same services to different groups of patients, offer different services to the same patients, or provide the same services to the same patients (Druss et al., 2003). In the first instance, APNs provide services in place of physicians, in the second they complement physicians, and in the third they compete with physicians.

Physicians and APNs have long provided a similar set of primary care and routine medical services to different groups of patients. Advanced practice nurses have historically thrived in rural, poor urban, or other traditionally underserved areas where, for a variety of reasons, physician services are unavailable. More advanced practice nurses and fewer primary care physicians will likely result in a growing number of people in underserved areas having an APN rather than a physician as their principal health care provider. The recruitment and retention of physicians in rural and other underserved areas has been an ongoing challenge. Though one fifth of Americans live in nonmetropolitan areas (and are, on average, older, poorer, sicker, and less educated and have a perception of worse health status than their urban counterparts), only 11% of the nation's physicians practice in nonmetropolitan areas. The experience for APNs in underserved areas has been more promising. In California, for example, recruiters have been able to use a variety of "carrots," including increased salary, professional challenge, and independence, to fill rural nurse practitioner slots, in sharp contrast to the state's intractable rural registered nurse deficiency (Tone, 1999).

EXHIBIT 5.2

Columbia Advanced Practice Nurse Associates

One model of an independent primary care practice staffed entirely by advanced practice nurses exists in a program operated by the Columbia School of Nursing in New York City. In 1997, the school opened (not without controversy and concern within the physician community) the first-of-its-kind nurse practitioner-run primary health care practice, the Columbia Advanced Practice Nurse Associates (CAPNA) in midtown Manhattan. CAPNA functions like any other primary care clinic:

- It makes available the same basic outpatient services but with an emphasis on prevention and wellness
- CAPNA accepts most forms of insurance: enrollees in managed care plans (with which CAPNA has a contract) and Medicare beneficiaries are able to choose CAPNA as their primary care clinic
- CAPNA's nurse practitioners function as the patient's primary care provider
- The nurse practitioners have hospital-admitting privileges at New York-Presbyterian Hospital

The fundamental difference is that CAPNA's clinicians are all nurse practitioners. They are also all faculty members at the Columbia University School of Nursing. In another first for nurse practitioners in an area that is not medically underserved, CAPNA's clinicians are paid by Medicare and commercial insurers as primary care providers at the same reimbursement rate as physicians.

Source: Columbia Advanced Practice Nurse Associates (CAPNA). www.capna.com/ (accessed July 28, 2003).

In many health care settings, APNs and physicians collaborate to expand the range of health care services available to patients beyond those traditionally offered by physicians. When APNs and physicians provide services to the same patients, their skills and competencies complement each other. In the care of chronically ill, frail elderly persons, for instance, advanced practice nurses have "demonstrated interest and expertise in helping [such patients] and their family caregivers manage the day-to-day aspects of their chronic conditions and treatments" (Aiken, 2003), an essential task for which physicians often do not have time. In these situations, the physician and advanced practice nurse (and often other health care professionals as well) typically collaborate as members of patient care teams. For one example of such team practice, see exhibit 5.2.

Even when advanced practice nurses provide the same services as and thus substitute for physicians, their different philosophy of care differentiates the care they provide. Advanced practice nurses are less rooted in the traditional medical model, with its focus on diagnosing and treating a disease; instead, they take a more holistic approach to care and pride themselves in spending the time needed to get to know the patient and to understand their needs and concerns. Moreover, advanced practice nurses concentrate on early detection of illness and emphasize prevention through patient education.[10]

Models

Models of care for patients with chronic conditions include several that have a single clinician function as the patient's principal care provider. This provider would, in essence, be at the gate of the health care system to direct and manage the patient's overall care, but little agreement exists about who should be the principal provider. Physicians have traditionally been, and have been viewed as, the providers with primary responsibility for patient care. Expanded clinical roles of clinicians without medical (i.e., physician) training will challenge the medical community to collaborate in new ways with other clinical disciplines. In each of the models below, physicians will need to collaborate with colleagues whose work not only complements but also sometimes competes with the practice of medicine. This will demand a sharing of clinical authority among health care disciplines. Alternative models include:

- A primary care setting, with an advanced practice nurse as the patient's principal care provider. The clinic established by the University of Columbia Advanced Practice Nurse Associates (CAPNA) is an example of this model (see exhibit 5.2).

- A primary care setting, with a physician as the patient's primary care provider. This is a workable model if there are enough geriatricians or other physicians with the requisite skills and competencies. Supply projections and the deficiencies in health care professional education outlined above may make this unlikely.

- A specialty-care setting, with a physician-specialist providing organ-specific or other specialized care and an advanced practice nurse as the principal provider for all the patient's other care (see exhibit 5.3)

EXHIBIT 5.3

Nurse Practitioner–Specialist Physician Collaborative Team Care

The nurse practitioner-physician collaborative practice model combines joint commitment to patient care with integration of talents and skills (Chmielewski et al., 1996) and shared goals, responsibility, accountability, and philosophy of practice (Kedziera & Levy, 1994). In specialty and subspecialty medical practice, the nurse practitioner-specialist physician collaborative practice model evolved to address the needs of patients with specific chronic diseases who require complex therapeutic interventions, close monitoring of clinical status, and extensive education and counseling. Research has demonstrated that site-specific, nurse practitioner-specialist physician collaborative practice models improve patient outcomes in ambulatory (Smith et al., 1997; Cintron et al., 1983), acute care (Dahle et al., 1998), and community settings (Applebaum & Phillips, 1990).

The Columbia University School of Nursing has expanded the site-specific, nurse practitioner-specialist physician model of collaborative practice. Faculty nurse practitioners, in collaboration with specialist physicians, provide direct care for a patient panel in ambulatory, hospital, and community settings. This model promotes continuity of care for patients during different stages of chronic illness across care-delivery settings.

In the Movement Disorder Center, a multidisciplinary team—consisting of a movement disorder neurologist, nurse practitioner, registered nurse, social worker, clinical geneticist, physical therapist, speech therapist, psychiatrist, and neurology house staff—provides treatment for patients with chronic neurological diseases. Even with optimal treatment, most of these patients experience impairment in performance of activities of daily living that requires lifestyle changes.

The initial patient evaluation occurs in the ambulatory setting. A patient is assigned to the nurse practitioner, who records the patient's health history, conducts the physical examination, and develops a preliminary diagnosis and treatment plan that is discussed with the collaborating neurologist. The nurse practitioner and neurologist review pertinent aspects of the history and physical examination with the patient and outline a plan of care. The plan is discussed with the social worker, who further assesses the patient's social and financial needs. The social worker's recommendations are integrated into the plan of care. Depending on the patient needs identified, specific team members evaluate the patient during the appointment to further develop the care plan. The nurse practitioner reviews the completed plan with the patient at the conclusion of the appointment. A consult letter is dictated to the referring provider.

Follow-up appointments are scheduled with the nurse practitioner. During these visits, the nurse practitioner requests consultation from members of the multidisciplinary team to assess changes in the patient's status. If medically indicated, home visits are scheduled to assess the patient's clinical condition and home environment. These evaluations are conducted by the nurse practitioner and social worker. Between appointments, the nurse practitioner assesses treatment interventions by telephone. The nurse practitioner is the primary point of contact, through the on-call pager system, when patients have questions. Changes in the treatment regimen are discussed with the collaborating physician.

If a patient requires hospitalization, the nurse practitioner and collaborating specialist physician see the patient in the hospital according to established protocols. When a patient is no longer able to live at home, the social worker and nurse practitioner assist the patient and family in choosing a skilled nursing facility (SNF) that best meets their needs. The multidisciplinary team provides the SNF with information to coordinate the patient's care. Patients residing in a SNF continue to receive treatment at the Movement Disorder Center.

This model combines the specialist physician's in-depth, disease-specific knowledge with the nurse practitioner's approach to comprehensive health care. This provides patients with state-of-the-art therapeutic interventions and health promotion in the context of changing needs that result from the interplay of environment and degenerative disease. The ongoing relationship with the patient and significant others allows the nurse practitioner to provide education about disease progression and the ability to develop a long-term plan of care, with input from team members, that addresses different aspects of quality of life.

Janice Smolowitz, RN, Ed.D., Assistant Professor of
Clinical Nursing, Columbia University School of Nursing

These three models are not mutually exclusive; each may be optimal for some patients with chronic conditions. The challenge is to decide which model is best for which patients and when. The third model may be most appropriate, for example, for patients with complex or multiple chronic conditions, such as transplant patients or patients with extensive neurological damage, for whom APNs may not have the clinical knowledge or experience to manage the patient's complex conditions on their own. In this model, the specialist would, for instance, provide necessary medical care during the patient's acute episode and the APN would then assume primary responsibility for the patient after the acute medical episode ends.

Some commentators aggressively argue that advanced practice nurses could assume the primary care provider role for nearly all patients with chronic conditions and that the second model listed above is therefore not needed. A study comparing nurse practitioners and physicians as primary care providers, for example, found no significant differences in patients' outcomes, health status, and health services utilization between patients randomly assigned to either a nurse practitioner or a physician (Mundinger et al., 2000). Others counter that physicians' broader base of clinical knowledge and diagnostic skills means neither nurse practitioners nor clinical nurse specialists can offer the entire range of services provided by physicians. Under this view, APNs would provide only a subset of more routine and less complex services and their care of patients with chronic conditions would focus on handling single-system disorders and not include managing the complex care for frail older people or other patients with multiple chronic conditions.

Whereas in all three models, a principal care provider, supported by health care professionals from various disciplines, has primary responsibility for managing a patient's care, in a fourth model, an interdisciplinary team would substitute for the single primary care provider. The interdisciplinary team would provide the patient with access to the expertise of all members on an as-needed basis. This model would promote greater continuity because one member of the team leaving or becoming unavailable would cause less disruption in a patient's care than if a new primary care provided is needed, who may not have the time or energy to thoroughly review the preceding history and start a new plan of care.

In one view of the interdisciplinary model, teams would have responsibility for a group of patients with physicians limiting their role to treating patients with exacerbations of chronic conditions or with acute problems, intervening in stubbornly difficult chronic cases, and training the members of patient care teams. Other clinicians would take the lead for the "planned management of chronic conditions" including arranging for and providing routine periodic tasks (e.g., laboratory tests for diabetic patients, eye examinations, and foot examinations), ensuring appropriate follow-up, and supporting patient self-management (Bodenheimer, Wagner, & Grumbach, 2002b). With the team model it is essential that the patient and family have one team member to whom they can turn for assistance and advice and who can speak for the entire team.

Barriers

Ensuring the right number of health care professionals with the right skills to care for patients with chronic conditions will require significant changes in the health care education enterprise. Altering health care professional education, particularly medical education, is a perennial topic that has become even more important in recent years as the pace of change accelerates in health care, the health care system, and the broader society. Despite numerous calls for health care education reform from the public and private sectors few significant changes have been adopted. Significant barriers to change include both factors internal to the health care education enterprise (from already crowded curricula to professional "turf" issues and faculty resistance) and external factors such as professional licensing and practice requirements.

The struggle to increase the number of geriatricians is illustrative. Despite medical schools' efforts in recent years to interest undergraduate and graduate medical students in geriatrics, relatively few physicians have chosen to specialize in geriatrics. Among the challenges that deter physicians from pursuing careers in geriatrics are "the growth of specialization, the growing income gap between specialists and generalists, managed care, and protechnology biases in fee-for-service payment, as well as economic dependence on the complex Medicare program" (Warshaw et al., 2002). Because their caseload makes geriatricians almost entirely dependent on Medicare payments for their income, poor Medicare reimbursement is viewed as a disincentive to enter this field. The median income of geriatricians in 2000 was $141,500, roughly the same as family physicians and other generalists and substantially below the $260,000 average for specialists. As a relatively new field in medicine, with closer links to primary care than to high-tech or procedure-heavy medical or surgical specialties, geriatrics continues to experience low professional and public recognition, making it a relatively unattractive career choice. The shortage of geriatric faculty may also contribute to the low number of geriatricians, because medical faculty often serve as role models or mentors who influence medical students' career choices.

Medical students have long expressed little interest in fields that focus on the chronically ill. Even though most students begin training with positive attitudes toward caring for elderly patients or those with chronic illness, their socialization experience throughout their training engenders more ambivalent or even negative attitudes. Studies show, for example, that during clinical rotations (typically starting in the third year of medical school) students become less idealistic and develop more negative attitudes toward the elderly, people with chronic pain, and chronically ill patients in general (B. E. Davis et al., 2001; Griffith & Wilson, 2001).

Students' attitudes are shaped in part by the culture of the medical education enterprise, which has traditionally exhibited a preference for dealing with acute as opposed to chronic health problems and in which the acute stage of an illness is typically viewed as more "interesting" and educational for students than "the long convalescent stage which generally produces no new increments of information or clinical experience" (Kutner, 1978). The positive attitudes of entering students toward patients with chronic conditions are repeatedly challenged and consequently erode as the training experience progresses (B. E. Davis et al., 2001). It is not the patients themselves, but trainees' observations of how those patients are treated by clinicians and the health care system, that underlie the change in the students' attitudes. Although nearly three-quarters of medical students enjoyed the relationships they had with chronically ill patients, significantly fewer students rated as positive their experience with residents or attending staff in managing the care of these patients. Some students, for example, perceive the quality of care received by chronically ill patients to be poorer than that received by other patients (B. E. Davis et al., 2001). The "role modeling by faculty and residents in the care of chronically ill patients" may be a factor contributing to the students' depreciating perception of caring for patients with chronic conditions (B. E. Davis et al., 2001).

One medical school dean noted that: "Medical school and residency training exposes trainees to the seductive qualities of 'high-tech' specialties, such as cardiology, critical care medicine, and transplant surgery, while simultaneously devaluing the treatment of the chronically ill. Procedure-oriented specialties present the allure of advanced technology and the perception that the physician's active role restores the patient to health. In contrast are the perceptions that the chronically ill are complex patient with multiple problems who are psychologically demanding and 'incurable.'" (Cohen, 1998).

Student attitudes are also influenced by the perceived lack of rewards in caring for patients with chronic conditions, whose health typically declines over time. The sustained care such patients need rarely offers the kind of immediate rewards achieved in surgery or emergency medicine. Instead, the rewards are subtler and take longer to accrue—such as avoiding an exacerbation by aggressively monitoring the patient's health or managing a patient's successful rehabilitation and return to his own home and community.

Negative attitudes toward particular groups of patients are important, as they influence students' choice of specialty, the quality of the physician-patient relationship, and the treatment strategies developed for chronically ill patients (Rezler & Flahertly, 1985). At the end of their senior year, nearly 25% of medical students (compared with only 9% of students in their first year) would seek another specialty if the incidence of chronically ill patients increased in their chosen field (B. E. Davis et al., 2001). Negative attitudes toward elderly and chronically ill patients have also raised concerns in nursing. Such attitudes have been documented among nursing students (graduate programs in gerontology nursing, for example, have long had difficulties recruiting students) as well as nurses, suggesting that external factors such as pay, poor organization, and lack of continuity of care may be more important in shaping attitudes than the profession's values and philosophy (S. Cooper & Coleman, 2001; J. Davis & Barnes, 1997).

Summary

A health care system capable of meeting the needs of all Americans with chronic conditions requires a workforce with the right number of health care workers with the right skills and competencies. The responsibility for ensuring such a workforce rests primarily with the programs for health care professional education. These programs must augment their exemplary training in the hard sciences and clinical knowledge with a greater emphasis on interpersonal, communication, and other skills and competencies that are central to good chronic care. The ACGME core competencies for medical residents are a step in this direction.

Expanded training in the skills and competencies reviewed in this chapter will equip students in the health care professions to provide high-quality chronic illness care. It will enable them, first as trainees and then as practitioners, to better respond to the unique challenges of chronic illnesses. Training that helps health care professionals adopt a patient-centered perspective promoting close partnerships with their patients, work more effectively on interdisciplinary teams, and use information technologies proficiently should serve to counteract pressures and negative perceptions commonly associated with chronic illness care. It should also relieve some of the "practice burdens and frustrations" that underlie the "discontent" that many clinicians, particularly primary care physicians, experience in their care for chronically ill patients (Mechanic, 2003).

Improving chronic illness care requires clinicians who know what to do as well as an environment that allows and encourages them to do the right thing. Ensuring that clinicians have the right skills and competencies thus requires changes both in training and in the practice environment—one without the other will not change clinician behavior. It remains to be seen whether the health education enterprise will lead the charge or whether changes in practice will create a demand that, in turn, will spur health care professional schools to catch up.

Regardless of the future supply and demand for various types of clinicians—and estimates on both vary widely—the roles and responsibilities of clinicians providing chronic illness care will change. The most dramatic change will likely be the broader responsibilities for advanced practice nurses in managing the care of people with chronic conditions. They may represent the chronic care primary providers of the future. They combine training from two relevant disciplines with a philosophy that is compatible with such care. They have been shown to provide reasonable levels of care, certainly adequate for ongoing patient management. It is not yet clear whether they will emerge as the dominant providers of such care or whether their threatened ascendance will stimulate medicine to become more committed to this aspect of care, much as the threat of competition from family practice motivated internal medicine and pediatrics to bolster their primary care activities.

The precise configuration of various clinicians' roles and responsibilities for optimal chronic illness care are not yet clear and several alternative models of care have been proposed. However, no single model is likely to fit all circumstances, necessitating decisions about which model is best for which patients. Whichever model is used, clinicians will need to be adept in providing patient-centered care, using health information technologies, and working on interdisciplinary teams. In managing chronic conditions, clinicians will also need to adapt to new and more expansive roles for informal caregivers and patients themselves, as discussed in chapter 6.

6.   Patients and Families

Patients, payers, and the public [must recognize] that patients them-
selves are truly the primary providers of chronic care and health main-
tenance, with all of the associated rights and responsibilities.

ETZWILER, 2003, p. 1508 (emphasis added)

Ultimately, formal health care services are only a small, albeit critical, component of care for chronic conditions. Patients and their families live with
chronic illnesses continuously, whereas health care professionals see them
only occasionally. It is naïve to expect that these periodic contacts would be
sufficient to manage daily events. Once a diagnosis is made, primary responsibility falls to the patient. Because by nature chronic conditions continue
for an extended or unlimited period, their management must be integrated
into patients' daily lives and their ongoing responsibilities related to their
families, workplaces, and communities. This reality extends the impact of
chronic conditions outward from the patient to other people, most notably
their families, in the broadest definition of the term. Moreover, good outcomes often depend on patient (and family) involvement in all aspects of care,
including goal setting, decision making, treatment planning, adhering to treatment, and monitoring. The challenge is how to involve patients actively and
meaningfully without making their illnesses the centers of their lives.

Patients and families already provide the yeoman's share of chronic illness care. Personnel shortages and other resource constraints mean their
role will likely increase rather than decrease. Proposing that chronic care be
patient managed and involve families is not advocating a radically new approach as much as it is acknowledging a central element of the nature of
chronic illness. It is perceived as radical only when contrasted with the current acute care-oriented health care system, which rarely recognizes the work
patients and families must do and often treats patient and family involvement as optional.

Patient Involvement

Terminology

   "Self-management" has been defined as "the individual's ability to manage the symptoms, treatment, physical and psychosocial consequences and life style changes inherent in living with a chronic condition" (Barlow et al., 2002, p. 178). The major program components of interventions designed to assist people with self-management include: providing information, symptom management, drug management, addressing psychological consequences, lifestyle changes, social support, communication, and other support ranging from career planning to addressing spiritual needs (Barlow et al., 2002, p. 180). Many who use the term specify that it encompasses the role of formal health care providers: "Self-management is an essential part of chronic disease care and includes both patient and provider responsibilities" (Rukeyser, Steinbock, & Agins, 2003). We will thus use the term "self-management" to refer to the range of tasks and responsibilities patients with a chronic illness or condition may undertake to promote their own health and quality of life. Moreover, we will use it in the most inclusive sense to include formal provider roles in these activities as well. This usage acknowledges that, although patients' active involvement in their care is necessary for successful chronic care, it does not imply acting totally independently of formal care providers.

What Patients Do

There are 525,600 minutes in a year. A person with chronic diseases must address the impact of the diseases and their treatment on his or her life and manage this for many of these minutes, and for most of this time this will be done without the presence of a health care professional. A patient requiring monitoring may need only a monthly (or less frequent) office visit. Even weekly visits, or the addition of an emergency department/urgent care visit, will not bring the total time in formal care to more than 520 minutes or less than one-tenth of 1% of the total time in a year. One or two hospitalizations may increase the patient's contact with the health care system to 1%. Thus, only very ill or unstable patients will have health care providers physically present when they must handle most of the issues related to their chronic illness or condition.

   What patients do for their own care and how much time this takes varies across individuals and illnesses. Nevertheless, with the exceptions of diagnosis and complex treatments, all activities surrounding chronic illness care may, and often do, become the responsibility of the patient, or the joint responsibility of the patient and his/her family (family involvement will be discussed in the next section of this chapter). Understanding these activities is the first step in considering how the health care system can better support patient self-management.

Because patients live with their chronic conditions 24 hours a day, 7 days a week, they are the only ones who can continuously monitor their symptoms and clinical signs. This monitoring may involve noting changes in function (such as a decrease or improvement in range of motion or ability to walk a specified distance without shortness of breath) or sensation (increased pain, blurred vision, tingling, or the development of pressure points or sores). Monitoring may require using tests or measures that can detect changes even before they produce symptoms. Examples of this type of monitoring include peak flow measures for asthma, blood glucose for diabetes, and increase in body weight for congestive heart failure (indicating retention of fluids). Frequently, monitoring includes recording and reporting the results to health care providers who can use them as an indicator of how well a treatment plan is working or trigger early intervention. In some cases, monitoring requires enlisting the aid of others, either because the patient is too frail or the changes render the patient unable to respond, such as when a person with diabetes can not recognize and respond to insulin shock, or a person with epilepsy does not perceive the changes that precede a seizure. Because an important goal of chronic illness management is to detect changes early and to intervene promptly to avoid crises, the health care system must provide a capacity for rapid response.

Patients also must mediate risk factors, avoid triggers, and reduce problems with comorbidities. In many cases this recognition includes lifestyle and behavior changes, which are also promoted as ways to stall or, in some cases, prevent the progression of the disease. Most chronic conditions require changes in diet and exercise. Other behavior changes may include not smoking, avoiding environmental irritants (pollution, animals, humidity, stressful situations), or undertaking new activities (meditation, joining a support group).

Increasingly, patients are responsible for "treatments," with medication management being the most common. A simple medication regime may only require creating reminders or linking the taking of the medication to another habitual activity. However, for patients with some chronic illnesses, such as HIV, or multiple conditions, self-administering medications involves a complex regime involving a large number of pills, liquids, or injections with complex and different scheduling. (Preventing problems associated with medication management is discussed in chapter 8.) Other treatments that patients or families may carry out include wound care and changing of dressings, inserting a catheter, or managing a ventilator.

As an illness progresses or leads to a disability, patients may need to take on more activities related to treatment and ideally become involved in care planning. In this situation, patients (along with their clinicians) must set treatment goals, prioritize these according to their own values, and then make decisions and choices among treatment options. For most chronic illnesses, several different approaches to treatment are feasible, making it possible for patients and their clinicians to work together to determine what approach best fits a patient's condition, living situation, personality, and a host of other factors.

It seems logical that a patient who not only agrees with his or her chronic care regimen, but has also participated in setting its goals and priorities, will be more likely to complete the necessary tasks. The results of randomized studies support this assumption. For example, an intervention designed to help people with diabetes interact more effectively with physicians resulted in improved blood sugar control, decreases in functional limitations, and improvements in patients' abilities to elicit information from clinicians (Greenfield et al., 1988). A self-management program for arthritis reduced pain, disability, and physician visits (Lorig & Holman, 1989); likewise, a program based on the same model for people with any of a variety of chronic conditions resulted in improved health status and reduced utilization of services (Lorig et al., 2001b). Conversely, lack of patient involvement in self-management activities has been linked to poor adherence and clinical outcomes.

Research on patient preferences and their perceptions of the health care they receive reinforces the need for continuity, coordination, and timely access. A series of focus groups held with primary care patients identified four major themes: need for information, desire for ready access to health care, dissatisfaction with the lack of coordination, and infrastructure issues (wait times, need to make multiple calls) (H. R. Holman, 1997, unpublished manuscript cited in Wellington [2001]). Another study had patients with chronic illnesses (chronic obstructive pulmonary disease [COPD], rheumatoid arthritis, or diabetes mellitus) and specialty physicians who treat these conditions rank nine aspects of care in the order of their contribution to quality. Although the patients and physicians were in close agreement on many items, patients ranked continuity second while physicians ranked it sixth (van der Waal, Casparie, & Lako, 1996).

Patients' involvement in care processes and planning is important, but they must also manage the psychological and social aspects of chronic illness. People with chronic conditions often experience depression, anger, disappointment, other emotions, and stress. For some patients, coping with the emotional component of the illness may be as great a challenge, if not a greater one, than dealing with the physical manifestations. A serious chronic illness can become a major crisis or trauma in a person's life (Lewis, 1998). The diagnosis or disease progression may trigger the need to adjust social roles, changing how individuals can function in their family, job, or community.

In sum, chronic illness care requires more of patients than acute care. The management of chronic conditions requires activities (self-treatment, behavior change, psychological and social adjustment) that cannot be contained in a delineated time and space, such as an office visit or a hospital stay. The patient is essentially the care manager and must assume a large portion of the responsibility for his or her own care, unless the patient's condition is severe, totally debilitating, or seriously compromises cognitive function. Especially when the patient is very frail, families must step in to play this active role as agents of the patient.

Family Involvement

Variation in Roles, Status, and Activities

The family is usually recognized as one of many environmental factors affecting the course of a chronic condition. Discussing the involvement of families, however, is difficult because, in health care in general and chronic care in particular, both the definition of family and the perceptions of their influence and appropriate roles differ across disciplines, cultures, and ideologies. Although families are usually assumed to be a positive influence, providing emotional support as well as indirect and direct care, this is not always the case. At the extreme, family members may physically, emotionally, or financially mistreat (up to and including actively abusing or neglecting) someone who is frail, impaired, or dependent (Fulmer, 2002). Family members may also knowingly continue to place patients at risk, such as when a family member smokes around a person with asthma or prepares high-salt meals for someone with hypertension. Such behaviors may reflect a lack of understanding of a family member's chronic condition, or an assessment that the personal benefits from the behavior are more important. In the most benign negative situations, family members may simply not realize the impact of their actions and unwittingly undermine their relative's health.

Families rarely receive the level of attention corresponding to their potential influence. In some situations, or by some providers, families may be perceived as tangential and are excluded from care planning and management. In a very few cases family members may not even be discussed (though this is hopefully rare). Questions from clinicians are often limited to determining whether the patient is in an abusive or dangerous situation, as this is becoming part of standard assessment for vulnerable patients. When the illness is mild and does not impair function, family involvement may seem unnecessary. However, given that most chronic illness management includes diet, exercise, and other lifestyle modifications, at a minimum those who share the patient's household are likely to influence adherence. Once a chronic illness begins to become disabling, families are often the first source of assistance, requiring discussions between providers and patients about informal caregiver availability and family members' willingness and suitability for this role. As severity and disability increase, roles may change, with a family member becoming the principal contact with the health care system and ultimately the decision maker.

There is no correlation between the level of family involvement and disease progression. Some families may be involved in a "mild" chronic illness, whereas others do not become involved even when the patient becomes disabled. This variation in engagement could be due to patient preferences, the family's culture or traditions, geographic proximity, competing obligations (such as child rearing or occupations), prior relationships, or a long list of other factors. Nevertheless, families are universally affected by the diagnosis and subsequent management of the chronic illness in one of their members (Rankin & Weekes, 2000).

With chronic illness may come fear of loss, changes to established routines, new activities associated with disease management, modifications to family members' responsibilities, reconsideration of expectations, and other emotions, reactions, and realities that have an impact on family function. How families are affected will depend on their individual history and resources. How they adjust will depend in part on the stage of the "family life cycle" during which the chronic illness is experienced (i.e., young adult independence, new couple, raising young children, families with adolescents, children leaving, and late-life families) or how the family has handled past transitions (Carter & McGoldrick, 1988).

Families, like individuals, need to perform various functions. Chronic illness care may be a threat to their stability and ability to perform these functions as family boundaries (privacy) and identity (race, ethnicity, history) are threatened both by the illness and the care. The chronic illness or condition can precipitate a crisis, and family function and individual health change in response (Pittman, 2003). "A member of the family with an established identity is suddenly given a new identity. Old unspoken family identity roles, and rules for living need to be rewritten. The fantasy of who the

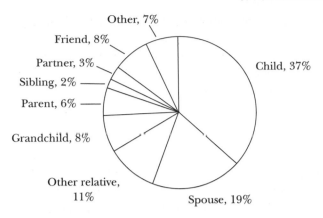

FIGURE 6.1.

Relationship of caregiver to person receiving care.

Data from Robert Wood Johnson Foundation, 2002.

family is and what the family will become is shattered. The premorbid identity, rule, and roles need to be left behind and new ones formulated (Lewis, 1998).

For persons with a chronic illness, families can be beneficial or detrimental, a source of care and support or a source of anxiety, even harm. This variation makes it difficult to generalize about the involvement of families and their activities. What can be said emphatically is that families are rarely irrelevant. Whatever the nature of their involvement and influence, family members need at least to be considered and likely involved in chronic illness care. In our individualistic society, the patient will always be the primary focus of health care. However, patients do not exist in a vacuum; health care providers must consider multiple elements of patients' environments in addition to their physiologic function. One possible way to reconcile any perceived conflict between the primacy of the focus on the patient and the need to consider the family in chronic illness is to have the patient define the level of involvement of his or her family.

Families as Informal Caregivers

Although family members can be involved in chronic illness care in many ways, one of the most important roles a relative often assumes is that of caregiver. "Informal caregivers" refers to people who are not paid to provide care, have little or no training, and are not licensed or recognized primarily

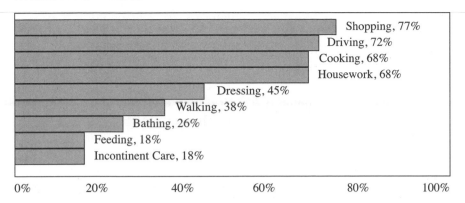

FIGURE 6.2.

Activities performed by informal caregivers.

Data from Robert Wood Johnson Foundation, 2002.

as health care clinicians. The term only includes health care professionals and workers when they provide care to their own family members and are not compensated. Informal care is not defined by the relationship between the caregiver and the care receiver and could be provided by anyone; however the overwhelming majority of informal caregivers are family members, as indicated in figure 6.1.

Caregiving includes many different activities, ranging from providing emotional support, coordinating medical care, to assisting with activities of daily living or ADLs (bathing, dressing, transferring, eating, and toileting). The less personal tasks performed by caregivers to manage a household, such as cooking, housework, and paying bills, are referred to as instrumental activities of daily living (IADLs). Figure 6.2 lists the percentage of caregivers who perform specific tasks. The most common activities are shopping (77%) and driving (72%), but many caregivers are engaged in intimate and demanding activities such as bathing (26%), incontinence care (18%), and feeding (18%). However, care does not include only bodily maintenance and household tasks. Eighty-three percent of caregivers report that the most frequent type of care they provide is emotional support and companionship.

When people with chronic conditions need help with household or personal care tasks, this work often falls to informal caregivers. Informal care may not be paid, but it is not free. Informal caregivers may reduce their working hours, quit jobs, retire early, or make other changes that negatively affect personal finances and productivity on a national level. Caregivers often "pay" for the care they provide in several ways. They experience emotional stress, increased financial obligations, and worsening of their own health. Even though caregivers may describe caring for a family member as a positive experience, the negative effects on their health (Baumgarten et al., 1994), specifically in terms of increased depression (Gallagher et al., 1989), morbidity (Schulz et al., 1995; Schulz, Visintainer, & Williamson, 1990), and suppressed immune function (Kiecolt-Glaser et al., 1991; Vedhara et al., 1999), are well documented. The concept of "caregiver burden" is discussed in more detail in chapter 2.

Negative effects of caregiving, combined with competing demands on potential caregivers, most of whom are women and in the workforce, and increases in life span and disability, could reduce the availability of informal care and increase reliance on formal care (Spillman & Pezzin, 2000). Any shift from informal to formal care will have an enormous impact on the costs of care. The value of care provided by unpaid family members and friends to ill and disabled adults was estimated to be $196 billion for 1997, which far exceeds the amount spent on formal home health ($32 billion) and nursing homes ($83 billion) for the same year (Arno, Levine, & Memmott, 1999). Also, most people prefer to receive care in their own homes from family members and friends, rather than in another setting (likely to be institutional) from strangers. Given the size of the dependence on informal care combined with a desire not to lose this resource, the concept of "chronic illness care" is beginning to expand to include the care of informal caregivers; the interest in protecting and promoting the well-being of such caregivers, particularly family members, is increasing.

Including Families in Chronic Illness Care

At a minimum, good chronic illness care demands that clinicians know and understand their patients' family situations and acknowledge that families are involved (whether positively or negatively) in determining care and outcomes. The wide variation in family structures and dynamics makes it difficult to propose exactly what health care providers should do relative to families; however, not ignoring them would seem to be a good start. Nevertheless, many programs and interventions designed to improve outcomes still focus only on the patient. For example, a review of diabetes programs found that only 17% of programs included family members (Elasy et al., 2001).

Going beyond simply acknowledging the importance of family involvement to including members in care planning and education or even treating family relationship problems as part of chronic illness care requires a significant shift in focus as well as additional skills. More comprehensive approaches to the participation and influence of family members exist in some current programs. One approach focuses on the naturally occurring processes of change in families to help build the resilience and improve the families' abilities to use their resources to respond to the challenges of chronic illness care (Shapiro, 2002). In other cases, family therapy may be used as an adjunctive therapy, which may improve the odds of recovery, increase quality of life, and help both patients and family members deal with the patient's chronic or recurring illness (Ryan, 2002).

The Committee on Health and Behavior and the Institute of Medicine created the National Working Group of Family Based Interventions in Chronic Disease to identify "potential mechanisms by which the relational context of the family affects disease management and how characteristics of family relationships serve as risk or protective factors" (Fisher & Weihs, 2000). This group also reviewed the available research on interventions that target the family setting as opposed to the traditional focus on the individual patient and concluded that:

> There is, therefore, sufficient evidence to support an expanded application of family-based approaches to chronic disease management. . . . Early and on-going attention by clinicians to the setting of disease management and the central figures involved in care can have a substantial clinical payoff. Attention to the level of family stress, emotional tone, amount of patient and family member disease knowledge, how the disease is managed in the home and by whom, degree of conflict in the family regarding disease management, and adequacy of disease-related problem solving may prevent exacerbation of the disease and keep comorbidities to a minimum. (Fisher & Weihs, 2000)

At the same time, there is a danger that families may overwhelm the patient's role. Especially with frail older patients, families may be too quick to step into the decision-making role and displace the patient. Likewise, harried clinicians undoubtedly find it much easier to discuss things with more alert and active family members than to actively involve older patients in the process.

Challenges and Issues

Clinicians' Attitudes and Influence

Self-management includes a different role for formal health care providers. Physicians, nurses, and other health care providers must first determine whether patients are engaged and families are involved in chronic illness care. Some patients may take an active role in their own care and involve their families, regardless of what their clinician does; however, most require encouragement and help. An extremely important function for health care professionals in chronic illness care is fostering the development of patients and families to become "experts" in the sense that they will then be able to manage their own chronic illnesses in a manner that minimizes decline and disability and maximizes function and quality of life.

Involving patients in managing chronic conditions differs considerably from clinicians' primary tasks in acute care. It requires translating scientific and medical knowledge about the condition for the patient and training patients for self-management. Comprehensive patient education is more complicated than simply giving information or handing patients brochures. Clinicians need to help patients develop self-efficacy and self-management skills and make sure patients know what resources are available and how to access them. Patient training needs to be customized so it can be provided when needed and when the patient is most receptive to the information and the need to change behaviors.

Chronic illness care can be ambiguous and frustrating for clinicians. They are not good at predicting which patients will self-manage well and which will not (Clark, 2003). Clinicians' expectations often do not match reality—the patient who the clinician thought understood and would adhere to treatment may, in fact, fail to control his or her disease and have poor outcomes. This discrepancy may help explain why only 36% of physicians surveyed were "very satisfied" caring for patients with chronic conditions (compared with 57% who were "very satisfied" with caring for patients in general [Partnership for Solutions, 2002b]).

Clinicians may also find working with empowered patients uncomfortable or threatening. Involved, empowered patients expect physicians to provide the information they need to make their own decisions. Although a clinician can rely on authority to obscure knowledge gaps, sharing responsibility means giving patients information and in many cases admitting the limitations of current medical knowledge. When such information is not available, it reveals how much of medical care still relies on practices derived from expert judgment rather than a strong evidence base. Sometimes patients may even have more current information then their clinicians, situations clinicians may find embarrassing. Other times patients may ask about or request inappropriate treatments based on what they have learned from other sources (advertisements, the Internet, or other patients).

Involving patients and their families changes the clinician-patient dynamic from one in which clinician experts treat patients who lack needed knowledge or skills, to a collaboration where expertise is shared and can be held by either party. Clinicians may encourage patient involvement in decision making when it leads to adherence or compliance with treatment, but their support wanes when it uncovers disagreements. The goals of clinicians may differ from the goals of patients, for example. This difference is perhaps the key to many treatment and management "failures." Studies in populations ranging from children with asthma (Juniper et al., 1996) to adults with chronic conditions (van der Waal, Casparie, & Lako, 1996) have demonstrated the gulf that exists between patient and clinician goals and priorities.

Maintaining a Balance

A person with a chronic illness rarely gives up work and family obligations and other major roles or activities completely. Rather, managing the chronic illness or condition is layered over the roles and responsibilities associated with work, family, and/or community life. The person with a chronic illness then faces the challenge of blending the activities of his or her "normal" life with those required by the treatment and management of the illness or its symptoms.

One manifestation of this tension is a potential conflict between the need to monitor the signs or symptoms of the chronic illness and the potential for a patient to become overwhelmed. Chronic illness management may require a variety of monitoring activities. For example, in the case of diabetes, blood glucose may need to be checked several times a day and sores or pressure points on legs and feet cleaned and protected; congestive heart failure may require charting of daily weights and awareness of changes in functional abilities; HIV may require a complex drug regime and attention to possible routes of transmission. These tasks require time and commitments that can be viewed as burdensome by both newly diagnosed individuals and those whose disease has progressed to the point that it requires additional changes. Struggles with these demands are voiced by patients who complain about "becoming the disease" or being reduced to a "diabetic", "asthmatic", or "hypertensive" rather than a person with many roles (parent, child, professional, neighbor) who happens to have a chronic condition. To avoid this sense of excessive involvement, people may reject some self-management activities as a way to assert independence and protect their identity.

Conversely, some clinicians worry that patients with significant self-management tasks may become obsessive, or at least compulsive, in their self-monitoring and see crisis and decline in the smallest changes. They fear that patients may overreact or develop an unhealthy fixation on their condition and, as a result, may require extra time, attention, and resources. Evidence of the development of "obsessive patients" remains anecdotal. Though any indication of this level of obsession has not been documented, some research has begun to quantify the extent to which these concerns affect clinicians' attitudes toward chronic illness care (Griffiths et al., 2001).

A related conflict concerns the intrusions and restrictions that accompany ideal treatment and management of many chronic illnesses, which may be unacceptable or accepted only grudgingly by a person trying to preserve the elements of life that are key to identity and enjoyment. Lack of adherence to treatment is often not understood by medical providers who strongly believe in the cause-and-effect relationships between failure to follow a prescribed plan and acute problems, decline, and ultimately death (even though the evidence may be weak in some cases). This frustration with their patients' lack of adherence is a reason why many clinicians do not enjoy caring for patients with chronic illnesses. At the same time, patients may face treatment regimes that may be, or at least seem, unrealistic and that conflict with their long-standing activities and habits. They may understand the potential for long-term benefits but prefer a present guarantee of enjoyment or accomplishment. Understanding and appreciating the risks and having an honest desire to follow a management plan may not be enough to help people make difficult changes.

People with chronic illnesses attempting to manage their own care often struggle to find acceptable balance between dependence and independence. Elements of diagnosis, monitoring, and treatment require technical expertise and training. Obtaining these means a person with a chronic illness must depend to some extent on professionals and technicians. At the same time, living with the disease for an extended period often makes patients experts on their own particular situation. Although dependence and independence in different areas may become complementary over time, achieving a proper balance can be difficult. Furthermore, the preference to be more-or-less independent in chronic illness care can vary from patient to patient. Some patients may be more comfortable deferring to a health care professional, whereas others prefer to have primary responsibility for and control over their own health care.

Toward a Patient-Centered System

Current Knowledge

Models, demonstration projects, and research studies suggest what elements need to be included in system reform to encourage self-management and how they could be implemented. Although "self-management approaches can provide benefits for participants, particularly in terms of knowledge, performance of self-management behaviors, self-efficacy, and aspects of health status," differences in effectiveness between different approaches to self-management are not yet clear (Barlow et al., 2002). Community-based self-management education programs have also been shown to be effective. For example, improvements in blood glucose levels have resulted from such education programs for adults with type 2 diabetes in community gathering places (centers, churches, libraries) and from home-based programs for children and adolescents with type 1 diabetes (Norris et al., 2002).

An example of a program that combines an innovative approach to developing patients' self-management capacity and a community orientation is described in exhibit 6.1. The Partners in Diabetes program represents a major divergence from traditional medical care in that it uses lay experts, explicitly places the patient and the health care professional on equal footing, and strives to be driven by patient concerns.

Changes to promote patient self-management are also occurring within traditional health care organizations, such as hospitals and outpatient clinics. In the Chronic Illness Care Breakthrough Series Collaboratives developed by the Institute for Health Care Improvement, health care teams sought to implement "rapid" changes in a variety of care settings to improve care for diabetes and heart failure. Feedback from the 21 organizations that participated in this program and preliminary outcomes data are encouraging; for example, the percent of heart failure patients reporting self-monitoring of weight went from a median of 19 to 93 and the median percent reporting documentation of diabetes self-management goals increased from 3 to 23 (Glasgow et al., 2002). This approach to making change in "real world" as opposed to academic or demonstration settings appears promising.

Clinical trials of self-management have found that this approach is more effective than information-only patient education in improving clinical outcomes and reducing costs for arthritis and adult asthma patients. These results suggest that programs bringing together patients with a variety of chronic conditions may improve outcomes and reduce costs (Bodenheimer et al., 2002).

Summary

The nature of chronic illness means that patients and families must be involved in the treatment and management of their condition more than in acute care. Greater patient and family involvement demands large-scale changes on two fronts. First, care needs to move to the setting of most self-management activities. Community-based programs, for example, can encourage and support patient and family involvement in ways that may not be possible in short, sporadic clinical encounters in physician offices. Second, health care delivered in hospitals and clinics needs to change. Organi-

EXHIBIT 6.1

Partners in Diabetes: A New Initiative in Diabetes Care

Partners in Diabetes (PID) (Mendenhall & Doherty, 2003) is an initiative in which patients and families who have personal experience with diabetes are connected with others who are struggling with the illness to provide support. As pioneered by Health-Partners (a Minnesota managed care organization), 14 PID "support partners" were nominated by their physicians to design and receive training and then reach out to other patients and family members (called PID "members") across a variety of contexts, including home visits and telephone calls. Sometimes members simply need a single pep talk, and other times members and support partners meet regularly for 3 months or more.

Support partners commit at least two hours per week toward the project, and all participating health care providers and support partners meet monthly to collaboratively consult and discuss challenges that support partners have experienced while working with members and to develop solutions to issues identified as warranting attention.

Partners in Diabetes is based on a model for civic engagement called the Families and Democracy Model (Doherty & Carroll, 2002), which was developed specifically for professionals who work with families in community settings by researchers at the University of Minnesota. Providers are viewed as citizens with special knowledge and skills who work actively with other citizens who also possess important knowledge and skills.

Participants in Families and Democracy initiatives self-consciously and explicitly avoid conventional provider-consumer dynamics by recognizing and valuing all members' contributions to a common mission. Accordingly, every aspect of Partners in Diabetes has been approached in a participatory, collaborative, and democratic manner, in which patients, family members, and providers share responsibility for creating a new initiative from the ground up. From designing the training curriculum, to establishing procedures regarding support partner-member connections, to coauthoring an informational pamphlet to distribute across clinic communities, everyone involved has functioned (and continues to function) as an active contributor.

For instance, the principal topics in the PID training sequence for support partners were identified collaboratively by support partners and providers alike. These topics include (1) living with diabetes: support skills: (2) medical information: giving advice versus providing support: (3) psychosocial issues: individual, couple, and family stress/resources: (4) boundaries and self-disclosures: and (5) resources and confidentiality.

The evolution of PID has been slow and messy, marked by a series of trials, errors, challenges, and successes. Sometimes providers unconsciously shifted away from the collaborative and flat hierarchy central to PID's guiding philosophy. In one instance, providers assumed a hierarchical role and unilaterally reversed an already-established group decision about how to conduct invitations to a large public PID-sponsored forum. The turnout for the forum was disappointing and support partners' enthusiasm waned. As PID has matured as an established democratic initiative, providers have worked hard to decenter their roles and consistently facilitate democratic processes in which citizenship functioning is both stable and enduring.

PID intentionally used (and uses) existing resources rather than relying on external funding, because external funding tends to bring with it the expectation of specific "outcomes" that are defined by the funders. This can undermine the democratic process of developing a project through citizenship participation.

HealthPartners (the HMO that owns the two Minnesota clinics in which PID was founded) is now considering expanding PID to other sites, as this initiative has gained visibility with increased system-wide attention to improving patient-centered care. Consistent with PID's guiding philosophy, support partners maintain a personal stake in PID's ongoing presence and replication. They believe citizenship work like this is only beginning to realize its potential and are advocating the utility of applying Families and Democracy principles to breast cancer, HIV/AIDS, and hospice care.

The greater vision for Partners in Diabetes is to create a model of health care by and for citizens, with all stakeholders working as active contributors. Citizens in PID show a sense of doing work of profound and far-reaching significance, and they are energized by this sense of broader vision.

Tai J. Mendenhall, Ph.D., Department of Family Practice and
Community Health, University of Minnesota
William J. Doherty, Ph.D., Department of Family Social Science, University of Minnesota

zational mechanisms that recognize and support the enormous role that patients and families play in chronic illness care and strive to give them the tools and support they need to carry out these responsibilities can be effectively used in clinical settings.

Self-management by patients, involvement of families, and support of informal caregivers must be the foundation on which we build a chronic illness care system. " The question is not whether patients with chronic conditions manage their illnesses, but how they manage" (Bodenheimer et al., 2002). The essential principles related to patient and family involvement are:

- Self-management and family involvement cannot be viewed as add-ons or optional services.

- Full patient and family participation in monitoring, treatment, and decision-making activities should be a goal of care.

- Patients and family caregivers need practical training on what to expect and what to do in various situations.

- Discussions surrounding health care reforms related to personnel, finances, and the organization of care must acknowledge what patients and families are already doing for themselves and focus on concrete ways to support their activities.

7. Innovative Technology

Americans are technophiles. Technology has been reshaping the organization, delivery, and financing of America's health care system since at least the end of the Second World War. New technologies have entered the system at a rapid pace. Not only is there more technology, but much of what is available is for most patients readily accessible and widely used. And the pace for developing and disseminating new techniques, drugs, equipment, devices, and procedures continues to intensify. These technologies have changed the face of chronic disease. Medical successes have allowed many more people to survive previously fatal illnesses and to function better. Some recent and forecasted advancements are summarized in table 7.1. Moreover, recent revolutionary advances in computer, Internet, and other communication technologies have added a new category—information technology, or IT—to the health care system's armamentarium. More than ever before, a wide range of existing and emerging technological innovations now has the potential to reshape all areas of health care, including dramatically improving chronic illness care.

Technology can improve chronic illness care in several ways. Information technologies such as electronic health records can facilitate the organization and retrieval of patients' clinical information. They can eliminate redundant paperwork, provide needed information or reminders, and present data in a way that more easily allows clinicians to manage the care of their chronically ill patients. Other information technologies allow clinicians to assess and consult with their patients at a distance, thereby cutting travel time for patients and reducing the number of in-person visits. Frequent contact with clinicians no longer needs to mean frequent visits to the doctor's office (Berwick, 2002). Patient care technologies, on the other hand, can change the actual care provided. Therapeutic devices such as pacemakers, for instance, extend the life of persons with abnormal heart rhythms. Diagnostic technologies such as computer-enhanced imaging devices can detect abnormalities long before the patient experiences any symptoms. Some patient care technologies not only treat the patient's condition but also integrate the medical device with clinical information, allowing clinicians to remotely monitor both the device and the patient's health status. Finally, assistive and environmental technologies may compensate for some of the functional impairments people with chronic conditions experience, en-

TABLE 7.1.
Selected Medical Advancements

Chronic Condition	Progress	Potential
Coronary artery disease	• Drugs to reduce risk (e.g., statins); to reduce symptoms (e.g., calcium channel blockers); to reduce mortality (e.g., beta-blockers) • Imaging modalities (e.g., cardiac echo, nuclear imaging, and angiography) • Surgical modalities (e.g., CABG, PTCA, stents, transplantation) • Improved management of acute disease (CCUs, thrombolytics)	• New medications to modify risk for disease, improved surgical modalities (e.g., better stents, CABG with less adverse impact)
Cardiac arhythmia	• Pacemakers, defibrillators • Drugs (e.g., amiodarone) • Surgical ablation	• Remotely managed implantable devices
Cerebrovascular disease	• Drugs to reduce the risk of stroke (e.g., antihypertensives) • Imaging modalities (CT imaging, angiography) • Surgery to reduce risk of stroke (e.g., carotid endarterectomy) • Better treatment for acute stroke (thrombolytics, stroke units)	• Better drugs to reduce the risk of stroke and possibly the morbidity with acute stroke
Cancer	• Radiation therapy and chemotherapy	• Improved chemotherapeutic modalities (e.g., highly specific agents from genetic engineering)
Arthritis	• Nonsteroidal anti-inflammatory drugs • Disease-modifying agents for inflammatory arthritis • Joint replacement	• "Living," self-repairing artificial joints
Diabetes mellitus	• Insulin pumps • New drugs	• Implantable self-regulating insulin pumps ("artificial pancreas") • Alternate means to deliver insulin (e.g., inhalation)
Depression	• New antidepressants (e.g., tricyclic antidepressants, SSRIs)	• Distance technologies (e.g., Internet, e-mail) to assess and deliver supportive interventions

Note: CABG is coronary artery bypass grafting (bypass surgery); PCTA is percutaneous transluminal coronary angioplasty; CCU is coronary care unit; CT is computed tomography; SSRIs are selective serotonin reuptake inhibitors.

abling them to remain in their own homes, delaying the need for hands-on care, or decreasing the quantity of direct care needed.

Nevertheless, technology's potential is easily exaggerated. In health care, in particular, Americans are prone to believe in the "technological fix," that technology can overcome almost every ailment or problem. Accordingly, a dose of caution is warranted: although technology may indeed significantly improve chronic illness care, it is not a panacea. Information technology, for instance, is only a tool, a means to help achieve important health care goals. Interest in expanding its use is largely driven by the promise of producing better care and providing care more efficiently. IT is expected to improve the flow of information by getting the right data to the right people at the right time—when decisions need to be made—thereby reducing medical errors, improving health care outcomes and patient satisfaction, and increasing efficiency. Generating clinically useful information is notoriously difficult, however, and many advances in health care information technology have focused more on the technology than on the information or meeting the needs of clinicians and others who will actually use the information. Moreover, many advances in IT are relatively recent and have not yet been widely disseminated and implemented. As a result, the potential of IT to improve chronic illness care remains by and large just that, a potential. It will take time to fully evaluate the impact of the many new information technologies on chronic illness care.

Caution is also warranted regarding patient care technologies. Here the primary concern is over costs and resource allocation. The wide dissemination and routine use of patient care technologies is often cited as the primary cause of the rapid escalation in health care costs during the past few decades. New technologies that enter medical practice may bring added benefits to patients, but they also come with added costs. In health care, new and improved usually also means more costly. Thus, continued advances in patient care technologies will exacerbate already difficult resource allocation issues. This danger is particularly true in chronic care where many of the new technologies transform acute, fatal diseases into chronic conditions or are "half-way" technologies that at best moderate the slow progression of a chronic condition (Thomas, 1974).

The implantable artificial heart illustrates the problem. Though still experimental, this device may one day be able to extend the lives of patients with chronic heart conditions for whom no alternative treatments exist. But the large number of patients who may be candidates for the device (about 100,000 Americans suffer from end-stage heart failure every year), combined with the cost (an estimated $70,000 to $100,000 for the device itself), will force the question: is the implantable artificial heart worth the cost? Paying for a large-scale artificial heart program will almost certainly take money away from other patient care technologies and other health care services. Costly technologies that may improve the diagnosis or treatment of chronic conditions, such as the artificial heart, will thus force us to confront difficult resource allocation issues, including how these decisions should be made, on what criteria, and by whom.

Similarly, joint replacement surgery, typically regarded as a "last resort" measure for persons who have exhausted other alternatives, has been shown to ease the pain and functional limitations of severe arthritis. But the projected increase in the number of people with arthritis—the number of older adults in the United States with arthritis or chronic joint symptoms, for example, is expected to nearly double by 2030—combined with the ability to replace nearly every joint in a person's body with artificial implants prompts the question: where do we stop? The continued development and use of patient care technologies may exceed our society's ability and willingness to pay.

This chapter examines four categories of health care technologies that can improve chronic illness care—information, patient care, assistive, and environmental technologies. It concentrates on information technologies, whose application cuts across all chronic conditions and health care settings. Their dissemination and use may have the greatest impact on health care outcomes and costs. In contrast, patient care, assistive, and environmental technologies are typically designed for specific conditions and thus affect comparatively fewer patients, limiting their impact.

Information Technology

Good chronic illness care requires timely, "actionable" information, that is, information that could influence the management of the patient's condition. Yet there is growing concern that such information is either not available or even when it is, that it is not being used as effectively as possible (Hersh, 2002). The current state of information collection and retrieval provides both too much and too little. Consider, for example, the patient with a long history of chronic health problems whose arrival in the clinic is heralded by four volumes of medical charts. Such a collection of information is of little use to the harried clinician. On the other hand, if multiple clinicians in disparate locations care for this same patient, each attending to a specific health problem, the patient may instead arrive at one clinic with no information regarding the drugs and other treatments he or she receives elsewhere. Such a dearth of information leaves the clinician without adequate guidance for making sound clinical decisions. The goal of information technology in these situations is to promote better clinical decisions by providing accurate, complete, and relevant information in a timely way and in a form that will focus the clinician's attention on the salient data.

In the context of health care, IT encompasses all forms of technology used to create, store, exchange, and use information in its various forms (including data, voice, video, and pictures) to support the delivery and processes of health care.[1] The IT toolbox in health care includes discrete devices, such as PCs and handheld computers (also called personal digital assistants, or PDAs), as well as complex technology systems that combine multiple components. These devices and systems can be designed to perform single tasks, such as computerizing patient health records, or meld together multiple tasks, such as billing, admission-discharge-transfer, pharmacy, and clinical matters. Mobile computing, for example, combines portable or handheld devices (e.g., a PDA, cell phone, or tablet PC^2), centralized storage information systems, and connecting technology that allows information to pass back and forth between the handheld devices and the centralized system. Mobile computing applications can link clinicians, regardless of their location, to all the clinical, administrative, and patient care information they need. Other IT tools include e-mail and Web-based applications that allow health care providers to communicate with patients as frequently as necessary, monitor patient care and, if necessary, intervene early in health care issues—without ever being in the same room as the patient.

The status of IT in health care is extremely fluid and characterized by rapid developments. Overall, however, the rate of adoption of IT in health care has been slow relative to many other industries. America's hospitals, for example, spent less than 3% of gross revenue on IT capital and operating budgets in 2002, compared with the 10% that is typical among hardware and software firms and the more than 7% in financial services. Despite what many believe is an enormous potential of information technology to improve chronic illness care (and health care, in general), there has been great reluctance within health care to invest in IT systems, outside financial accounting and billing.[3] As a result, "while information technology is advancing rapidly in other sectors of the U.S. economy, the U.S. health care system remains mired in a morass of paper records and bills, fax transmittals and unreturned telephone messages" (Goldsmith, Blumenthal, & Rishel, 2003). But that situation may be changing. In April 2004, for example, President Bush announced the Health Information Technology initiative, setting among other goals the widespread adoption, in both the public and private sectors, of electronic health records within 10 years.[4] A growing number of health-care firms are taking an interest in IT. Among the stimuli for expanding the role of information technology in health care are the shortage of nurses, technicians, and other health care workers; increasing pressure for pay-for-performance from big employers, whose health-insurance costs are soaring; rising concerns about quality and medical errors; and consumer pressure.

Information technology can serve as a building block for reforming chronic illness care. But IT must do more than facilitate communication; it must restructure information. Among its myriad uses in health care are translating science into practice, tracking changes in a patient's health status, highlighting salient data, helping to structure the clinician's attention, alerting the clinician to potential problems, issuing prompts or reminders to clinicians and patients, juxtaposing the expected and actual course of a patient's condition, and educating and informing patients about health and medical issues. These uses of IT can be categorized into five key functions:

1. Provide clinical decision support.

2. Collect and share clinical information.

3. Reduce medical errors.

4. Enhance patient-clinician interactions.

5. Empower patients and consumers.

Some of these functions overlap. For example, providing clinical decision support and collecting and sharing clinical information are both aimed at reducing medical errors, among other objectives, and both combine, to some extent, medical knowledge with patient-specific information. Nonetheless, it is helpful to distinguish among them and to examine some of the distinct information technologies used to advance each function.

Provide Clinical Decision Support

Clinicians' primary clinical task is to apply knowledge about medications, treatments, and other health care interventions to the care of their individual patients, recognizing each patient's distinctive health status, background, and care preferences. The vast number of new drugs, devices, and procedures for diagnosing and treating chronic conditions that are now available or under development fuels the exponential growth in medical knowledge. In light of this expansive and constantly increasing volume of knowledge, it is virtually impossible for clinicians to always be aware of the best current evidence regarding the safety, effectiveness, and cost-effectiveness of health care interventions. Compounding this problem, the increasingly competitive health care market puts new pressure on clinicians to reduce the amount of time spent to gather information about the patient and then to apply the growing body of medical knowledge to the patient's care.

One form of information technology, clinical decision support systems, or CDSS, includes "any software designed to directly aid in clinical decision making in which characteristics of individual patients are matched to a computerized knowledge base for the purpose of generating patient-specific assessments or recommendations that are then presented to clinicians for consideration" (Hunt et al., 1998). CDSS can assist the clinician in determining the most appropriate intervention for a given patient. Providing clinicians with instant access to computerized patient care protocols at the point of care enables them to more readily render decisions consistent with evidence-based recommendations, thereby increasing the quality of care. In a study to improve medication management, for example, a computerized CDSS helped clinicians use antibiotics more effectively and appropriately, reduced costs and adverse drug events due to antibiotic therapy, and decreased overall use of antibiotics (Pestotnik et al., 1996). Similarly, electronic drug databases can alert clinicians to patient drug allergies, potential drug-drug interactions, and possible excessive dosages. They can even relate laboratory abnormalities that may affect the metabolism of the drugs being prescribed.

In addition to guiding clinical decisions, CDSS could integrate medical knowledge and patient information with other functions to generate alerts and reminders. Computerized algorithms could generate reminders or prompts to clinicians to collect all needed information when performing routine patient care tasks such as drug ordering, bedside charting, and note writing. For patients who have access to the Internet or are connected electronically with their providers, similar reminders could be used to prompt them, for example, to regularly monitor their blood pressure, weight, and medication regimes and adjust their medications, if necessary, or to perform other tasks to manage their condition. These applications of clinical decision support systems provide clinicians and their patients ready access to the information they need to make appropriate care management decisions.

Clinical decision support systems could also include insurance eligibility information. This would allow the clinician to verify that the prescribed intervention such as a particular medication is included in the patient's health plan's drug formulary and thus is covered by the plan. Including insurance benefit information could decrease for clinicians the "hassle factor" in providing patient care in accordance with health plans' administrative processes such as requirements for prior authorization.

Despite the general consensus that clinical decision support systems have the potential to improve care, most studies evaluating CDSS in a clinical setting have focused not on health care outcomes but on system accuracy and on how clinical performance changes (Kaplan, 2001). A 1998 review concluded that although CDSS can improve "clinical performance for drug dosing, preventive care, and other aspects of medical care," their impact on patient outcomes had not been studied sufficiently (Hunt et al., 1998). Moreover, because of their narrow focus, studies of CDSS so far "tell us little about whether clinicians will incorporate a particular CDSS into their practice routine and what might occur if they attempt to do so. Such studies cannot inform us as to why some systems are (or will be) used and others are not (or will not be), or why the same system may be useful in one setting but not in another" (Kaplan, 2001). As a result, relatively few clinical decision support systems are in general use in clinical settings and the potential for CDSSs to advance clinical practice and improve chronic illness care has not yet been realized.

Collect and Share Clinical Information

Information technology can streamline the collection and sharing of clinical information between the clinician and the patient or among various members of the health care team. A variety of tools can help clinicians quickly document clinical activities, enable them to track patient information from one encounter to the next, and provide easy access to such information. Small computers or handheld devices can be placed either at the point of care or carried by a clinician to record patient data and transmit it to a central information system. The clinician can later retrieve the data, as needed; other clinicians can access the data as well.

A popular example of this type of information technology is the electronic health record (EHR).[5] Storing medical records electronically, instead of on easy-to-lose or -misplace and sometime illegible paper records, can ensure that each clinician treating a patient has all relevant information readily available and that the same information, such as a medical history, need not be collected multiple times from the patient (Dick, Steen, & Demeter, 1997). EHRs could include complete, longitudinal information about a person's health status and care, simultaneously displaying the relationship between the treatment and the clinical course. Such electronic records may be particularly useful for patients with chronic conditions, who typically see a variety of clinicians in different settings, all needing access to the same information about the patient's health history, test results, allergies, diagnoses, and treatment orders, including all active medication orders.

Ideally, EHRs should do more than simply replace paper records with a more accessible and legible computerized version. They should include simple mechanisms for recording and displaying needed data, for analyzing the data, and for sharing them among clinicians and patients. Indeed, investing in EHRs that simply allow the current level of information to be transferred squanders an opportunity that may not come along for some time. Changing the fundamental structure of the medical record can produce enormous benefits for medical practice. Electronic records should structure data entry to encourage complete and accurate recording. They should collect data in ways that allow them to be tabulated and plotted over time. And they should use data elements to focus clinicians' attention on pertinent aspects of a patient's health, such as deviations from the expected course of the patient's condition.

Developing an electronic medical record system that is able to perform all these tasks has so far proven elusive. Consider the following record of a patient's medical visit:

> Mrs. Jones returns today to follow up on her congestive heart failure (CHF) and diabetes. She states that she has been doing relatively well since her last visit although her sister has been ill and because of the stress of this she has not been as diligent in following her diabetes. Most of the values of her fingerstick record are within normal range, although a number around the beginning of the month were in the 200s. She denies any significant CHF symptoms; specifically no PND, orthopnea or edema. She says she was having some dizziness last week but that it is similar to the symptoms that were thoroughly worked-up last year and felt to be BPV.[6]

Interpreting complex free text such as this is tricky (and most medical information is in similar free-text form). Imagine that before the next visit, Mrs. Jones' clinician wants to get a clear idea of how often she was having dizziness in the past year. It would be extremely difficult, if not impossible, for a computer to tell from this paragraph that she was having dizziness. The mention of "dizziness" by itself is not helpful—the sentence could have been "She denies having dizziness." Multiple mentions of the term "dizziness" would be similarly unhelpful. Because of the many pitfalls in designing computers capable of understanding the English language, it has so far not been possible to develop EHRs that can interpret written clinical records, flag potentially important passages, and present concise actionable information to clinicians. Instead, electronic health records require that data be entered in a structured format that facilitates later manipulation and comparisons.

Although few question the need for a new record-keeping paradigm, except for a few medical centers and physician practices that have used electronic health records (some for up to 20 years), the EHR is entering the mainstream of health care delivery relatively slowly. Fewer than 10% of institutions such as hospitals and about 17% of physicians in office-based practice have adopted EHRs (Goldsmith, Blumenthal, & Rishel, 2003). Overall, the benefits of EHRs, particularly their promise of greater efficiency, have been difficult to achieve (Hersh, 2002). Some successes have been documented. Integrating a set of alerts and reminders into an electronic medical record system, for example, resulted in "significantly faster and more complete adoption of practice guidelines" by clinicians treating patients with HIV infection (Safran et al., 1995).

Recent private and public initiatives may speed up the adoption and use of EHRs. The Kaiser Permanente system, for example, began implementing a systemwide electronic health record in the fall of 2003. The Medicare Prescription Drug Improvement and Modernization Act (MMA) of 2003 requires the Centers for Medicare and Medicaid Services (CMS) to develop standards for electronic prescribing, an essential step toward the widespread use of electronic health records. In July 2004, Department of Health and Human Services (HHS) Secretary Tommy Thompson announced a 10-year plan to transform the delivery of health care by building a new health information infrastructure, including electronic health records and a new network to link health records nationwide, and released a "Framework for Strategic Action" to guide the nationwide implementation of interoperable EHRs in both the public and private sectors.[7]

Reduce Medical Errors

A number of IT applications in health care specifically target the reduction of errors or other aspects of the quality of care. Such applications may, for example, prompt the clinician to consider various treatment options or warn of possible conflicts with the patient's current treatment or condition. One such application is computerized physician order entry, or CPOE, which refers to the direct entry of orders into a computer or other electronic format by a clinician. This technology can be used for all types of orders, including drug, laboratory, hospital discharge, and nursing orders.

CPOE has been used for more than two decades. Prototypes can be found in pharmacy benefits management programs, which help identify potential drug-drug interactions or use algorithms to assure that the proper steps, such as checking on allergies, have been taken before allowing a drug to be ordered. Medication errors are among the most common preventable mistakes, and the more drugs a patient is taking and the more people involved in the delivery of a drug, the greater the chance of a mistake. The Institute of Medicine recently recommended CPOE as one strategy for reducing medication errors (Institute of Medicine, 2001). Similarly, the Leapfrog Group, a coalition of some of the country's largest employers, endorsed CPOE as one of its three initial methods to improve patient safety.[8] The expectation is that CPOE will improve quality of care by intercepting errors when they most commonly occur—at the time medications, laboratory tests, or other services are ordered.

Once entered, CPOE orders can be processed more quickly than handwritten, paper-based orders. An electronic order can be moved instantaneously to a nursing station and pharmacy, whereas a written order must be physically transported from one location to another. Other advantages of

CPOE are the orders' accuracy, clarity, and completeness. Misplaced decimal points, clinicians' legendarily illegible handwriting, and misreading a "u" (short for units) as a zero have all been cited as causes of medication errors.[9] CPOE should minimize, if not eliminate, each of these types of errors. Computerized ordering systems can also help prevent accidental overdoses and make it virtually impossible for a clinician to prescribe a drug to which the patient has a known allergy.

Despite "having very real, potential benefits," CPOE systems have not yet proven their effectiveness, except in reducing the rates of certain types of medication errors. They are most useful in identifying patient allergies to new medications and potential interactions of new medications with current medications (Institute for Clinical Systems Improvement, 2001). Other researchers see broader benefits and argue that there is already "an important and growing body of evidence [that] shows that CPOE . . . can influence physicians to order medications and tests in a more clinically appropriate and cost-effective manner" (Doolan & Bates, 2002). Beyond such disagreements, there is consensus that further research should be conducted to evaluate CPOE. Specific issues include evaluating the use of CPOE in conjunction with other IT, such as clinical decision support systems or electronic health records. Preliminary data suggest that CPOE is more likely to be effective when it is part of an EHR system that allows full access to a patient's clinical information (Institute for Clinical Systems Improvement, 2001) and when it is combined with clinical decision support systems (Bates et al., 1999).

As with electronic health records, CPOE systems have had only limited acceptance to date. According to the Leapfrog group, only about 7% of U.S. hospitals had a computerized order entry system up and running in 2002. Among the reasons for the relatively slow adoption rate of CPOE systems are the systems' high cost, their uncertain benefit-cost ratio, physician resistance, and the complexity of designing and implementing such systems in light of "the variety of information technology systems present in different organizations" (Institute for Clinical Systems Improvement, 2001).

Enhance Patient-Clinician Interactions

In a world of chronic disease, information technology is critical in facilitating full and efficient communication between clinicians and their patients. For patients with multiple chronic conditions timely, easy access to medical expertise is essential; periodic office encounters may not suffice to monitor disease states. Continuous monitoring must be coupled with mechanisms for identifying early changes in patients' health status and prompt notification of clinicians. Likewise, the concept of team care relies on effective communication. Frequent face-to-face meetings among team members may be too costly and time consuming.

Information technology can change the way in which patients receive care and interact with their clinicians. Electronic communication such as telemedicine may become a substitute for some face-to-face encounters. Telemedicine includes a broad continuum of equipment and services that can be used for medical diagnosis, treatment, consultation, monitoring, and health maintenance. The term is used to describe something as simple as using a fax machine to transmit medical information from one provider to another. At the other end of the continuum, telemedicine refers to a complex and sophisticated network of equipment that enables clinicians to see, hear, examine, question, and counsel patients from miles away. A remote monitoring system linked to a clinician's office, for example, can gather and transmit information on a patient's vital signs and other physiological information, giving clinicians the ability to quickly and easily respond, if necessary.

Potential applications of telemedicine include the following:

- Conducting patient interviews; obtaining medical histories

- Performing follow-up assessment of functional status (physical and mental)

- Monitoring vital signs; screening, monitoring, and tracking patient responses to prescribed treatment regimens

- Monitoring medication and treatment compliance

- Facilitating case management

- Providing education to facilitate shared responsibility between patient and provider

- Consulting among clinicians

Multiple and varied benefits accrue from these applications of telemedicine. For example, telemedicine may improve patients' quality of care by expanding their "access" to specific services. Telemedicine may permit more aggressive patient monitoring, increasing both the opportunities for early intervention and the responsiveness of clinicians to changes in the patient's condition. It may also improve efficiency by reducing travel time for both patients and clinicians and limiting unscheduled visits to clinicians' offices.

Telemedicine may be of particular benefit for certain populations, including older adults, people with chronic conditions, and rural residents. Telemedicine can connect such patients with their clinicians from their own homes or other remote sites, thereby overcoming transportation and similar barriers to care. Preliminary studies indicate that telemedicine can promote independence among older adults as well as provide needed support for their informal caregivers (Goins, Kategile, & Dudley, 2001). Telemedicine also enables, for instance, the primary care clinician of a rural, elderly patient with multiple chronic conditions—sometimes a generalist with little training in geriatrics or chronic illness care—to consult with various specialist clinicians to develop and implement a coordinated care plan for the patient's complex, interrelated conditions (Goins, Kategile, & Dudley, 2001).

Telemedicine facilitates regular monitoring of a patient's clinical parameters. Information collected and transmitted by the patient can either be processed by a midlevel health care professional or interpreted by using computer algorithms programmed to identify changes in patterns and generate appropriate alerts. The patient's primary care provider could then become involved, if necessary. The abundance of programs now written for PDAs also make it is easy to envision a new approach to home care in which home care workers will be equipped with such devices that are programmed to guide them through making targeted observations. Linked to a central station through modems, these workers can be directed about the indicated next steps in a patient's course of treatment. The very same technology can be used with family members and other informal caregivers and even with patients themselves.

For telemedicine to be used effectively, clinicians need to be comfortable with it and have confidence in their abilities to diagnose and manage care without direct contact with the patient. In a study conducted by Kaiser Permanente, early resistance by nurses to a study of tele-home health care was resolved as data began to show that it did not decrease the quality of care or patient satisfaction and did not increase the use of health care services (Johnston et al., 2000). In addition, clinicians may need to examine their own beliefs about what constitutes care and the benefit of face-to-face contact. In a study of tele-home care videoconferencing, the home care nurses reported that 94% of "virtual visits" were as useful clinically as actual face-to-face visits (Veen et al., 2002). Similarly, patients, family members, and other informal caregivers must feel comfortable with the telemedicine system and have the needed skills (ideally, the system should require only minimal skills), or be trained to use it appropriately.

The impact of telemedicine has been most thoroughly studied in home health settings. A "TeleHomeCare" system developed by researchers at the University of Minnesota, for example, linked patients in their own homes with clinicians by videoconferencing and the Internet. The system used (1) videoconferencing equipment, including the patient's TV and telephone, a videophone, and a camera; (2) home-monitoring devices to measure vital signs such as blood pressure and pulse; (3) a home health care agency work-station, including videophone and camera; and (4) an information system to store and analyze patient-specific information. In a study of patients with CHF, chronic obstructive pulmonary disease, and those requiring chronic wound care, fewer patients were transferred to a hospital or a nursing home when they had received TeleHomeCare. Patients using the home monitoring equipment were also more satisfied with the home care they received (Veen et al., 2002). Outside tele-home care, few studies have evaluated patient or clinician satisfaction with telemedicine or its cost-effectiveness.

Empower Patients and Consumers

The final set of IT tools in health care are intended more for consumers and patients who are accessing information and services than for clinicians and other health care providers. Various information technologies, but especially the Internet, provide consumers and patients with unprecedented access to health information. On the Internet, consumers have immediate access to a staggering array of commercial and noncommercial Web sites including those of academic health centers, drug companies, government agencies, health care providers and insurers, disease-specific advocacy groups, and many other stakeholders.

Much on-line information is not personalized; rather, it is designed principally to educate and inform people about health and medical issues. Most people who use the Internet for health purposes seek information about particular physical or mental ailments. These on-line searches often precede or follow visits to a clinician (Fox & Rainie, 2000). A small but growing set of on-line health care activities are more patient specific. For example, many Web sites provide individual patients with salient targeted information about their chronic conditions or with access to advice from health care professionals, online personal coaching, and virtual pharmacies. However, only a small fraction of consumers use the Internet for such nonresearch or reference purposes. Only about 10% of people who use the Internet for health purposes have purchased vitamins or drugs on-line, 10% have described a medical condition or problem to get advice from an on-line doctor, and 9% have communicated with their own clinician via e-mail. In contrast, 91% of those who use the Internet for health purposes have looked for information related to a particular illness (Fox & Rainie, 2000).

Consumer use of the Internet for health information is growing, though researchers disagree over the extent of such use. A national survey indicated that about 40% of Americans with Internet access used the Internet to look for information or advice about health or health care in 2001 (Baker et al.,

2003). Because only about half the American population uses the Internet at all, this means that about one in five Americans use the Internet for health purposes. Other estimates suggest that use of the Internet for health purposes may be higher (Fox & Rainie, 2000). Reasons why consumers like the Internet include the convenience of being able to get health information at any hour, the wealth of information online compared with other sources, and the appearance of giving the user anonymity. The belief in anonymity may be misplaced, however, because many health-related Web-based business models depend on identifying and tracking users for a variety of purposes, often without the user's knowledge or consent (Goldman & Hudson, 2000).

Even though consumers increasingly use the Internet for health information, they complain that what they find online still falls short. Consumers are mainly concerned that there is too much data to sort through and they are unsure what they find is credible. Nearly 80% of consumers say it would be helpful to have health care professionals such as nurses available via the phone to assist with questions and validate the information they found online.[10] Critics agree that, because much of the information on the Internet is not screened or delivered to patients by health care professionals, there are problems with its quality and accuracy. There is no quality control for health care information on the Internet, and studies confirm such information is sometimes not reliable or up-to-date (Eysenbach et al., 2002). Others note that most health-related Web sites require a high school level or greater reading ability, which undercuts their usability by some lay persons (Berland et al., 2001).

Some expect expanded consumer access to health care information to profoundly affect patient-clinician interactions, though the precise impact is not yet clear. Proponents argue that these IT tools empower individuals by providing information that enables them to make more informed decisions regarding their own care. Increasingly, as consumers gain equal access with health care professionals to information sources online, they come to their clinician's offices armed with information they found on the Internet, seeking answers. Although some clinicians welcome such initiative on the part of their patients, others are leery that this will upset the long-standing balance of power and authority in their patient-clinician relationships. To date, the use of the Internet or e-mail seems to have had a negligible impact on the utilization of health care services. About 95% of people who used the Internet for health purposes said such use had no effect on the number of times they visited or telephoned their physician or other health care provider (Baker et al., 2003).

Patient Care Technology

Health care may lag behind other industries in developing and adopting in-formation technology, but it is often at the cutting edge in other areas of technological innovation. Each year thousands of new diagnostic or thera-peutic medical devices are developed and disseminated throughout the health care system. New equipment and techniques have safely moved sur-geries that once required days in the hospital to the outpatient setting. New imaging devices have increased the speed and accuracy of diagnostic proce-dures. The full range of patient care technologies includes, for example, glu-cose sensors that can be worn as a contact lens,[11] infrared ear thermometers that record body temperature in one second, tiny drug-coated stents that are implanted in a patient's body to keep arteries from clogging, and huge, multi-million dollar imaging devices such as positron emission tomographic (PET) scanners that must often be housed in their own separate buildings.

Patient care technologies for chronic illnesses can be separated into two categories, depending on their effect on the roles of clinicians and patients, particularly with respect to patient self-management. We call technologies that help patients play a more active role in their own care and reinforce pa-tient self-management by keeping the patient in the information and care management loop "patient-enhancing technologies." Patient care devices in the second category, in contrast, manage a patient's chronic condition by bypassing the patient's involvement altogether. We call such devices "patient-supplanting technologies."

Patient-Enhancing Technologies

Some patient-enhancing technologies help patients monitor their health conditions in their own homes. For example, in-home electronic scales that track the weight of patients with chronic conditions can be programmed to routinely ask the patients a series of questions about their symptoms, which the patients then answer by using a simple numeric pad. The patients' re-sponses, along with the weight data, are transmitted back to their clinic, where they are interpreted and, if necessary, used to help the patients bet-ter manage their own care.

Other patient-enhancing technologies are therapeutic devices that in-tegrate information and medical technology. Already, patients can have a pacemaker or other cardiac device implanted in their bodies that collects a variety of data monitoring the device itself. Newer devices such as an im-plantable hemodynamic monitor collect physiologic data on the patients' condition as well and then allow transmission of the data—on both the patient and the device—to their clinician. These new monitoring devices allow heart patients, for example, to use the Internet to relay up-to-date cardiac data from their homes to clinicians' offices. A small monitor held over the patient' chest, close to the implanted device, records information transmitted by the device on the patient's health status (e.g., heart rate, right ventricular diastolic and systolic pressure) and on the implanted device (e,g,, battery status). The patient then transmits the data to a clinician over a secure Internet link. The clinician could call the patient in for an office visit, if needed, or discuss with the patient by phone or e-mail changes to better manage the condition, such as modifications in medications or diet.

Because such devices can provide clinicians with detailed information about the patient's condition, they can relieve the anxiety some patients and their caregivers experience in not being sure when to report symptoms to their clinician. Focus groups conducted by the manufacturer of the implantable hemodynamic monitor, for example, found informal caregivers to be particularly receptive, anticipating that the information capabilities of the device may lighten their burden of having to make health decisions for a chronically ill family member. They viewed the devices as a "safety net."[12]

Patient-Supplanting Technologies

Technologies that take patients out of the care and information loop include devices that monitor the patient's physiological parameters and use that information to automatically adjust their own performance. Such self-regulating devices already exist. For example, heart pacemakers to detect abnormal heart rhythms and administer electric shocks to treat arrhythmias are also capable of performing their own self-diagnostics to ensure their calibration is adequate. Along the same lines, ongoing research is exploring the feasibility of an insulin pump that continually monitors blood sugar (and other parameters) and adjusts the insulin dose accordingly. In essence it would function as an artificial pancreas. Similar devices could monitor blood levels of various drugs and dispense dosages in response.

Alternatively, patient-supplanting technologies could bypass the patient by linking the device directly to the clinician. In this situation, a clinician receives data on a patient's therapeutic device and, without notifying the patient or the patient even being aware of it, remotely adjusts the device. Both types of patient-supplanting technologies permit "remote patient management" without the patient's participation.

One basis for patient-supplanting devices is to increase patient compliance (though "compliance" may a misnomer if the patient has no choice but to comply). Another rationale for circumventing the patient's involvement is that new patient care devices may become so complex that it is impractical to involve the patient in any significant way. However, by taking the patients out of the decision-making process regarding the management of their care, such devices may undercut the trend toward empowering patients and disregard informed consent requirements.

The sheer complexity of many new patient care technologies will affect ongoing patient care management in other fundamental ways. Many implantable devices require a specialist or subspecialist to place the device in the patient's body. For example, cardiovascular electrophysiologists now implant most pacemakers and similar cardiac devices. The patient's subsequent care is then provided by other clinicians, such as the patient's primary care physician and nurse practitioners. As a result, the relative roles and responsibilities of the specialist who implants the device, the generalist who manages the patient's chronic condition, other health care professionals who provide additional health and supportive services, and the patient may need to be redefined.

Assistive and Environmental Technology

Assistive technologies are "products, devices, or equipment that are used to maintain, increase or improve the functional capabilities of individuals with disabilities."[13] These technologies, which compensate for a person's physical and sensory deficits, range from everyday items, such as walkers, wheelchairs, and hearing aides, to elaborate prostheses and cutting-edge mobility devices. As these aids improve and more are developed, individuals whose functions are impaired by chronic conditions may be able to perform more self-care and activities of daily living, whether at home or in a health care facility. This may reduce the number of hours of help from another person or eliminate the need for such personal assistance altogether. For example, a van can be equipped with a hydraulic lift and modified so that it can be driven safely by a person in a wheelchair, providing the person greater mobility and reducing the need for assistance from someone else. New wheelchairs are able to "climb" stairs, expanding the places people in wheelchairs can get to on their own. The use of a wide range of assistive technologies (mostly low-tech devices such as railings, walkers, shower seats, and grab bars in bathrooms) has been associated with the use of fewer hours of personal assistance (Hoenig, Taylor, & Sloan, 2003).

Environmental technologies seek to improve the care and quality of life for persons with chronic conditions by using automation and other technological advances to alter the person's living environment. A principal goal of these technologies is to promote independent living, especially by allowing individuals, such as elderly persons with chronic conditions, to continue to live in the familiarity and comfort of their own homes, enabling them to "age in place." To combat safety concerns and loss of independence, technology can be used to create "smart" living environments that monitor or remind residents of unsafe conditions, such as alarms and alerts indicating a stove or iron is left on, guests are at the front door, or intruders are in the home (Tran, 2002).

The technologies to remotely monitor the health status and living environment of people with chronic conditions may include relatively simple sensors. Researchers in Japan, for example, used a combination of low-tech, readily available devices to monitor the health status of elderly patients through their daily routines in their own home. The devices included infrared sensors to detect human movement, magnetic switches to detect the opening and closing of doors, wattmeters embedded in wall sockets to detect the use of household appliances, a flame detector to detect the use of a cooking stove, and a CO_2 sensor to detect the presence of a person in a room. A networking system combined the sensors and each day automatically transmitted the data to a clinician. This data set enabled the clinician to observe daily behavior patterns, such as the length of sleep, absences from the house, use of the stove, and the time spent watching television. Deviations from the daily behavior patterns would prompt the clinician to telephone the person to ask about health issues or other problems (Ogawa, Suzuki, & Otake, 2002).

The Independent Life Style Assistant, or ILSA, developed by Honeywell Laboratories, represents another home-based automation system using a diverse set of sensors, medical devices, and "smart" appliances to enable users to live and function safely at home.[14] The three-year ILSA project, which ended July 2003, was a system of integrated sensors and control devices throughout the home that interpreted the data collected and responded appropriately. ILSA could be used, for instance, to alert the resident of any potentially unsafe conditions, remind the resident of essential tasks (e.g., when regular medications are to be taken), and record data over a period of time and generate reports (e.g., on patterns, trends, or changes in the occupant's behavior or activities).

Users of environmental technologies include noncognitively impaired, nonhomebound persons who are able to live independently, but who are on the threshold of needing assistance due to chronic conditions, frailty, or other impairments. The technologies are designed to extend the period such persons can safely live at home by themselves. The technologies can also provide "reassurance" to the user's children and caregivers regarding their safety and security. Other applications of such environmental technologies include monitoring the functioning of individual to efficiently schedule home-care or home-health visits or using the system in homes of people with moderate disabilities, dementia, or propensity to "wander." The systems also have temporary uses, including assessing hospitalized patients' readiness to be discharged or assessing persons with chronic conditions for appropriate placement in a nursing facility, assisted living, or home setting.

Environmental technologies can be designed to specifically collect a variety of clinically useful data. For example, a person's ability to get out of a chair and walking speed are good predictors of future clinical problems. Currently available sensors can be used to collect such information in a way that could be analyzed and tracked over time. Other "wearable" sensors, such as a device that clips on a belt or is worn on the wrist, could detect falls. Sensors to collect physiologic information could also be embedded in clothing.

Barriers

Barriers to the expanded use of information technologies in health care include:

- Financial barriers, including the high cost of building and maintaining an information technology infrastructure and the lack of reimbursement;

- Concerns over patient privacy, confidentiality, and security;

- Resistance to technology among patients and clinicians;

- Legal issues, such as state licensure laws; and

- Lack of standardization.

Financial Barriers

Financial barriers to expanded use of information technology in health care include the cost of purchasing, installing, and maintaining the equipment or information system. For hospitals and other large facilities the costs for a new information system can be millions of dollars. The cost of developing and implementing a CPOE system at Brigham and Women's Hospital in Boston, for example, was estimated at $1.9 million, with an additional $500,000 annual maintenance cost (Bates et al., 1998). The total, 10-year cost of implementing the electronic health record throughout the Kaiser Permanente health system (8.4 million members) is estimated at $3 billion.[15] The majority of these costs are incurred up-front, for training and initial lost productivity, which is expected to be repaid as clinicians become more familiar with using the EHR.

A health care facility typically would make such a major capital investment expecting to recover their costs for the technology. Under current reimbursement systems, however, the anticipated cost savings of implementing and using a new information technology system may not accrue to the facility purchasing the system. In fact, under fee-for-service reimbursement the cost savings achieved, for example, by a CPOE system as a result adverse drug events avoided or fewer tests ordered may, perversely, reduce the income for the health care facility. Even under prospective or capitated payment systems, "the investment can be hard to justify when there are powerful short-term cost pressures and the benefits [of the technology] are unsure and occur in the medium and long-term" (Doolan & Bates, 2002). Given the uncertain financial incentives, many health care facilities balk at spending money on information technologies when it is easier and more popular with their staff to buy a new diagnostic or therapeutic device that clinicians want and that could also attract patients.

Physicians also cite high initial cost as a major barrier to expanding IT in their practices (Miller & Sim, 2004). Large group practices, which have deeper pockets and are thus better able to absorb implementation costs, typically take the lead in adopting and using IT innovations. In the absence of clear productivity gains, physician practices find the cost of many new information technologies prohibitive. Up-front costs for implementing EHRs, for example, ranged from $16,000 to $36,000 per physician, whereas financial benefits varied from "none in practices that made few work practice changes and retained paper processes to more than $20,000 per physician per year in the few practices that eliminated most paper processes" (Miller & Sim, 2004). The fragmentation of the current system, in which many patients with chronic conditions receive care from a collection of independent or loosely affiliated physicians and other health care organizations, also makes it difficult to implement clinical information systems capable of providing access to complete patient information to all providers rendering care. No single organization may have the financial incentives or wherewithal to invest in such a system. The trend toward larger health plans and integrated health systems may provide a needed correction to such fragmentation and reduce these financial barriers. The alignment of financial incentives in integrated systems such as Kaiser Permanente may explain why these organizations, which combine the insurer and provider functions, are at the forefront of implementing costly information technologies. In such integrated systems, the savings that result from the use of a new technology accrue to the same organization that incurs the cost of its adoption and implementation.

Another financial barrier is that the current financing system specifically excludes some information technologies from reimbursement. Even though telemedicine, for example, has made it easier to deliver health care services to patients in distant locations, coverage of this technology by public and private payers is inconsistent. Similarly, under the dominant fee-for-service reimbursement system, clinicians' use of email communication with their patients is typically not covered, although some insurers are beginning to pay for e-mail encounters.

Privacy, Confidentiality, and Security

Concerns over the privacy, confidentiality, and security of health care information are not unique to the adoption and use of new information technologies. Restricting access to personal health care information to only appropriate users is a ubiquitous challenge for all health care organizations, regardless of the format of the information. However, many of the new IT tools raise unique privacy-related concerns. For instance, portable and hand-held devices are at much higher risk than fixed desktop computers for theft and loss, raising the risk that confidential patient information becomes accessible to unauthorized users. On the other hand, the concerns over some information technologies may be exaggerated. For example, the National Academy of Sciences has noted that the major threats to the confidentiality and security of electronic medical records are related to inappropriate use of patient-specific information by health care workers who have access to the information as part of their regular work (National Research Council, 1997). These risks apply equally to patient-specific information stored on paper records.

Personal health care information stored in various electronic formats is also susceptible to security breaches. In 2000, for example, a computer hacker stole about 4,700 electronic patient files containing treatment information from the University of Washington's computer network (Eng, 2001). This and other publicized breaches of computer or Internet security, whether related to health care information, have undermined the confidence among Americans that their online health information is secure—from hackers and other unauthorized users. In one survey, 75% of those seeking health information on the Internet indicated that they were "concerned" or "very concerned" that sites where they have registered may share their personal health information with a third party without their permission (Eng, 2001). Despite strides in encryption and other security measures to guard personal health information, the practices at many health-related Web sites provide some justification for the public's concern about the lack of privacy protections. Some Web sites, for example, have strong privacy policies but then do not hold their business partners, with whom they may share information, to the same privacy standards they espouse (Goldman & Hudson, 2000).

The most far-reaching legal requirements to address privacy concerns in health care are in the federal Health Insurance Portability and Accountability Act of 1996 (HIPAA). The act's core privacy provisions require providers and health plans to disclose how they use, store, and share health information; ensure patient access to their own medical records; and obtain patient consent before releasing patient information. To implement these provisions, HIPAA mandates the development and adoption of a number of national electronic health information standards, including standards for electronic data exchange of health information; standards for the privacy of individually identifiable health information; a national provider identifier; an employer identifier and secure electronic signatures. Regulations to implement HIPAA's privacy requirements went into effect on April 14, 2003 and apply to the use and disclosure of personal health information, regardless of the form in which the information is kept, the methods of transmission, or the way it is communicated. Security standards for computerized health care information will take effect as part of the HIPAA in 2005. Even after HIPAA's regulations have been implemented, however, a host of unresolved issues regarding the privacy and security of personal patient information remain, including:

• Clarifying the relationship of HIPAA and more stringent state law governing medical privacy

• Developing mechanisms and strategies to overcome the real or perceived lack of security of online personal health information

• Developing appropriate protections among the burgeoning on-line activities that are not covered by HIPAA and are "beyond current privacy law, since they operate in the nascent gray zone beyond 'traditional' health care" (Goldman & Hudson, 2000)

• Assessing the impact of HIPAA regulations on clinicians and providers who use information technologies designed to ease the sharing of patient-specific information

Resistance to Technology

Information technologies can alter the traditional way of doing business. Thus, adopting a new IT system may require a cultural change on the part of everyone involved. The traditional face-to-face visit or consultation between patient and clinician, for example, is so ingrained in our health care system that both clinicians and patients are hesitant to consider electronic communications (whether by phone, e-mail, or Internet) as an equivalent substitute. The "virtual visits" made possible by the new forms of communication may supplement office visits, but few patients or clinicians believe they can fully supplant them. Likewise, insurers have been reluctant to pay for consultations unless the patient is physically present.

One might wonder why clinicians, who embrace new technologies in areas of diagnosis and treatment, are reluctant to use IT. What is different about magnetic resonance imaging (MRI), for example, which clinicians embrace as an important diagnostic tool? The answer may be that IT is not seen as offering any immediate additional benefit. Indeed, many clinicians fear that IT will only add to their already demanding workload, particularly if it slows, rather than enhances, productivity at the outset (Bodenheimer & Grumbach, 2003; Miller & Sim, 2004).

Certain types of information technologies raise specific concerns. Shifting from paper prescriptions to CPOE, for example, is a giant leap for clinicians, made more difficult if the benefits are not readily apparent. Using a computer and scrolling through a series of screens to select the right drug and dosage typically takes longer than dashing off a prescription on a paper pad. This time quickly adds up for clinicians who must "write" numerous orders per day. Several large medical centers have scrapped their CPOE systems in the face of physician resistance. Physicians complained that the paperless systems were slower, cumbersome, and did not follow physician workflow (Chin, 2003).

Physician resistance to CPOE and other information technologies can often be traced to how the technologies have been implemented. Implementing new information technologies requires numerous parties to change the way they work. The keys to successfully implementing such technologies, in particular, if they directly affect patient care, include involving clinicians (as the technology's primary users) in the implementation process and providing features of benefit to them, widespread adoption and implementation across the organization, and strong involvement of the organization's clinical leadership (Hersh, 2002). Health care organizations that have successfully implemented CPOE have involved clinicians in all phases, from initial design or purchase to testing to final implementation.

Physician resistance to new information technologies may reflect a basic disagreement on IT's benefits and goals. Many of these technologies, including electronic medical records and computerized physician order entry, are championed by the IOM and other organizations as strategies to help reduce medical errors. Such errors, according to the IOM, are due primarily to failures of institutional systems rather than the failures of individuals

(Institute of Medicine, 2001). Information technologies, it is thought, address such "system failures" by improving decision-making processes and the flow of information within organizations, or systems. But physicians view medical errors differently, citing individual failures, such as "overwork, stress, and fatigue on the part of health professionals," as the primary causes (Blendon et al., 2002). These differences regarding the nature of the problem extend to disagreement on possible solutions. For example, only 19% of physicians believe that increasing the use of computerized medical records would be a "very effective" strategy for reducing the number of medical errors, whereas 51% believe increasing the number of nurses in hospitals would be very effective (Blendon et al., 2002).

Legal Issues

Beyond patient privacy and confidentiality concerns, information technologies raise a variety of other unresolved legal issues, many related to licensure of health care professionals and the provision of services and consultations across state lines. The expanded use of the Internet (which knows no boundaries) for sharing health-related information between clinicians, consumer purchasing of prescription drugs, and online interstate consultations creates many new legal issues. For example, if a patient in one state sues a clinician in another state who has provided consultations to the patient via a Web site, it is not clear which state has jurisdiction. This situation also highlights the difficulty for the state where the patient resides to enforce its state health licensure laws (which are, in part, designed to protect patients from fraudulent or unqualified providers) if the clinician providing the consultation is not licensed in that state.

Most states now have laws regulating out-of-state telemedicine practice by physicians. The majority of these states require full licensure of out-of-state physicians who provide telemedicine services to a patient located in that state. The lack of laws in the remaining states continues to restrict interstate telemedicine practice. Interstate telemedicine practice by nurse-clinicians is permitted by states that have adopted the Interstate Nurses Licensure Compact (at least 12 states as of 2002). The compact is based on mutual recognition across states, creating uniform standards for nursing licensure and permitting interstate practice by all states that adopt the compact. An unresolved issue beyond licensure concerns the need for any additional validation of (licensed) clinicians' competency to engage in telemedicine. Some suggest that clinicians also need certification or some sort of credentialing mechanism to ensure that they are trained, proficient, and safe in using telemedicine technologies.

Lack of Standardization

Technologies that store or transmit electronic information use different methods for transferring and synchronizing data. Some devices are physically connected to others by wires, others are wireless and use radio frequency technology to transmit and receive data through the air. Because the methods used to send and receive data (e.g., the specific radio frequencies used) differ across devices, not all devices are able to communicate with each other. In some circumstances there are information exchange protocols to translate, for example, the signals a handheld computer sends to a gateway server into language the Web can understand so that the Web, in turn, can forward the information to another user. But these protocols add to the complexity and cost of IT devices.

There are also no standards for the ways in which patients' health care data are recorded by today's commercially available EHR software, including the structure of the record itself, level of detail, coding, and the nomenclature. Currently, the only way to convey EHRs between health care providers using different vendors is to "write costly custom interfaces to move clinical information between different clinical software platforms" (Goldsmith, Blumenthal, & Rishel, 2003). The lack of standards across different types of EHRs is compounded by the lack of adequate electronic data exchange between EHRs and other clinical data systems, such as clinical decision support systems (CDSS).

Uniform standards would allow various information technologies and systems to operate and interoperate in a smooth and seamless manner. They alleviate the time and effort spent on ensuring that the terminology used in different health care settings to identify the patient and to record clinical information is consistent and they enable the seamless flow of information among different IT systems, even those developed by different vendors. Without widely adopted standards and guidelines, interoperability and interconnection between the multitude of information technologies and devices will be difficult and the potential for advances in IT to improve chronic care will be hard to achieve. Some call for uniform federal standards, without which, it is argued, "clinical information will be trapped inside vendor-constructed boxes and cannot follow the patient from institution to institution or from practitioner to consultant and back" (Goldsmith, Blumenthal, & Rishel, 2003). As required by the Medical Modernization Act of 2003, there are now several federal initiatives to develop national standards to achieve interoperability among various types of health information technologies.

Summary

The continued development and dissemination of new technologies will reshape the process of care for people with chronic conditions as well as the care itself. The integration of therapeutic devices with information capabilities will enable people with chronic conditions to become more involved in the management of their own conditions. Some devices will facilitate remote monitoring and, in some cases, allow clinicians to remotely adjust treatment without the patients' involvement. Assistive and environmental technologies will provide greater independence to people with chronic conditions, reduce their need for assistance, and allow more of them to continue to live in their own homes. Of the four types of technologies discussed in this chapter, information technology (IT) is likely to have the greatest impact on chronic illness care. Information technologies are designed to improve the flow of information in health care by getting the right data to the right people at the right time—when decisions about a patient's care and treatment need to be made. Information technologies redress deficiencies in the processes of care that cut across various chronic conditions. They can be used for any patient in any setting.

Information technology is seen as a vital tool for improving health outcomes, reducing costs, and achieving other important health care goals. The potential of information technology, however, has so far exceeded its proven worth, as a number of questions regarding the ability of IT to improve health care outcomes, reduce costs, or both, remain unanswered. Still, its potential is such that substantially greater use of IT is almost universally cited as an important component of a health care system capable of providing optimal chronic illness care. Some even suggest "a modern health information architecture is an indispensable precondition of safe and effective clinical practice" (Goldsmith, Blumenthal, & Rishel, 2003). Yet significant barriers continue to impede widespread adoption and use of IT in health care. Of these, financial barriers and resistance to technology (ironically, often from health care professionals) may be the most formidable. More evidence showing the effectiveness and cost-effectiveness of various types of information technologies may be needed to reduce these barriers. Despite the unanswered questions, however, the push for expanded use of IT is accelerating, in both chronic care and the health care system in general.

8. Prevention

The best way to manage chronic disease is to prevent it from occurring, but accomplishing that goal is not easy. Lifestyle factors including diet, exercise, tobacco-alcohol-drug use, and environmental exposures all contribute to the development of chronic conditions. Appropriate actions can reduce and, in a few cases, completely eliminate the incidence of chronic illness. Similarly, these types of behavior changes may prevent another episode or the progression of an acute problem into an chronic illness, as when diet and exercise changes made by a person after experiencing a heart attack reverse coronary artery disease. Second, early detection may render some diseases more treatable. Preventing the development of chronic illness and screening for presymptomatic disease are combined in the first part of the discussion that follows.

Prevention continues to play an important role even after a person is diagnosed with a condition such as diabetes, asthma, or arthritis. Good care for any chronic condition involves an effort to prevent decline and disability. As one group of researchers observed, "the goals of effective chronic-disease management are preventive in orientation: to prevent exacerbations, complications, treatment side effects, and emotional distress" (Glasgow, Orleans, & Wagner, 2001, p. 602).

Another important aspect of prevention is avoiding iatrogenic illness, or illness caused by treatment. This includes avoiding drug interactions and/or side effects. Medications are an important tool in the treatment of chronic conditions and as conditions progress or as people develop multiple conditions, the number of both prescription and over-the-counter medications used increases. With this comes a significant increase in the risk of illness or death related to the drug treatment rather than the original illness. For this reason, it is also important to examine how preventing medication problems is an element of chronic illness care.

Preventing the Development of Chronic Disease

Getting to the Causes

The landscape of chronic disease has changed considerably, at least in part because of successful prevention initiatives. The prevalence of chronic diseases is influenced by two offsetting activities: preventive efforts (including fundamental behavior changes) will reduce the rate at which the disease occurs, whereas the success of various treatments once a problem actually arises may increase the number of persons surviving with chronic illnesses.

Although declines in some diseases have been observed in recent years, the effect on the prevalence of disability seems to be mixed. Declines have occurred in mild disability, but not in the rates of more severe disability that result in a need for assistance with personal care. For instance, among older persons, the prevalence of chronic disability has declined significantly, from 22.1% in 1984 to 19.7% in 1999. Most of this decline is the result of lower rates of elderly persons receiving human assistance only for instrumental activities of daily living, or IADLs (such as preparing meals and managing money).[1] In contrast, the mean number of activities of daily living, or ADLs (more basic activities such as bathing or dressing) per older person actually rose slightly (Spillman, 2004). That is, among older persons, the rate of mild disability is declining, but the rate of severe disability has remained nearly constant. Some observers have predicted a compression of morbidity as a result of prevention, whereby people would delay the onset of chronic illnesses and, as a result, experience only a short period of disability prior to death (Fries, 1980), but so far this prediction has only been seen in limited areas and to a limited extent (Fries et al., 1998). However, the growing rate of obesity threatens to dampen any trends for reduced disability (Flegal et al., 2002).

The decrease in the prevalence of several chronic illnesses has been shown to be a product of both better prevention and better medical care. For example, an analysis of the decline in mortality from coronary heart diseases suggests that only 25% of the decline was explained by primary prevention, whereas 29% was explained by secondary reduction in risk factors in patients with coronary disease and 43% by other improvements in treatment in patients who already had the disease (Hunink et al., 1997). Likewise, a review of stroke mortality gains suggests that most, but not all, of the benefit comes from improved treatment of strokes after they occur (Sarti et al., 2003). Other estimates give more credit to prevention. During the period from 1981 to 1990 reductions in risk factors such as smoking, high blood pressure, and high cholesterol reduced the rates of heart disease and stroke—which are the first and third causes of death in the United States as well as the cause of disability for over 10 million Americans—by an estimated 7–11%, thereby adding an estimated 1.9 million quality-adjusted years of life (Centers for Disease Control and Prevention, 2003).

Some improvements in health behavior have already had widespread consequences. For example, declining rates of cigarette smoking are associated with reductions in mortality from several conditions. In California, the largest tobacco control program in the United States has improved the health status of the population. Between 1989 and 1997 the per capita consumption of cigarettes declined faster in California than in the rest of the country and is estimated to have resulted in 33,300 fewer deaths from heart disease (Fichtenberg & Glantz, 2000). Smoking-attributable cancer deaths for 1995–1999 compared with 1990–1994 declined for men in California while they increased in the rest of the country, and rates for women increased more slowly in California than nationally (Centers for Disease Control and Prevention, 2002).

Efforts to prevent chronic disease are anchored to two areas of inquiry. One is the vast amount of biomedical and epidemiological research into the causes of many chronic conditions. The other is the development of models of population health that attempt to generate an understanding of how socioeconomic factors such as the distribution of wealth, the environment, and culturally constructed categories and roles interact with personal characteristics to affect health. Both areas of inquiry suggest that actions taken by individuals, communities, and societies can decrease the incidence of many chronic illnesses.[2]

Epidemiological research has linked a variety of behaviors and exposures to chronic disease whereas biological research has, in some cases, precisely explained how a range of physiologic functions, from chemical reactions to organ function, cause or are affected by chronic illness. The overwhelming evidence linking smoking to lung cancer and other diseases is the basis for including smoking cessation in public health education campaigns and in individual medical care. Diet and exercise are also increasingly acknowledged as key contributors to several chronic diseases (diabetes, cardiovascular disease) and cancers (colon, stomach). For other behaviors, such as alcohol consumption, the evidence is weaker or contradictory (Belleville, 2002; Ellison, 2002; Rehm, Sempos, & Trevisan, 2003).

Epidemiological and biomedical research has led to recommendations with which most people are now familiar: do not smoke, get regular exercise, watch your weight, eat more vegetables, fruits, and whole grains, and drink alcohol in moderation (maybe). These lifestyle choices and related behaviors are the predominate focus of efforts to prevent a wide range of chronic illnesses. This emphasis does not discount the fact that there are important genetic components in some chronic diseases.

Research in population health has added to this biological and epidemiological knowledge by seeking a more comprehensive explanation for variations in health. Broad models of population health developed in the past two decades have added income and social status, social support, education, working conditions, community norms, and physical environment to the list of contributors to health that previously included only biology-genetics, personal health practices, and health services. These population health models contain many similar features and all are based on the ideas that (1) in addition to individual characteristics, social, economic, cultural, and physical environments play important roles in determining health; (2) the interactions among these factors are complex; and (3) a focus on medical care and how to make people well must be balanced by concerns about why they became ill (Evans & Stoddart, 2003).

Reducing Risk Factors

Estimates abound of the potential reduction in medical care expenditures or how many years would be added to life if people would adopt healthy behaviors. For example, the leading causes of death can be recast in terms of the underlying causes, which are often preventable behaviors. From this perspective, the cause of death is not simply the chronic disease (such as heart disease or type 2 diabetes) but rather the behavior (poor diet or lack of exercise) that contributed to the development of the illness and ultimately death. Table 8.1 reproduces the results of such a calculation, suggesting that nearly 50% of deaths in the United States are actually caused by lifestyle factors and behaviors.

Presented in this somewhat simplistic manner, people's failure to follow recommendations that could prolong life and/or delay disability seems difficult to understand. Given that adherence to these recommendations appears to be the exception rather than the rule, realizing the possibility of prevention requires an understanding of the issues surrounding, and barriers to, risk reduction on a societal level. For example, the obesity epidemic

TABLE 8.1
Actual Causes of Death in the United States in 2000

Cause	Estimated No. of Deaths*	% of Total Deaths
Tobacco	435,000	18
Diet/activity patterns	400,000	17
Alcohol	85,000	4
Microbial agents	75,000	3
Toxic agents	55,000	2
Motor vehicles	43,000	2
Firearms	29,000	1
Sexual behavior	20,000	1
Illicit use of drugs	17,000	<1
Total	1,159,000	49

*Composite approximation drawn from studies that use different approaches to derive estimates, ranging from actual counts (e.g., firearms) to population attributable risk calculations (e.g., tobacco). Numbers are based on McGinnis & Foege (1993) as updated in Mokdad et al. (2004).

has been attributed (in part) to environmental factors that encourage eating and discourage physical activity (Hill & Peters, 1998). Influences on diet and exercise include food supply trends, advertising and promotion, food pricing, trends in transportation and occupational activity, and the availability of sedentary versus active leisure-time activities (French, Story, & Jeffery, 2001).

Some risk reduction activities are designed to affect an entire population, whereas others need to focus on specific high-risk groups to be effective and efficient. The decision depends on a combination of logistics and available resources. In some cases, such as reducing air pollution or water fluoridation, it is illogical if not impossible to aim the efforts at a particular subgroup. In other cases, those at greatest risk should be the focus of attention; such as when diabetics or persons with a family history of heart problems need to be especially diligent in avoiding the risk factors associated with heart disease.

Once the target population is identified, preventing the onset of chronic diseases still faces two enormous hurdles. First, the causal links between an individual behavior and disease (e.g., obesity and type 2 diabetes) or between the characteristic of the social environment and disease (e.g., stability of the social hierarchy and cardiovascular disease) are not deterministic. Everyone knows someone who smoked, drank, ate bacon everyday, or grew up in chaotic poverty and lived to be ninety in good health. They also know of a health-food nut and runner who died young. Risk factors are rarely the direct causes of disease; therefore, changes in behavior or environment can only increase or decrease the risk of developing a chronic disease or condition.

The second hurdle is that chronic disease prevention requires difficult decisions and actions from individuals and societies. Setting up a vaccination program or ensuring completion of a course of antibiotics to prevent an infectious disease may be challenging, but this task pales in comparison with the effort required to sustain a change in a person's eating habits or empower a disenfranchised member of a society. Without both a definitive reason and an obvious mechanism, neither individuals nor societies are likely to change. Advancing chronic disease prevention requires still more research to accumulate and refine the evidence about the causes of chronic conditions. Equally, if not more important, prevention requires understanding how to facilitate the processes of change on multiple levels, ranging from individuals to families to communities to entire cultures. Examples of how towns, cities, states, and the federal government are working to prevent chronic illnesses by reducing one major risk factor—obesity—are included in exhibit 8.1.

Acknowledging that behavior is influenced by environment and that social values and norms shape individual attitudes can lead to the conclusion

EXHIBIT 8.1

Community Approaches to Preventing Chronic Disease

More and more people are acknowledging the role that social forces and the environment play in influencing diet and exercise behaviors. At the same time, obesity and its negative effects (increased rates of chronic diseases, higher health care costs, lost productivity, and individual pain and suffering) are increasing at an alarming rate. In response, communities and their leaders are developing programs and policies to encourage physical activity and good nutrition.

Here are some examples:

- After Philadelphia was named the fattest city in 1999 by *Men's Health* magazine, the mayor put his city on diet. He appointed a health-and-fitness "tsar," and the city has encouraged city residents to walk or bike to work, instituted a variety of programs for people who are obese or overweight, and organized community events such as a New Year's Eve replicating the run in the movie *Rocky*. More information is available at http://phila.gov.fitandfun/fitness.html

- A pilot program in Boston, Sisters Together, targeted young black women in three intercity neighborhoods. A coalition of community organizations and residents developed programs to encourage physical activity such as walking and dancing and programs on nutrition planning, shopping, and cooking to promote healthy eating. Additionally the coalition participated in larger community-wide efforts to advocate for safe, pleasant places to exercise and access to fresh food at reasonable prices. http://hsph.harvard.edu/sisterstogether/

- In Madelia, Minnesota, 250 people lost 2,340 pounds by the end of a 10-week community-wide diet. People paid $10 to participate and attended weekly meetings of the "Fight the Fat" program that included diet and exercise advice and a weekly weigh-in. Teams competed to lose the most collective weight, local restaurants added healthy menu items, the grocery store provided signs and recipes near healthy food items, and people exercised in groups. The community support, social nature, and the accountability of teams (and a small town culture where participants were known) all seem to have contributed to the program's success. Burcum, Jill. 2003. "Taking a load off," *Star Tribune* (Minneapolis, MN) May 12, p. 1A.

- California Project LEAN (Leaders Encouraging Activity and Nutrition) began in 1987 as a Henry J. Kaiser Family Foundation public awareness campaign to promote low-fat eating. In cooperation with the Public Health Institute, the project conducts programs throughout California that target different populations ranging from school children to low-income Latino mothers. www.californiaproject lean.org/

- The mayor of Madison, Wisconsin, recently announced his "Fit City Madison" plan. This citywide effort includes regular fitness events with the mayor, a partnership with restaurants to develop standards for healthy menu items, and weight-loss challenge competitions. www.fitcitymadison.com/

At the federal level, the Centers for Disease Control and Prevention (CDC) are developing and disseminating Guides to Community Preventive Services. These guides provide public health and policy decision makers with information about population-based interventions to improve health. They cover a variety of topics in three broad categories: changing health risk behaviors (tobacco use, alcohol abuse, and physical activity), reducing diseases (cancer, diabetes, mental illness, oral disease), and addressing environmental challenges. www.thecommunityguide.org/

that unhealthy behavior is not only an individual problem, but a community responsibility as well (Thompson et al., 2003). Changing views about what behaviors are acceptable and the resulting social pressure on individuals may be influenced by mandates as well as scientific proof. Perhaps the most vivid example can be found in smoking, which has gone from a socially desirable behavior to one that is shunned in part due to antitobacco policies that include taxes and prohibitions on smoking in more and more places.

For an individual with a chronic condition, the condition itself may shape risk reduction efforts. Although we tend to think about eliminating risk factors before an illness develops, getting sick can also be a great motivator to change behavior. Some of the strongest converts to heart-healthy regimens are those who have suffered their first heart attacks. However, having a chronic illness also may interfere with some positive preventive activity or make it inappropriate. For example, severe arthritis may interfere with the ability to exercise. In other circumstances, enthusiasm for prevention must be weighed against the person's overall health and situation. Consider how a woman with severe congestive heart failure who asks her physician whether she should be taking medication to prevent osteoporosis differs from an otherwise healthy woman asking the same question. Whether the patient with heart failure is likely to survive long enough to benefit from such a preventive course has to be considered.

Screening

Screening for disease that is present but not yet causing problems is preventive in the sense that it facilitates early treatment. Most screening programs are based on the belief (and sometimes evidence) that although disease may already be present, early diagnosis and the appropriate follow-up may make it more treatable, and in some cases curable. This is the rationale for many cancer-screening programs, such as those designed to detect breast, cervical, and colon cancer.[3] Other screening activities seek to identify markers of clinical risk such as high blood pressure, high cholesterol, or low bone density before they cause strokes, heart attacks, or broken bones.

Although screening by itself will not prevent the development of disease, screening and primary prevention are similar in many ways. In both cases people who have no current complaint are asked to do something now relative to a possible, but far from guaranteed, future (for screening it is to have a test which may be uncomfortable, expensive, or entail some risk; for prevention it is to change a behavior or lifestyle). Because both involve addressing an issue that is not currently problematic, the acute-care focused medical care system has historically treated both primary prevention and screening as sidelines or add-ons rather than integral to patient care. These similarities make it possible to merge them when talking about how they are currently incorporated into health care and they are often grouped together under the label "clinical preventive services."

Clinical Preventive Services in Health Care Today

There are two principal explanations for why primary prevention and screening have not been incorporated into the mainstream of health care. First, the division between public health and medical care, combined with the focus in medical training on problem solving, have relegated these activities to the margins of care. Primary prevention and screening are lower in terms of both priority and prestige than treating a trauma or making a difficult diagnosis. Second, prevention and screening activities have historically not been well reimbursed; presently, many such services are under-covered by both private and public health insurance. It is unclear whether coverage is minimal because medical care has not emphasized these activities or whether the lack of reimbursement has encouraged medical care to focus elsewhere.

Both private and government insurance have steadily added clinical preventive services, but in a less than systematic way. For example, Medicare, which finances health care of most Americans over age 65, was designed to cover only diagnosis and treatment. Preventive services were specifically excluded from the original coverage plan. However, some changes have been made since its inception in 1965. Although hundreds of bills to add specific clinical preventive services have been introduced in Congress, none passed until 1980 when pneumococcal pneumonia immunizations were added. In the subsequent decades, Congress approved adding nine more preventive care services to Medicare coverage. These inclusions have come in response to the advocacy efforts of specific groups rather than a planned expansion of the program (Kamerow, 2003).

All the same, a consensus has developed around what prevention and screening services are components of good care. The Canadian Task Force on Periodic Health Examination and later the U.S. Preventive Services Task Force (USPSTF) developed a means to evaluate individual services and have published and periodically updated lists of recommended preventive services. These recommendations have become the standard for health care professional training and practice in their respective countries.

Comparing Medicare coverage and the USPSTF guidelines for someone older than 65 years vividly illustrates the persistent lack of congruence between coverage and consensus guidelines for prevention and screening. Table 8.2 lists the preventive services that (1) are recommended and covered by Medicare Part B, (2) are recommended but NOT covered, and (3) are not recommended but still covered. Covered clinical preventive services

TABLE 8.2.
Comparison of USPSTF Recommendations and Medicare Coverage

Recommended and covered
  Pneumococcal pneumonia vaccine
  Hepatitis B vaccine
  Influenza vaccine
  Pap smears for cervical cancer
  Mammography for breast cancer
  Screening for colorectal cancer
  Bone mass measurement for osteoporosis
  Eye doctor screening for glaucoma
Recommended but NOT covered
  Diphtheria-tetanus vaccine booster
  Eye chart screening for visual acuity
  Screening for hearing impairment
  Blood lipid screening
  Screening for depression
  Tobacco cessation
  Diet counseling for high-risk patients
  Motor vehicle injury prevention
  Household and recreational injury prevention*
  Sexually transmitted disease and HIV prevention*
  Discussion of aspirin to prevent cardiovascular disease
  Discussion of tamoxifen or raloxifen for high breast cancer risk
NOT recommended but covered
  PSA† test and digital rectal examination for prostate cancer
  Pelvic examination for vaginal cancer

Source: Adapted from Kamerow, 2003, p. 40.
*Lesser level of evidence used to support this recommendation (per USTSTF).
†PSA, prostate-specific antigen.

include vaccines and screenings for cancer and other conditions. The services not covered include some items that could be part of a moderate office visit (e.g., questions about hearing difficulties or depression) and counseling activities.

Organized programs of health education can also reduce disease burden among older persons. In one randomized study, a low-cost program for retirees resulted in a reduction of risk factors and lower health care costs (Fries, Bloch, et al., 1993; Fries, Koop, et al., 1993). Health promotion programs have been found to reduce health care charges by 20% (Fries et al., 1998). Based on this evidence, legislation has been introduced to expand Medicare coverage for health promotion to cover services provided by firms with established track records in bringing about desired health behaviors.

Difficulties Preventing Chronic Illnesses

Many people do not have insurance coverage for the recommended screening services or the training and support they might need to change behaviors and prevent chronic illnesses. This lack, coupled with the fact that the necessary behaviors often involve fundamental lifestyle changes, helps to explain the wide gap between recommendations based on current knowledge and the actions of both health care providers and the public. Closing this gap is likely to require major changes in both reimbursement and the delivery of health care.

Significantly increasing prevention and screening activities in the health care system would be only one step in preventing chronic disease. Other changes would need to be made at the level of communities and society. Recommendations that people exercise are less likely to be followed when there are no community centers, gyms, parks, or even sidewalks. Asthma will continue to be a problem where air quality is low. Making changes to our physical environment and our communal lives that would reduce the incidence of chronic disease requires both a level of awareness and commitment that are often difficult to achieve.

Although understanding the similarities between primary prevention and managing chronic illnesses might aid in explaining why both have received less attention than acute care, there are also significant differences (see table 8.3). The differences mean that an optimal system for managing chronic illnesses will not, in and of itself, allow us to maximize prevention of chronic diseases. Focusing on approaches to organizing care that serve multiple purposes (i.e., promote prevention and improve chronic illness care) may be one way to justify change. However, given these differences, there likely will always be a separate need for prevention programs.

TABLE 8.3.
Similarities and Differences between Chronic Illness Management and Prevention

---

Similarities
- Involve regular (non-symptom-driven) screening and counseling for health behavior change to prevent disease.
- Require being able to identify a defined population of patients
- Require ongoing planned care with proactive follow-up
- Are complex, require addressing multiple health behavior changes or risk factors, and need decision guides for priorities.
  - Bulk of intervention needs to be in primary care
  - Providers often work without adequate information
- Acute illness-reactive care model is inadequate for both.
- Require active patient involvement in adherence to complex screening, behavior change or treatment regimes; patient activation, tailoring, and shared decision making are important for both.
- Providers are inadequately trained for their roles.
- Require links to community resources outside the health care setting and benefit from supportive community policies and programs.
- Policy maker / decision maker fears that both are costly and may not be cost-effective.

Differences
- Visits for patients needing primary prevention are less frequent than visits for patients with chronic illness
- Patients with diagnosed chronic illness (and the providers treating them) are likely to have stronger motivation to change health behaviors.
- Patient and provider demands are greater for chronic-illness care since, in addition to regular screening and health-behavior change, there are issues involving adherence to prescribed medical care for the disease.
- Prevention is more outside the medical culture and less often tracked or reimbursed.
- Perceived health and economic benefits of prevention in healthy populations may be less than among patients with chronic illness.
- There are fewer health care specialists and greater reliance on community/centralized programs for prevention.

Source: Glasgow, Orleans, & Wagner, 2001.

Preventing Decline and Disability

Prevention and the management of chronic conditions overlap because the elements of good chronic care are essentially activities designed to prevent negative outcomes. After a chronic condition has been diagnosed, the focus typically shifts to preventing or reducing morbidity and delaying mortality. While there is currently no cure for diabetes, asthma, or arthritis, proper management can prevent some of the negative effects of these conditions. For example, blood sugar control lowers the risk for vascular disease in diabetics, knowing and avoiding triggers prevents asthma attacks, and exercise increases range of motion and decreases pain in arthritic joints. Some chronic illnesses may cause impairments that put persons at high risk for serious, yet preventable problems. Persons suffering from dementia may need oversight to be sure that they eat and drink regularly, thereby avoiding common but preventable complications such as malnutrition and dehydration.

Similarly, a minor foot injury may become the first step in a chain reaction that puts a diabetic at risk for a lower leg amputation. For all these examples, the "treatments" are not the time-limited, location-specific, technology-based procedures that most people associate with medical care. Rather, "treatment" for chronic conditions becomes the long-term management of physiologic processes, symptoms, and any resulting impairments or disability. This care cannot be accomplished within the walls of a clinic or hospital in a limited amount of time using a specific drug, procedure, or surgery.

Guidelines or protocols for managing many chronic illnesses specify timetables for tests designed to monitor either the control of the disease (such as the blood test for HgA1c that measures long-term glucose control for diabetics), its progression (tracking peak-flow ventilation in chronic lung disease), or the side effects of treatment (monitoring of liver function for patients taking some blood pressure medications). These also include medication and counseling recommendations, and algorithms or decision trees that aid with the detection and resolution of side effects. These guidelines are made available to providers and patients and serve as a template for good care. (Examples are included in table 8.4.)

Knowledge from clinical medicine and public health make it possible to prevent a significant amount of the disability and morbidity caused by chronic disease. There is a reasonable level of consensus on what to do; the

TABLE 8.4.
Examples of Guidelines for Chronic Illness Care

Topic	Producer	Reference/Electronic Source
Detection, evaluation, and treatment of high blood pressure	Joint National Committee including 39 professional, public, and voluntary organizations and 7 federal agencies	Chobanian et al., 2003 www.nhlbi.nih.gov/guidelines/hypertension/
Diagnosis and treatment of asthma	National Asthma Education and Prevention Program, coordinated by the National Heart, Lung, and Blood Institute	National Asthma Education and Prevention Program, 2002 www.nhlbi.nih.gov/guidelines/asthma/index.htm
Aspirin for the primary prevention of cardiovascular events	U.S. Preventive Services Task Force	Aspirin for the Primary Prevention of Cardiovascular Events: Recommendation and Rationale, 2002 www.ahcpr.gov/clinic/3rduspstf/aspirin/asprr.htm
Medical care for diabetes	American Diabetes Association	Standards of Medical Care for Patients With Diabetes Mellitus, 2003 http://care.diabetesjournals.org/content/vol26/suppl_1/

greater problem is figuring out how to do it. The existing acute care system is ill fitted to the activities that are critical to preventing the negative effects of chronic illness. Specifically, the management of chronic conditions requires continuity and coordination, emphasis on behavior change, support of patient self-management, and timely access to appropriate providers and services. These principles of chronic illness care are discussed in detail in several sections of this book, but it is worth emphasizing how they are linked to the idea of prevention

For instance, after diagnosis, preventing decline and eventual disability from chronic conditions requires that care be organized to respond to the ongoing needs of the patient. Care needs to include continuity, at least of information, if not of clinician. The various clinicians a patient may see need to be able to share information and treatment plans. Perhaps most importantly, both the clinicians and patients need a system to monitor the chronic condition, enabling them to recognize decline at a point where it may still be reversed or at least slowed and make changes in treatment. Information technologies that facilitate this type of monitoring are discussed in chapter 7.

Still, the relative value of reversing decline and preventing further loss remains controversial. For example, the Medicare reimbursement policy for rehabilitation does not acknowledge any value in maintaining function or delaying decline. Evidence of continuous improvement is required for payment, effectively denying services that might have preserving function as a goal. This runs counter to research that has shown that even modest rehabilitative efforts directed at very frail persons can prevent functional decline and may even result in modest improvements (Fiatarone et al., 1994). More research to demonstrate that these improvements are cost-effective and efforts to change these policies are needed if patients are to realize the benefits of optimal chronic illness care.

Promoting Health and Well-being in the Face of Serious Illness

Care of the frail or seriously ill is not routinely associated with prevention. However, even when chronic conditions become serious and cause disability, a critical component of care remains preventive in nature. The need and emphasis switch from preventing decline and disability to preventing pain, emotional distress, and unnecessary limitations. Care at this point in the chronic illness progression aims to maximize quality of life and the ability of the patient to maintain physical function and social roles.

Interventions designed to accomplish these goals might be more accurately described as health promotion and descriptions of these efforts often include phrases that at first may seem contradictory, such as "healthy ill people" or "wellness for cancer patients" or "quality of life with advanced disease." In this usage, health promotion "is concerned with enabling people to maximize their health potential" and is based on the assumption that "from whatever point one starts in life, . . . health and well-being can be enhanced and developed" (Kickbusch, 1992).

Systems of acute care often place health promotion as the first step in a linear arrangement. Health promotion is followed by disease detection, diagnosis, treatment, and rehabilitation. For chronic illness, this sequence does not make sense and health promotion can occur at any stage and is categorized as "the search for new quality of individual health, independent of the specific form of illness" (Milz, 1992).

One example of the growing emphasis on health promotion for patients with serious or multiple chronic conditions is the recommendation for exercise programs for people with cancer. Exercise can improve physical function (Segal et al., 2001) and psychological well-being (Segar et al., 1998) in either programs designed around a specific cancer or for patients with different types of cancer (Young-McCaughan et al., 2003). While exercise is often part of rehabilitation or care following treatment, it is increasingly seen as an integral part of treatment or an adjunct to therapy, such as when an in-hospital exercise program was designed and evaluated for patients receiving high-dose chemotherapy (Dimeo et al., 1999).

Health promotion in the face of serious disability or frailty is particularly relevant for elderly people with chronic conditions. Frequently, the combination of age and chronic conditions has resulted in an assessment that certain types of care are inappropriate or that certain services are futile. The Canadian Association on Gerontology adopted a policy in October 2000 to demonstrate its support of health promotion and counteract this stereotype. The Association "rejects the societal myth that proactively promoting the health of older individuals does not have an impact in old age and believes that health promotion is a justifiable priority even for those who are already frail and chronically ill" and "encourages . . . the integration of health promotion with traditional illness-oriented care" (Canadian Association on Gerontology, 2000).

Prevention at the advanced stages of a chronic disease process is difficult to accommodate in the acute care system. The tasks may require the expertise and involvement of a team of different types of providers. Continuity becomes increasingly important as the patient's needs become more complex. Perhaps most importantly, not only cure, but also improvement in clinical indicators may be impossible, making definitions of success and justification for payment problematic. However, health promotion for the frail and seriously ill is an important component of a chronic illness care system.

Preventing Iatrogenic Complications

A major aspect of prevention in chronic illness care is the reduction of problems caused by health care itself. These problems are referred to as iatrogenic illnesses or complications. A recent report from the Institute of Medicine has alerted the country to the dangers of medical errors (Kohn, Corrigan, & Donaldson, 2000). Frail older persons with complex or multiple chronic diseases may be especially susceptible to these types of problems for several reasons. They appear to have a smaller therapeutic window, the time during which treatment can do more good than harm, and they can be harmed by care in several ways. Also, relying on stereotypes can convert a temporary problem like confusion into a permanent diagnosis of dementia, with all its unfortunate consequences. Patients with serious or multiple chronic diseases are at risk of complications, no matter their age. General poor health or treatments that suppress the immune system may increase the likelihood of contracting infections while in the hospital; treatment for one condition may aggravate another; or the side effects of treatment may become serious or life threatening.

Medications and Iatrogenic Complications

There are many possible causes of iatrogenic problems, but most are related to the use of medications. The over 87 million Americans with a chronic condition receive an average of 11 prescription drugs a year. People with three or more chronic conditions (22.3 million people) receive 28.3 different prescription drugs a year on average. This climbs to an astounding 46.8 drugs per year on average if a person has more than three chronic conditions, a severe disability, and severe functional limitations (Anderson & Knickman, 2001).

Prescription and over-the-counter drugs are used in all phases of treatment and management of chronic conditions. Drug therapies now exist that decrease or eliminate symptoms, slow or stop disease processes, improve quality of life, and in some instances cure. The appeal of medications and their increased use can be attributed to a variety of factors, including their effectiveness and acceptance by clinicians and patients, their noninvasive nature, and the increase in direct-to-patient advertising. Medications have eliminated or reduced the need for some more invasive procedures, extended life spans, and relieved symptoms for many people, although the extent to which this is true depends on how specific drugs are used and with what alternative treatments they are compared (Neumann et al., 2000). These positive outcomes are the goal of pharmaceutical therapies. Negative outcomes of drug therapy include therapeutic failure, reactions, or side effects, interactions among drugs, or adverse response to drug withdrawal.

Reasons for the negative drug outcomes are varied. Polypharmacy—taking multiple drugs—can cause problems, especially when care is not coordinated across the many clinicians often involved in the care of one patient. Drugs may interact with other drugs or with factors such as diet, environmental exposures, or disease processes—either the disease being treated by the drug or comorbidities. The way the body processes the drug (pharmacokinetics) and how the drug works (pharmacodynamics) may change according to age, gender, or health status. Drugs may be overused or underused given the severity of symptoms, the cost of the drug, or poor understanding by clinicians or patients. Also, treating a person with multiple chronic illnesses may require the use of a drug that addresses one condition while making another worse (i.e., using prednisone improves a person's asthma, but worsens diabetes). In these complex cases, choices need to be made between the lesser of two evils, or trial and error may be required before optimal therapy is determined.

Examining these negative outcomes is important because side effects, drug interactions, and the clinical consequences of noncompliance, are significant causes of illness, disability, and death. A study of adverse drug events among people older than 65 years treated in ambulatory settings (not in hospitals or nursing homes) estimates that there are 50.1 adverse drug events per 1,000 person-years. An "adverse drug event" is defined as an injury resulting from the use of a drug and does not include errors that did not result in injury. More than 27% of all injurious events were considered preventable, whereas 42.2% of the serious, life-threatening, and fatal adverse drug events were considered preventable (Gurwitz et al., 2003). Inappropriate prescription drug use is also often linked to negative drug outcomes. In one study approximately 20% of community-dwelling elderly persons who were surveyed had at least one prescription that was inappropriate, meaning that it was contraindicated due to disease, had a known interaction with another prescription, or the dosage and/or duration did not correspond to current guidelines. The most common problems involved benzodiazepines (the class of drugs that include sedatives and antianxiety medications) and NSAIDs (nonsteroidal anti-inflammatory drug) (Hanlon et al., 2002). Medication errors are also an important factor in hospitalizations, as both the cause of the hospitalization and the reason for an extended length of stay (Peyriere et al., 2003).

Prescribing errors are not the only source of medication problems. Given the pervasive use of drug therapy it is not surprising that medication management is a major patient activity in chronic illness care. Realizing the benefits of drugs requires that patients understand the recommended therapy and find a means to translate often-abstract instructions ("take as needed," "twice a day," etc.) into their widely varied schedules and lifestyles. Table 8.5 offers an example of the medication regime and schedule for a

TABLE 8.5.
Sample Medications Profile: 82-Year-Old Woman with Multiple Chronic Conditions

Condition	Drug Name	Prescribed Dosage
High cholesterol	Lipitor	40 mg, 1 per day
High blood pressure	Atenolol	50 mg, 1 per day
	Lotensin	20 mg, 2 per day
Congestive heart failure	Lasix	40 mg, 1.5 per day
	Zaroxolyn	2.5 mg, ½ every 4 days
Angina	Isosorbide	20 mg, 6 per day
	Nitro	1/150, as needed
Breast cancer (posttreatment)	Tamoxifen	10 mg, 2 per day
	Evening primrose	2 per day
Peptic ulcer	Prevacid	1 per day
Ulcerative colitis	Asacol	3 per day
Leg cramps	Vitamin E	400 iu, 1 per day
	Multivitamin	1 per day
Blood thinning	Baby aspirin	1 per day
Back pain	Glucosamine/chondroitin	3 per day
Constipation	Stool softener	1 per day
Insomnia	Temazepan	1 as needed for sleep
Pessary maintenance treatment	Betadine	weekly
	Replens	after Betadine douche

Current Schedule for These Medications

Breakfast   10½ pills
　　Lotensin　　　1
　　Isosorbide　　2
　　Tamoxifen　　1
　　Primrose　　　1
　　Asacol　　　　1
　　Lasix　　　　1½
　　Atenolol　　　1
　　Prevacid　　　1
　　Gluco　　　　1
Noon　5 pills
　　Isosorbide　　2
　　Multivitamin　1
　　Gluco　　　　1
　　Stool softener　1
Supper　7 pills
　　Isosorbide　　2
　　Lotensin　　　1
　　Gluco　　　　1
　　Baby aspirin　1
　　Asacol　　　　2
Bedtime　4 pills
　　Tamoxifen　　1
　　Lipitor　　　　1
　　Primrose　　　1
　　Vitamin E　　1

person with multiple chronic conditions. From this illustration it is easy to imagine how much time and effort is needed to plan and adhere to this treatment; why people might feel they spend their days taking pills; and how easy it might be to forget or mix-up medications.

The deficiencies in the current system reviewed in chapter 3 are also potential causes of adverse drug events. A fragmented, uncoordinated system may have several clinicians prescribing drugs for one patient, and without a centralized record or system of easy information exchange they may be unaware of the other prescriptions. Overwhelmed and confused patients may not understand their drug regimes or be able to incorporate complex regimes into their every-day life. Patients' priorities may differ from those of their health care providers, and if this discrepancy is not acknowledged and discussed, poor adherence is a likely outcome. Faced with paying out of pocket for an expensive medication, a patient may not fill the prescription, take less than the prescribed dosage, or skip days to make the medication last longer. This lack of compliance limits effectiveness and may also have serious clinical consequences (Hughes et al., 2001). Given the amount of communication possible in short out-patient visits, patients may not tell providers about medication problems or their concerns about cost. Likewise, clinicians may not be able to provide information about possible side effects or spend time teaching practical approaches to medication management.

A final potential source of adverse drug events is that research on interactions and the effects of medications sometimes does not parallel clinical reality. The drug approval process has historically been based on testing in comparatively young men and in people with a single condition. Testing of drug interactions has been limited. However, growing evidence that some drugs' effects vary by age and gender has resulted in the broadening of drug testing. Despite these important changes, the people most likely to have chronic conditions (the elderly and women) may still be prescribed drugs at dosages based on relatively limited testing on patients like them.

Potential approaches to preventing medication problems mirror the reforms proposed to improve chronic illness care. Coordinating a patient's care with an electronic information system or by a care coordinator could reduce the potential for drug interactions and establish priorities among multiple medications. Including pharmacists in team care for complex patients or encouraging patients to use a single pharmacy might facilitate the periodic review of medications and the identification of potential problems. Group visits or self-care groups could allow patients to share the expertise they have developed in medications management, such as the use of dispensers and reminders. Patients can be given specific information on the major side effects of their medications and encouraged to watch for these and report their occurrence. Ongoing patient support systems such as phone access to a nurse, pharmacist, or health educator could provide immediate answers to questions about how to handle missed or duplicate doses or how to adjust medications to changing circumstances (e.g., a flu that causes vomiting or a change in diet related to a special event). A recent review by the World

Health Organization of both the level of adherence to long-term therapies by the elderly and means to improve this concluded that promising interventions include individualized education, medication review, long-term pharmacist counseling; simplifying treatment, targeting high-risk patient (particularly those with cognitive or physical deficits that affect medications management), providing access to needed drugs, and developing better reminder and pill organization methods (DiPollina & Sabate, 2003).

Summary

The acute-care-focused health system separates prevention and treatment. Maintaining this separation in a reconfigured system that provides good care for chronic illnesses is simply impossible, given that essential principles of good chronic illness care incorporate prevention on many levels. That this traditional division between prevention and treatment cannot be maintained in a chronic illness care system may be a reason that implementing reforms and developing new programs for chronic illness care continues to be challenging.

A focus on prevention is important at all points in the trajectory of chronic conditions. Although preventing the onset or development of chronic conditions presents an opportunity to alleviate some of the burden they place on individuals, the health care system, and society, the heart of prevention in the context of chronic care is preventing exacerbations and the transition from disease to disability. The essence of effective management after the diagnosis of chronic diseases is preventing decline and disability. For those patients with advanced illnesses, health promotion is the means to prevent further functional decline and poor quality of life.

Although medications have become the most common mode of treatment, they can cause serious problems, in particular, for persons with chronic conditions, who typically take multiple prescribed and over-the-counter drugs. As a result, the prevention of adverse drug events must be included in any plans to reform health to address the needs of patients with chronic illnesses.

Prevention and chronic disease care not only overlap, they share a common problem. Both have difficulty demonstrating their effectiveness. In essence, the benefits of both are often reflected in nonevents. Good chronic care means that catastrophes do not occur. Prevention means just that, avoiding (adverse) events.

9. Paying for Chronic Care

The way we pay for care should reinforce the goals of that care. Several parties are involved in shaping the payment system to address chronic illness, and each party has its own agenda. They include the payers, the health plans, and the actual providers of care. However, the approach to paying for medical care has not been utilized primarily as a strategy to achieve preconceived ends. Reinforcing a social agenda, to say nothing of reforming a faulty health care infrastructure, has been a low priority.

Central tenets of chronic care include:

- Emphasis on illness episodes, not discrete encounters (or incidents)

- Active patient participation

- Active monitoring of a patient's clinical status

At a minimum, the payment system should not impose disincentives to pursuing them. Unfortunately, the current dominant approach to paying care providers does just that. The predominant payment approach is fee-for-service (FFS), which emphasizes individual encounters and pays for each separate billable service. The resulting gap between what we have (an encounter-based approach) and what is needed (an episode-based approach) could hardly be larger. Paying for encounters encourages more reimbursable (but not always necessary) services and less use of communications approaches that are harder to bill for. Paying for episodes rather than encounters would provide a means to encourage providers to make investments in patient management, monitoring, and education efforts that they might not otherwise make.

America's patchwork health care system leaves about 15% of the population without any health care coverage, and another large group with only partial coverage. Paying for chronic and other health care services for the 43.6 million uninsured Americans is a complex topic beyond the scope of this chapter. Here, we focus on the slightly less complex though still daunting challenge of paying for chronic care for the majority of Americans with some form of health insurance. Most of that insurance is managed by private firms, but the government also plays a significant role through the Medicare and Medicaid programs. Medicare, which serves primarily older persons, has a great stake in chronic illness.

183

TABLE 9.1.
Payment for Chronic Care

Level	Chronic Care Elements		
	Episodes vs. Incidents	Active Patient Involvement	Monitoring
Program	Medicare beneficiaries usually enrolled for life. Private health insurance enrollees may be enrolled for finite periods. However, Medicare beneficiaries can move in and out of MCOs more easily than private enrollees.	Could pay for such, but do not	Could pay for such, but do not
Plan	Fears that beneficiaries may leave before investment recouped. May use rewards or profiles to reward lower costs or less use of services	May contract separately for disease management	Folded into disease management but not coordinated with primary care
Provider	FFS emphasizes incidents, i.e., visits and services	Takes more time; paid on basis of in-person services/productivity; counseling may not be a specifically reimbursed service	Not usually covered, especially contact and communication not done in person

Payment for health care can be thought about at several levels. At the highest level are the basic programs that underwrite much of this care, such as Medicare and private health insurance. At the next level are the individual health plans or managed care organizations. Both plans and programs are ultimately implemented at a third level, by paying individual providers (i.e., hospitals, doctors, or clinics). Table 9.1 summarizes how the current system fails to adequately address chronic care at each level of payment. Based on insurance models, Medicare payments cover incidents of care. For both private health insurance programs and the Medicare program, reimbursement is targeted toward traditional clinical activities grounded in an acute care context. Essential components of chronic care, like employing strategies to increase active patient participation and continuous monitoring, are not reimbursable services. Health care plans may hesitate to make investments in chronic care if they fear that patients will leave when the next round of benefit negotiations causes employers to change their insurance carriers, that is, disenroll before the plans can recover their investments. Individual clinicians and medical groups are reluctant to deliver services that are not reimbursed.

Even a cursory examination of the current situation reveals that the payment system fails to support a chronic care delivery approach. Indeed, it presents major roadblocks and disincentives. Fee-for-service payments encourage activities that are reimbursable and especially those that pay well. The current fee-for-service payment scheme does not pay nearly as much for talking with patients as it does for doing things to them. It favors in-person visits over other means of communication. Actions, rather than outcomes, are rewarded. If the health care system is to change, so too must the payment system. Neither change will be easy. A great deal is invested in the status quo.

In the end, the ultimate limiting step is how we pay clinicians. Whether the money comes directly from public programs or indirectly through health plans, the payment message that the person or entity who is actually providing care receives will greatly influence what that provider does. It boils down to two basic choices: (1) pay the provider for specified services that reflect what is believed to be needed in good chronic care or (2) pay the provider some fixed amount to take responsibility for ensuring that good chronic care is provided (or tied to achieving defined objective outcomes), leaving the means to achieve this goal to the discretion of the provider. The former strategy requires clearly articulating which services under which circumstances are appropriate. The latter requires a method of accountability to ensure appropriate care is provided or the desired outcomes are achieved.

The way we pay for care and the way we think about care are closely linked. Much of our current medical care vocabulary is built around units of service. We talk about hospital stays, doctor visits, and emergency room visits. These familiar concepts have, in turn, shaped the way we view care. If payment does not shape provider behavior, it certainly reinforces it. A payment system that rewards individual services, for instance, will not encourage spending time on activities that are not reimbursed, even if those services result in substantial benefits in the future.

Paying Providers

Health care workers can be paid in various ways. Most physicians are paid for each unit of service they provide. In a fee-for-service payment system, they submit a bill for each service. The size of the fee may be set by prior contractual arrangement or it may be set by the provider; in either case it is a reward for a specific activity. The more activities performed (or the higher the payment for each activity), the greater is the reward. Such an approach fits well into an acute care delivery system, where each office visit, hospitalization, or health care intervention can be paid for as you go; however, it will not support the sort of approach to chronic illness care that was described earlier.

Some physicians are salaried employees of a medical care group, which may either hire them outright or may be a partnership of the physician employees. Most other medical workers are also paid salaries, although many have continually agitated for some form of fee-for-service payment. Those who do not bill directly for each service are monitored for productivity, using so-called relative value units (RVUs), whereby each activity is effectively assigned a dollar value. Here too, activities not covered by RVUs (often the very same ones not directly reimbursed) are not rewarded

Applying fee-for-service payments to chronic disease would involve paying for many vague services, such as counseling or tracking a patient's health status. Such payments are not without precedent. Psychotherapists are certainly paid to talk to patients. Routine checkups and monitoring visits are generally covered only when they are provided as part of a face-to-face encounter with a clinician. Expanding the scope of coverage to include expanded off-site versions of such services would likely contribute to a rise in medical costs, unless there was strong reason to believe that such care would ultimately lower costs by preventing expensive catastrophic care. The major question then is who is willing to bear this risk.

Although prospective payment systems seem more immediately conducive to the principles of chronic care, it is possible to harness fee-for-service payments in the cause. Just as managed care organizations have been willing to pay for disease management as a specific service, they could cover on a fee-for-service basis (perhaps with performance bonuses) specific actions such as monitoring and counseling, thereby encouraging such practices. (Indeed much of disease management is just such care.) As with disease management, new entities might spring up specifically to address these new lines of business. Primary care providers might find themselves reorganizing to cope with this competition. All these changes could create welcome new approaches to chronic care delivery.

However, it may prove difficult, and even undesirable, to make every act a basis for payment. Although the most direct way to change providers' behavior would be to pay for every increment of care, it may prove cumbersome to pay for each care element every time it is offered. It would be counterproductive to penalize those providers who find more efficient ways to deliver care or to achieve the same ends.

Institutions like hospitals and nursing homes are increasingly paid some form of preset, prospective rates, which may not necessarily correspond to the actual amount of care provided, but rather reflect an average level of expected care needs. This prospective payment approach was designed to eliminate temptations to increase payment by giving more care than was needed. But a payment system that pays a fixed amount can produce the opposite effect of a fee-for-service system. The incentive is now to provide as little care as necessary.

Whatever the particular payment arrangements, they all have a common focus on specific services. The payment system reinforces the concept of medical incidents, whether measured as doctor visits or hospital stays. The new prospective Medicare payments can be viewed as a step in the right direction. They provide a fixed amount to cover a bundle of services for a predetermined period. For example, in the case of the hospital diagnosis-related groups (DRGs), a set amount is paid for each hospital stay (illness episode) based on the patient's diagnosis, regardless of how long the patient stays or how many services he or she receives.[1] For home health care it covers a fixed period (60 days). For nursing homes, however, Medicare's payment is made for each day of care and more closely resembles FFS.

Some medical practitioners also accept bundled payments for an episode of care. For example, obstetricians are often paid a fixed amount that covers prenatal care, the delivery and some postdelivery follow-up visits. Surgeons' charges often cover pre- and postoperative care. Extending this approach to primary care would not represent too large a leap, but it would require defining areas of responsibility. For example, how would referrals be handled?

Insurers versus Providers

Although programs like Medicare and private insurance companies operate at different levels, and insurance companies can even contract with Medicare, the two operations face similar challenges. Whatever the insurer, be it a private company or a government agency, that organization must distribute funds to the providers of care.

The insurers and the providers of care (e.g., hospitals and doctors) have different financial goals. Whereas the providers want to achieve the greatest return for their individual efforts, the insurers want to minimize overall costs per enrollee. These costs are a function of two elements: the number of services provided and the price per service. Thus, one way to hold down costs is by reducing the volume of care.

The critical issue is the timeframe. It is easy to appreciate an immediate reduction in costs, but a delayed benefit may be more subtle. If a service today reduces the need for additional service in the future, it may be worth paying for, even if it costs more than a service that does not produce the latter saving. In addition to calculating the time-delayed pay-off rate, insurers who continuously enroll new and lose existing clients may reasonably worry that their investment will be lost if the clients do not remain enrolled long enough. With much private insurance linked to employment and employers continually shopping for better deals, the individual enrollee may no longer be able to enroll with a given insurance company, or the costs of that insurance may be higher than that of a competitor, who did not make the initial care investment. In either case, the savings that could result from the enrollees' reduced need for future services would not flow to the plan that incurred the expense.

Insurers may opt to bear the financial risk (and capture the benefits) themselves, or they may engage in some sort of risk sharing with the providers through a variety of payment arrangements. Many are based on fairly immediate results, but some may reflect thinking in terms of investments. In paying providers for each service, the insurers may employ strategies to reduce subsequent costs to themselves by using the fee structure to encourage certain provider behaviors. An example of an investment would be paying an extra fee for preventive services that they believe are beneficial, whereas an immediate offset would be paying a rate higher than costs for an outpatient service that could substitute for more expensive inpatient care. Insurers can create payment systems that link providers' payments to financial results (or financially linked outcomes like utilization). They can develop risk-sharing arrangements whereby the providers share some of the financial risks for future costs and derive some of the benefits from future savings. For example, they can pay bonuses if the total utilization at the end of a year is less than what was forecasted, or conversely they can hold back some portion of the provider payments to use as a hedge against cost overruns. They can pass on the risk altogether by paying the providers a fixed amount for all care to be provided over a defined period, leaving the providers to take the risk whether this amount will be adequate.

Each of these strategies has its strengths and weaknesses. Many require fairly extensive data systems to track provider behavior and outcomes. The more complex the approach, the less likely are clinicians to seek the incentives. Complicated formulas, which concatenate a variety of activities, are difficult to interpret and do not point clearly to desired behaviors. Most of the current payment incentives reward clinicians for accruing fewer costs, by reducing the use of laboratory tests and hospital admissions. In many respects it is easier to link rewards and penalties to utilization data than to outcomes.

Utilization-based incentives can come in two forms. The simplest is to concentrate on services such as laboratory tests and prescriptions. It is fairly easy to reward clinicians for ordering fewer (or less expensive) tests and drugs. The second level, which is more desirable but more causally complex because it is more indirect, involves utilization of emergency care and hospitals. Here, the rewards come from patients making fewer emergency room visits or being hospitalized less often. If it is hard to assess the effects of care on health per se, it may be feasible to show that good care reduces the use of services, especially those that are theoretically sensitive to such care. Clusters of so-called "ambulatory care sensitive conditions" have been identified (Billings, Anderson, & Newman, 1996). Admissions for these diagnoses are believed to represent hospital usage that might well have been avoided (at least on average) by more aggressive primary care. Examples of such conditions include chronic illnesses such as asthma and congestive heart failure.

In the past, most health care insurers were, in effect, financial conduits. They took in premiums and paid for care. If the payments exceeded the intake, they raised their rates accordingly. Over time these insurers were pressured to play a more active role in limiting costs (even though they ultimately benefited from these cost reductions). They began to exert more controls over how care was provided. They tried a variety of strategies, including requiring prior authorization for certain health care services, contracting only with providers who agreed to control costs and/or accepted a discounted payment for services, and limiting care to only those treatments deemed to be cost-effective or at least orthodox. A more direct approach to controlling costs was to financially reward those providers who used fewer ancillary services or prescribed fewer or generic medications. Ultimately, some insurers resorted to various forms of subcapitation, passing the risks directly on to the providers. To the extent that the insurance companies began to assume a direct role in controlling the costs of care they became managed care organizations.

Some managed care organizations (MCOs) have taken on chronic disease by contracting with external firms to carry out disease management initiatives (see chapter 4). In some cases, the payment to these firms reflects the extent to which utilization is reduced. However, because they do not have direct access to patients, and because patients may be seen by various clinicians and these clinicians may work with various insurers, some MCOs are forced to approach this task inefficiently. A common model is to contract with an independent disease management company that employs personnel (usually nurses) who contact beneficiaries identified from administrative data as having or being at high risk for developing a targeted chronic condition (usually on the basis of having specific diagnoses or a history of heavy utilization). These nurses use various strategies to educate and motivate the beneficiaries to take better care of themselves. They may give them advice. They may monitor the status of clinical parameters.

Contracting with an independent company has a major disadvantage; namely, it carves out care for the chronic condition and operates in parallel with basic primary care. The patients may receive conflicting suggestions and can become confused about whose advice to adopt. Although the disease management nurses will attempt to keep the primary care physicians updated on their patients' conditions, the physicians may resent this interference and fail to use the information effectively. Managing a patient with one chronic disease may be feasible under a separate system, but it becomes less tenable when the patient has several interactive problems. Simple protocols no longer apply. Actions taken on behalf of one problem may exacerbate another. For example, diuretics used to control blood pressure may complicate control of blood sugar. In that case, direct coordination with the primary care provider is critical.

A better approach would incorporate disease management into primary care rather than layering it on top. A barrier to using this strategy is the lack of participation of any single primary care clinician in a given insurance company's program. The average clinician works for several insurers. It would be cumbersome and inefficient for the clinician to set up multiple strategies to accommodate each insurer. If, however, disease management becomes standardized and routinely covered by all insurers, then practitioners might be motivated to establish such services for all their patients who needed them. Ironically, insurers seem willing to pay for disease management if it is contracted out, but they are less willing to cover such services if they are implemented at the level of clinical practice, where they might be even more effective.

As noted earlier, the government is an insurer. Programs like Medicare and Medicaid are health insurance programs that use tax money (and some premium money) to pay for the care of designated groups (i.e., the elderly and the poor). During the past four decades these federal insurance programs have attempted to transfer financial responsibility to private insurance organizations, such as managed care organizations. Rather than attempting to function as managed care organizations themselves, they opted to delegate that function to the private sector. This decision to use the private sector achieved several goals. It allowed the government to limit its obligations each year to a contracted amount and transferred the burden (and negative political fallout) of denying claims for care to another party. However, this transfer also meant that the government could no longer exert as much direct influence on the shape of health care. There are some indications that this position is changing. As described in chapter 4, Medicare is beginning to develop strategies that would allow it to recover savings from disease management efforts.

To the extent that the government represents the interests of the public, this loss of influence may prove significant. These government programs could be redesigned to encourage and reward good chronic care. Medicare is a national program with enormous potential to shape the way care is provided. It should foster greater attention to methods and practices conducive to such care Rather than looking for ways to disencumber itself, Medicare should use its buying power to lead the necessary reforms.

The Provider's Perspective

Health care providers, both clinicians and institutions, are accustomed to being paid for each service they provide. Their incomes are linked to staying busy. Perversely, the less effective is the care they deliver, the busier they can be with repeat trade. The present arrangement does not encourage real efficiency. Although much of what is currently done in physicians' offices could be done in less expensive venues (e.g., over the telephone or by computer), such an approach is not presently billable outside an office visit. For example, many return office visits to monitor chronic illnesses are not necessary, or at least they are not needed as often as they are scheduled. Some chronic illness might be better managed by regular monitoring phone calls or other distant communications, but the current billing approach rarely reimburses such contacts. Clinicians who implement such a strategy would be doubly penalized. They would be providing uncompensated care and they would forgo the income from the office visits that were displaced. At the same time, simply adding such services to the list of reimbursable services could be inflationary. A more radical change is needed.

Medical care could be paid for in some prospective manner, where the payment would cover all outpatient care (perhaps including emergency room care) for a defined period. The providers would then be left to distribute their efforts as they see fit. They might substitute other professionals for much of what has historically been performed by physicians. They might monitor more and see patients in person less. Under such an arrangement it might pay to keep a close watch on the clinical course of the patient's chronic illnesses and intervene at the first sign of a deterioration rather than schedule arbitrary return visit times.

However, implementing such a payment reform presents its own set of risks. The biggest risk in any prospective payment arrangement is always the threat of underservice. A better system of accountability would be necessary. At present, insurers have no way of assigning the responsibility of a patient's care to a given provider. The same patient may see many doctors and hence there is no single agent with whom the payer can contract for all medical care. Unlike in the United Kingdom (U.K.) and other countries, there is no designated primary provider through whom all care must be coordinated. However, the problem is not insoluble. Models point in the right direction.

Some managed care organizations have instituted variations of the gate-keeper model that imposes such a role by requiring that every patient designate a primary care physician who must authorize all other medical care (Hurley, Freund, & Gage, 1991; Kapur et al., 2000). Medicaid programs have experimented with paying physicians an additional case management fee to hold down the costs of care for clients with a record of high utilization. Under the basic primary care case management (PCCM) model, each Medicaid client is assigned to a primary care physician (PCP). The PCP provides or authorizes the client's primary, specialty, and hospital care. PCPs receive a monthly case management fee for each client, regardless of the amount of service they receive, plus the normal fee for each medical service they themselves provide (Smith, DesJardines, & Peterson, 2000).

One approach to getting plans to pay for interventions that reduce service fragmentation, that is, to help move the system from discrete patient/clinician encounters to episodes of care, uses capitation payments that are linked in some way to outcomes.[2] The capitation payments could be offered to providers. Instead of getting paid for what they do, the providers would receive a fixed amount per person in advance. By linking it to outcomes, the capitation payment could be used to focus attention on the end results, a major advantage because it is not feasible to monitor or observe all the details or processes. The details of such a payment structure remain a challenge, however. For example, should the program pay only for outcomes? Should it pay for services and track outcomes? Should it pay for some combination of process and outcomes, or employ some form of profit sharing? Any of these approaches can be done for one condition (i.e., construct a flat-rate payment for diabetics with add-ons), but it may be much more difficult to do this for patients with multiple conditions.

To be most useful, the capitation approach should be targeted at those who require more or different care. High-risk cases would be the best target, because higher payment rates would be justified and outcome differences would be greater. Eligibility criteria could be developed from data on diagnoses and disability.

However, covering new services could be inflationary unless they can be shown to ultimately reduce the need for other care. Monitoring patients with chronic conditions could be aligned with forgone office visits and a payment adjustment made to reflect such a change. Counseling raises more challenges. Just adding an additional fee for counseling will likely not work. It is hard to assess what constitutes a counseling session, or how many sessions are needed. Nonetheless, we have managed to wrestle with these service definition questions in mental health; they might be similarly addressed here. One approach would be to pay only those organizations that have demonstrated successful track records in achieving the desired behavior change. Such a strategy would move counseling out of primary care (if it was ever appropriately there in the first place) and establish it as a separate service.

Taking a more direct approach by moving away from FFS payment may have extreme political consequences. Providers are not likely to be happy with any efforts to dramatically reshape the way health care has been paid for and delivered. For a long time, they have done quite well financially with relatively few constraints on their actions. Although they express dissatisfaction about being inadequately paid, physicians as a group are financially secure and many specialties are very wealthy. Any moves to restructure what has been a basically comfortable and lucrative situation are not likely to be embraced.

Role of Managed Care

Managed care (and here we include Medicare and Medicaid) seems potentially more compatible with the premises of chronic care than does FFS (Kane, 1998). To the extent that managed care organizations (MCOs) can expect to retain their enrollees over the long term, they have a reason to invest in their enrollees' health. Because MCOs are responsible for people over time, they are more likely to think about episodes of care rather than incidents. Furthermore, because MCOs cover all care, the specific mode of care is less of an issue. Nontraditional services, if they work, are as valuable from the MCOs' perspective as the more familiar forms of care. Interactions (such as e-mail) that are not traditionally billable may prove very valuable and worth paying for in new ways.

A first step toward creating a more chronic-disease-oriented approach to care through managed care lies in aligning the health plans' incentives so that they promote desired goals in chronic illness care (e.g., improved outcomes, better integration and coordination of care). If plans determine that providing a specific type of service is in their long-term interest they can pay more for those specific care processes, such as preventive activities within an office visit, as done by the National Health Service in Britain. But the service has to be quantifiable. In principle, it is possible to reimburse for non-office-based services under a similar philosophy, but again such services must be financially justified (i.e., there must be evidence of their cost-effectiveness) and measurable. Chronic care services such as counseling and monitoring may fail one or both of these tests. It is hard to determine just how much counseling is effective. How does one distinguish just telling a patient to mend his/her errant ways from actually engaging with that person?

Despite the theoretical compatibility of managed care and good chronic disease management, the managed care industry has shown little inclination to establish expertise in the management of chronic illness. A major problem in encouraging MCOs to become active purveyors of chronic care is inadequate case mix adjustments in calculating the capitation rates. The term "case mix" is used to address the characteristics of clients that can affect the costs of care. A basic medical aphorism is that "every doctor treats the toughest cases." At present, MCOs do best when they enjoy favorable selection, that is, when they are paid the average cost for caring for healthier-than-average enrollees. They especially seek to avoid adverse selection, as would happen if they attracted chronically ill enrollees. Even allowing for hyperbole, however, there is a risk that those plans that become more skilled at treating persons with chronic conditions will attract a clientele that is sicker. It would be perverse to ask them to be paid at an average rate, which would represent less than the true costs. Imagine a plan that developed an approach to manage diabetes effectively (although it may be more expensive to do so). As word of this success spread, persons with diabetes would be attracted to the plan, but they have higher health costs on average than those without that disease. An average payment would penalize the plan that became effective in treating diabetics. Conversely, those plans that market to healthier clients should not be allowed to profit from that strategy by getting average costs. Setting rates fairly and accurately, however, is difficult.

The Medicare Advantage (formerly Medicare+Choice) program illustrates the perverse incentives to avoid enrollees with chronic conditions. Under Medicare Advantage, MCOs receive 95% of what is termed the adjusted average per capita cost (AAPCC). This payment calculation uses some simple demographic or administrative data (e.g., age, Medicaid status, nursing home residence) to adjust the average amount paid under Medicare's traditional FFS approach to create a payment. Partly in recognition of the disincentives the present model creates, this method of calculating the rate is being changed to incorporate data on each person's prior utilization. Under the original AAPCC system MCOs are much better off attracting healthy enrollees than sick ones. If they are paid at an average rate and can attract healthy customers, they will do well financially even if they do nothing different. The last thing they want to do is to attract a sick clientele. Adjusting the payment based on prior utilization history will help to remove this substantial disincentive.

However, the overall utilization pattern of almost every population is so skewed that even statistical adjustments are difficult. The upper 10% of care utilizers account for about 70% of all health expenditures. If one adjusts the rate to capture the risk of this heavy use, one runs the risk of paying too much overall. If payments target the rest of the utilization curve, the model tends to dramatically underpay for those high users. It remains to be seen whether the new AAPCC payment calculations, which include adjustments for both prior usage and diagnoses, will suffice to induce MCOs to become more predisposed to developing expertise in chronic disease care. The problem of such risk adjustment is complicated because, although prior utilization is an important risk factor, it by no means distinguishes those at risk of heavy utilization in the subsequent year.

Medicare Advantage MCOs face another disincentive to support chronic care. Because the Medicare program allows beneficiaries to disenroll at any time, the MCOs worry that beneficiaries may incur the front-end costs under their responsibility but then disenroll, causing the MCO to forfeit its investment. If there is a substantial time lag between the investment of resources (e.g., in prevention programs or better care) and the payoff (e.g., reduced utilization/hospitalizations), the MCO incurring the cost may not be the one that realizes the benefit; the enrollee who participated in the prevention program may have left the plan. In general, the incentives for Medicare and for private plans (MCOs) are largely the same, although the timeline is different. The problem is exacerbated for Medicare Advantage, where beneficiaries may disenroll at any time in contrast to the mandatory year-long enrollment in the private sector. Some sort of lock-in provision, at least to extend enrollment to the same annual basis used in other health insurance, may help to assuage some of these fears. It may not be enough to encourage long-term investments in counseling or behavior changes, but it could support short-term payoffs like more aggressive monitoring of patients' clinical status.

The problem of transient enrollees, however, affects private plans (including Medicare Advantage MCOs) more than the overall Medicare program. Once a person is in Medicare, he or she will stay in. The problem with changing health plans, which plagues private firms, does not apply. Even though beneficiaries may move in and out of managed care, they remain the ultimate responsibility of the Medicare program.

Medicare has opted to emphasize managed care as a means to control its costs, but it could also behave like a large MCO itself. The very same strategies proposed for MCOs could be used, perhaps through some sort of contracted intermediaries. Medicare could direct care at a regional level to avoid the problems of a single national bureaucracy. There are already precedents for Medicare to contract out the administrative aspects of the program to private insurance companies. Indeed, the arguments against adverse selection would not hold, because Medicare is virtually universal.

Summary

Paying for care should reinforce the goals of that care. Paying for chronic care should encourage an emphasis on episodes of care and active efforts to monitor patients' status. These ends can be accomplished under the traditional fee-for-service payment system but they will require special administrative steps. These new payment structures can encourage new forms of care provision for many of the newer tasks. Alternatively, primary care payments can be changed to move toward some merged form that combines aspects of capitation with prospective payment. Such an approach would have the advantage of maintaining the centrality of primary care, a prominent component in delivering high-quality chronic care.

PART III

Prospects for Change

10. The Context for Reform

The chronic disease revolution is a quiet protest more than a revolution. Although patients regularly bemoan the care they receive, they have not taken to the streets with demands to behead the current system. Sages and philosophers wax eloquent about the need to change the way care is given (Berwick, 2002; Institute of Medicine, 2001; Wagner, Austin, & Von Korff, 1996a), but progress is glacial.

In general, the debate over health care in the United States has continually rotated around three axes: cost, quality, and access. The 1960s can be seen as the period when access was of greatest concern, leading to the passage of both Medicare and Medicaid. Since that time the emphasis has shifted toward cost, although there have been sporadic bursts of concern over the plight of people without health insurance. Maintaining and improving the quality of care has come to the fore only in the past few years and, although the focus has primarily been on problems caused by medical errors (Kohn, Corrigan, & Donaldson, 2000), there is at least some sensitivity to the more pervasive implications of having a health care system that fails to address the most prevalent problems. The series of reports from the Institute of Medicine's initiative on quality improvement has been especially helpful in linking quality with failures to provide adequate chronic care.[1] Until these reports, however, little attention had been directed toward the fundamental infrastructure underlying chronic illness care.

As part of the IOM's initiative, the Committee on Identifying Priority Areas for Quality Improvement has identified 20 specific topics for quality improvement (Adams & Corrigan, 2003).

- Asthma
- Children with special health care needs
- End-of-life care with advanced organ system failure
- Frailty associated with old age
- Immunization (child and adult)
- Major depression

- Care coordination
- Diabetes
- Evidence-based cancer screening
- Hypertension
- Ischemic heart disease
- Medication management

- Nosocomial infections
- Pain control for advanced cancer
- Self-management/health literacy
- Stroke

- Obesity
- Pregnancy and childbirth
- Severe and persistent mental illness
- Tobacco-dependence treatment in adults

Many of these topics align closely with chronic illness management. The federal government is also preparing to issue a National Healthcare Quality Report modeled after the Healthy People reports that set objectives for improving the health of the nation. Last, the Medicare Modernization Act of 2003 includes a large-scale demonstration project to improve chronic care under Medicare's traditional fee-for-service program (see exhibit 4.1).

Despite the potential shift in health care reform efforts that these recent events portend, the various reforms proposed or enacted during the past four decades typically have accepted as given that the core function of our health care system was to diagnose and treat patients with acute conditions. The reforms did not seek to alter this core function but were aimed instead toward resolving various cost, access, or quality concerns to help the system provide acute care services more effectively and efficiently. In contrast, improving the care for patients with chronic conditions by addressing the deficiencies in the system reviewed in the preceding chapters has been consistently overlooked. Even today, health care reform policy discussions still seem preoccupied with how to pay for medical care, seemingly without questioning just what kind of care we are buying. Infrastructure reforms take a back seat to financing. A brief review of major health care policy reforms illustrates the range of issues addressed and health care reform strategies adopted in the United States and how these reforms have failed to address chronic illness care.

Public Sector Initiatives

Federal policies and programs, such as Medicare and Medicaid, have historically had the greatest influence over America's health care system. Medicare was established in 1965 as a social health insurance program for the elderly and was modeled after the private health insurance system at that time. Its primary goal was to provide elderly Americans with financial access to health care services. Medicare is now the largest federal health insurance program, covering about 40 million Americans. Beneficiaries include about 34 million persons age 65 years and older, about 5 million people of all ages who are permanently disabled, and 300,000 people with permanent kidney failure.[2]

Medicare was initially designed to provide health insurance coverage for acute illness (Iglehart, 1999). Notwithstanding several noteworthy but relatively minor additions, including home health care and hospice care, Medicare's covered benefits have changed little since 1965.[3] Still, as a result of these minor benefit changes and, more importantly, the aging cohort of beneficiaries and the numerous new technologies and other advances in health care that treat but do not cure, the majority of Medicare expenditures now pay for services for people with chronic health conditions. Almost 80% of Medicare beneficiaries have at least one chronic condition and they account for nearly 79% of the program's expenditures (Berenson & Horvath, 2003). Nevertheless, the underlying structure of Medicare has not changed and it remains a program that emphasizes acute care services. Precisely because the program continues to reflect indemnity insurance coverage and benefit principles, Medicare "is poorly positioned to improve service delivery for patients with chronic conditions" (Berenson & Horvath, 2003). The extent to which the three-year chronic care improvement demonstration initiative, scheduled to go into effect by early 2005, will reorient the Medicare program remains to be seen (see exhibit 4.1).

Medicaid, also enacted in 1965, is a public health insurance program that covers basic health and long-term care services for three groups of low-income people: parents and children, the elderly, and the disabled. About half of Medicaid's 51 million enrollees are children, but they account for fewer than 20% of Medicaid dollars spent. Disabled beneficiaries younger than 65 years of age account for an estimated 40–43% of all Medicaid expenditures, and elderly beneficiaries account for an additional estimated 27–30% (Iglehart, 2003). A significant portion of these expenditures is for long-term care (mostly nursing home care). The remaining balance goes to low-income adults who are neither disabled nor elderly. Though its covered benefits include many non-acute care services, Medicaid, like Medicare, accepts the health care system's core function as a given and is not designed to shift the system's focus away from acute care. By and large, long-term care has traditionally been separate from and rarely integrated with acute care. The Medicaid program has not sought to change this situation, even though it is the single largest payer of long-term care services.

Unlike Medicare and Medicaid, which were enacted primarily to expand access, reforms in the 1970s and 1980s were mostly designed to curtail increases in health care costs. For example, the Federal HMO Act of 1973, passed in response to a sustained period of health care cost inflation, established the legal framework and provided financial incentives for the establishment of health maintenance organizations (HMOs), the prototype for managed care organizations. Though the legislation's immediate impact was relatively minor, it put in place the foundation for managed care, the then relatively untried alternative way to pay for and deliver health care services that now dominates America's health care system. In the mid-1980s, Medicare adopted a new reimbursement system for hospitals to contain rising Medicare costs. Under the "diagnostic related group" or DRG system, hospitals are paid based on patients' average expected use of health care services rather than for actual services used. This shift in payments from piecemeal or fee-for-service reimbursement to a fixed or capitated prospective fee has since been adopted in other areas of our health care system, including many nonhospital settings. Like the access-oriented reforms before them, however, these cost containment reforms made no attempt to shift the health care system's principal focus away from acute conditions and acute care.

Private Sector Initiatives

Following the failure of President Clinton's health care reform initiative in the early 1990s to provide universal health insurance (Johnson & Broder, 1996), the momentum for health care reform has shifted to the private sector. Shortly thereafter, large employers took the lead in pressing for change in the financing and delivery of health care. The result was a rapid expansion of managed care, believed by many to be capable of delivering cost-efficient, high-quality health care. "Managed care" was originally defined with reference to organizations, such as health maintenance organizations, or HMOs, that integrated the financing of health care with the provision of care. Today, however, "managed care" is a much broader term and is most often used to refer to "a set of techniques used to influence the delivery of health services to a defined population" (i.e., the enrollees of a health plan) (Christianson et al., 2001). Such techniques, typically designed to ensure the quality and efficiency of health care, include, for example, various financial incentives to influence provider behavior, utilization review and management, health promotion and patient education, and restricted panels of health care providers. The enthusiasm for these strategies seems to be waning (Robinson, 2001).

By 2001, the majority of insured Americans were enrolled in a managed care organization (MCO) of one form or another, including HMOs and preferred provider organizations (PPOs). Traditional indemnity insurers, such as Aetna, Cigna, and the Blue Cross and Blue Shield plans, have also adopted many of the managed care techniques pioneered by the MCOs. Consequently, managed care is now the norm in the United States, covering 93% of all those who receive health insurance coverage through a plan sponsored by an employer (Dudley & Luft, 2001).

Although managed care has the potential to markedly improve the care for people with chronic illness by, for example, "developing comprehensive, integrated systems capable of providing health care that is both more effective and less costly than today's fragmented fee-for-service care" (Boult, Boult, & Pacala, 1998), the managed-care-dominated health care system has largely failed to capitalize on that potential. Despite numerous disease management and other programs within managed care organizations designed to expand the range of services and better integrate and coordinate care for people with chronic conditions, the organizations themselves, like the health care system, in general, remain oriented to providing acute care for urgent problems. The dominant view is that "managed care has failed to catalyze fundamental changes in how health care is delivered" (Grumbach & Bodenheimer, 2002).

Chronic Care Reform: Missing in Action

Health care reform in America has generally been reactive. The pattern has been to respond to one "crisis" or another in cost, access, or quality. Most often policy initiatives address the most pressing concern of the moment, which is sometimes an unforeseen consequence of a previous initiative. But, as this review illustrates, the core focus of these reform initiatives has always been on acute conditions and the acute care system. Any effort to target chronic conditions or to shape, modify, or direct chronic illness care has been conspicuously absent throughout the entire four decades of health care reform.

Given the prevalence of chronic conditions in the U.S. population, the cost of care for persons with such conditions, and the noneconomic burdens of such conditions for patients and their families, improving chronic illness care must now become the number one priority for health care reform. The time is right for refocusing our health care system on chronic illness. After several years of relatively low health care cost inflation, the cost of health care began to climb rapidly again in the late 1990s (Levit et al., 2003; Strunk, Ginsberg, & Gabel, 2002). Problems in access to health care, often a consequence of increases in health care costs, are escalating as well. By 2002, the number of Americans without health insurance had climbed to 43.6 million, eroding access to needed health care services. These cost and access problems have helped to once more place health care reform near the top of the national policy agenda, creating an opportunity to redirect our health care system toward chronic illness care.

Too often in the past, similar opportunities have been missed. For example, the National Bipartisan Commission on the Future of Medicare, the latest and most ambitious in a long series of efforts to reform the Medicare program, disbanded in early 1999 without reaching agreement on any reform proposal.[4] Moreover, its deliberations and proposed recommendations, like those of earlier efforts, focused only on the program's financing and avoided the difficult decisions, such as changes to the program's covered benefits and its overall structure, that would have been needed to refocus Medicare on chronic illness care. The Commission's cursory approach thus mirrored past health care reform initiatives by avoiding the real issues at stake.

Similarly, since the mid-1990s, much of the Congressional effort to reform private sector health insurance was dominated by the debate over various versions of a so-called Patients' Bill of Rights. The central concern behind the competing versions (none of which have been enacted into law) was the fear that some of the strategies used by managed care organizations (MCOs) to control health care costs may harm patients by, for example, denying them needed care. Though the details vary, the consensus remedies included provisions such as giving enrollees more opportunity to challenge treatment denials, assuring access to emergency care, expanding access to out-of-network specialists, and allowing enrollees to continue to receive care from a provider who has left the MCO. Aside from the fact that the only patients the various versions of the Bill of Rights were designed to protect were those fortunate enough to already have insurance, these legislative initiatives failed to the same extent as the Medicare Commission in addressing the fundamental issue, namely, the need to reorient the health care system to improve the care for people with chronic conditions.

When reorienting the system toward chronic care, the diversity among groups of consumers should not be overlooked. Major disparities exist in health status among racial/ethnic, age, and socioeconomic groups. Some of these are fostered by coverage policies, which affect access to care. But others involve risk factors related to both genetics and behaviors. Policies designed to improve chronic care may not work equally well across all these groups. Discretionary (or out-of-pocket) spending, for example, affects the poor much harder than the rich. Moreover, as the nation's population grows ever more diverse, the criteria for what constitutes good care will likely change. Different subgroups may look for different key attributes. Approaches crafted to meet the expectations of white middle class consumers may not be embraced by those from other cultures.

Failure to place chronic illness care at the forefront of health care policy reform will likely mean that policymakers will once again respond to the current crisis only by shifting costs among various stakeholders while ignoring the need for more fundamental systemic changes. Such changes demand that our health care system is finally brought into line with the population's chronic care needs. A transformation of our health care system is needed; minor changes at the margins of the current system are not enough. Whereas acute care will always be necessary (even chronic conditions have acute episodes), the health care system must now fully embrace the concept of caring for long-term health problems (World Health Organization, 2002). This can only be accomplished through a fundamental shift from a health care system concentrating on acute conditions to a system that gives chronic illness care top priority.

Barriers to Reform

We already know a great deal about what needs to be done to implement the changes in health care delivery that would facilitate chronic illness care, but we have generally failed to take the appropriate actions. Why? Several factors come readily to mind. These include financial issues, such as misaligned and perverse incentives, which lead to the failure to invest sufficient resources in changing the infrastructure. This reluctance can be traced to the lack of a business case for chronic care. Those in a position to make changes are not yet convinced that the investment is financially justified (Coye, 2001; Leatherman et al., 2003). Nor is chronic care a priority for key stakeholders, such as medical education leaders and professional organizations. By contrast, most would view the acute care model as a stunning success. What discontent there is currently focuses on cost and medical error rates (Kohn, Corrigan, & Donaldson, 2000). Not surprising then is the lack of consumer demand. Medical care consumers are generally still uninformed and unaware of what is possible. A general sense of inertia exists. Despite its relentless growth, health care overall is a conservative industry, and medicine is a conservative profession. Change happens slowly.

There is no groundswell of demand for reform. The media occasionally offer an expose but do little to raise public awareness about the extent of the problem or the potential solutions. (See Appendix A.) Although people complain individually, they fail to act collectively. Nor has chronic care become a political rallying point.

The most obvious barrier to changing the health care system is the difficulty in changing the mindset of an industry that has done quite well (on a number of levels) by following the traditional path of acute care. Health care is a big and profitable business. Generations of practitioners have been trained to deliver this sort of care. They view it as the heart of their professional practice. They have absorbed its culture and its tenets almost unconsciously. They equate them with how to practice their craft. Convincing them to undergo a major change in their modus operandi is no easy task. Indeed, the burden of proof is likely greater on those who advocate major change than on those who continue to work within the dominant framework.

Making a strong case for a shift in practice style will require powerful evidence of effectiveness, to say nothing of efficiency. We celebrate our new commitment to evidence-based medicine, but alas our knowledge base is incomplete: We know some things, but many questions are still unanswered. We have only fragments of the mosaic, individual studies that point to the benefits of improving aspects of care, but there is no major body of evidence that can conclusively demonstrate the benefits of making such a change. Instead, like most revolutions, the heart of the argument is based on an appeal to logic, driven by epidemiological data and bolstered by theory. The appeal has been made to believers, who can accept the logic of the arguments and are willing to undertake the interventions that form the advance wave of this social change. As a result, the movement, as such, is growing but still fragmented. The banner has been taken up by some leaders in some large organized practices, but the underlying situation is not yet ripe for major reorganization.

At the same time, more work is needed to develop the infrastructure and tools needed to facilitate this practice transition, but such developmental work has not been high on the research-funding agenda. A few private foundations, notably the Robert Wood Johnson Foundation, have made substantial commitments to chronic illness care, but their projects have been more directed to stimulating change than to creating an infrastructure. There is no sign that the federal government has made chronic care a priority for research funding. Admittedly, given the ubiquity of chronic conditions, the various institutes within the National Institutes of Health (NIH) are funding chronic disease research, but little of this enormous resource is directed specifically at creating the tools that will be needed to support the necessary changes in practice delivery. Instead, far more effort is directed at finding ways to treat (or some would still claim "cure") specific diseases than in testing how to organize chronic care better.

The difficulties in bringing about a fundamental change in the American health care system should be viewed in the context of making more discrete changes in medical practice. There is a long line of only limited successes in introducing best practices. The efforts to introduce the pronouncements of the NIH consensus documents designed to change clinicians' practice patterns were largely unsuccessful (Kosecoff et al., 1987). More recent efforts to induce practitioners to follow guidelines have encountered similar resistance (Grimshaw & Russell, 1993; Grimshaw et al., 2001; Gross et al.,

2001; J. Lomas et al., 1989; J. Lomas, Enkin, & Anderson, 1991; J. Lomas, Sisk, & Stocking, 1993; Woolf et al., 1999).

Another influence noted earlier is money. Health care in the United States is a big business. Much of the large incomes derived from it are directed at providing technologically intense acute care. At the same time, chronic care represents an enormous market opportunity. Developing more efficient ways to deliver such care could readily become a major business opportunity. However, a heavy demand for such products does not yet exist. Major stakeholders, including health care providers and health plans, have approached chronic care more by avoidance than by active engagement. However, some segments of the industry have seized this opportunity, particularly the medical device companies. For instance, Medtronic, a leading medical technology company, defines itself as a chronic care company. By contrast, the provider community has shown little enthusiasm for chronic care.

One might expect a strong consumer demand for better chronic care, with migration of patients to those practitioners and organizations that can demonstrate (or at least promise) improved outcomes for people with chronic conditions. But such a demand has not yet arisen. In part, consumers may not be aware of the art of the possible. Although they may be discontented with the existing system and regularly bemoan the care they receive, they may view the status quo as inevitable. They may have strong attachments to their current medical practitioners and be reluctant to consider a shift without a strong belief that such a transfer is worth the discontinuity. There certainly has been no direct-to-consumer advertising to raise awareness about what good chronic care might look like in any way comparable with what the drug industry has undertaken to market its products. Nor have the media played a substantial role in describing either the problem or the potential solutions. As a result, consumers remain largely uninformed.

The current deficiencies in chronic illness care can in large measure be blamed on the failure to create a compelling chronic care mythology. In contrast to acute care, there is no strong belief in the efficacy of chronic care. There is no strong sense that such an investment has the potential to pay large dividends in terms of physical or social benefit. Whereas society seems very willing to invest vast resources in pursuing interventions that offer, at best, only marginal benefits in areas like oncology and neurosurgery, it is far less interested in making even modest investments in chronic care. A belief system has grown up around acute care services that suggests that even if the likelihood of benefit is small, it is nonetheless worth the investment. Much like buying a lottery ticket, people seem willing to bet against the odds if the payoff is large enough. In truth, the acute care system reflects the "rule of rescue"—a socially valuable (but economically inefficient) tenet that leads us to expend enormous resources to rescue someone in peril when there is any chance, however small, of success.

By contrast, chronic care is seen as an investment that can yield only modest effects, if any. Although it has the capacity to make major contributions to improving both clinical outcomes and quality of life and lowering medical costs, these benefits are harder to recognize. As noted earlier, the test of chronic care's success becomes largely evident only when it can be contrasted to other care or to no care at all. Unlike acute care, where the patient's clinical course may make a dramatic recovery, the general pattern for chronic care is much more subtle, and hence much harder to sell. Chronic care requires investments at several levels. Not only must organizations create new infrastructures, with new equipment and new roles, operationalizing chronic care programs implies spending more resources up front in expectation of later savings.

Given the lack of market demand and associated costs, it is not surprising that few medical organizations—neither physician groups nor managed care organizations—have sought to develop a reputation for expertise in this area. Indeed, managed care faces a real disincentive to establish such a reputation in the current funding climate. In the absence of adequate case mix adjustment methods, becoming known as an organization that is proficient in managing chronic illness threatens to attract the very enrollees the MCOs seek to avoid, namely those with complex (and typically more costly) problems. Put another way, there is no strong business case for MCOs to pursue chronic care (Coye, 2002). A reputation for better quality in this area is not likely to be financially rewarding. The availability of sophisticated technology to treat medical emergencies is more likely to attract business.

Nonetheless, given the epidemiological realities, MCOs find themselves with a growing number of enrollees who do have chronic illnesses. However reluctantly, they will be forced to confront this growing group and to adopt techniques to address their needs more effectively.

These techniques will include both approaches that overlay new forms of care coordination onto extant practice and more integrative efforts to change the basic way care is provided. The choice of strategy will depend on opportunity and belief. Given the relationship between enrollees and MCOs, and because most MCOs work with large numbers of physicians, each of whom may have only a few enrollees of a given MCO, the MCOs have a hard time exerting direct influence on physicians' practice. For the same reasons, many of the MCOs' efforts to reach their enrollees through the physicians will fail because the physicians are unlikely to change their practice patterns for the small subset of their patients belonging to a given MCO. Although it may be preferable to use techniques that integrate clinical care and patient management, it is hard for MCOs to achieve sufficient influence over individual practitioners or groups if these providers can contract with a variety of MCOs.

A similar situation pertains in the United Kingdom, where the National Health Service (NHS) has moved to a new organization, which resembles many aspects of managed care without the profit-making incentives. Perhaps because it is more centralized, the NHS has overtly adopted chronic disease management as part of its fundamental reform strategy. It may prove feasible to implement some of the failed programs of the United States in this U.K. environment. (Appendix B describes some of the programs being tested in the United Kingdom.)

Motivating individual practitioners will require financial incentives, or at least the elimination of disincentives. Clinicians constantly complain about not being paid for elements of the work that they do, even if their overall compensation is reasonable. It is not totally clear that the payment system must reward every aspect of good chronic care practice, but at a minimum it must align the incentives with the goal of pursuing the activities that comprise good chronic care. It certainly cannot penalize practitioners for doing the right things. So long as clinicians make more money from cutting off a gangrenous diabetic foot than they make providing the best diabetes care, optimal diabetes care will be more wish than reality. Ideally the basis for payment will shift from the current emphasis on incidents to some form of payment that recognizes episodes of care, thereby allowing clinicians more leeway in how they manage their time and what activities they pursue.

Clinicians will be more likely to consider adopting chronic disease practices if they have access to tools that can simplify the task and increase their sense of empowerment to manage such cases. The availability of tools thus has a twofold effect. To the extent that these tools can structure practice and focus clinicians' attention on salient elements of care, they will change the way such care is provided. Simply making available a tool that is believed to be effective may also, by itself, help to change the beliefs about the value of chronic illness care and, hence, to reshape its mythology.

Some time ago investigators showed that people develop strong negative feelings about strangers they feel impotent to help (Lerner & Simmons, 1966). In the context of medical care, clinicians who view chronic illness as an overwhelming burden that has little likelihood of improvement despite one's best efforts may develop negative feelings toward the very patients who need their assistance most. Providing these clinicians with tools, even minimally effective tools, may give them a sufficient sense of empowerment to overcome and reverse these negative feelings toward their patients.

Necessary Steps

The first step toward implementing more effective chronic care is to create a demand for such care. Several routes might work. Consumer demand could become a strong motivator, but first consumers need to be educated about the art of the possible and the benefits of good chronic care. At present, consumers may recognize the limitations and frustrations of the current system but they do not appreciate how it could be improved. This educational role could be played by the media, or by some combination of the media and public health education. We have informational campaigns about various diseases. Why not use a similar strategy for chronic disease in general, since many of these diseases share similar management challenges? The media must be convinced that endemic health problems are newsworthy. The media's role will have to extend beyond the traditional news media to include the equivalent of an advertising campaign. It will take at least as much repetition to get across even an awareness of the ubiquity and threat of chronic disease, let alone any real behavior change in response to this danger, as is required to get consumers familiar with brand names. Nonconventional approaches can be tapped, including making chronic illness care a popular talk show topic.

Health care professionals need their own education. They need to be shown that something can be done to improve chronic care. They need to be taught simple behaviors that can empower them. Health care professional schools must take up the challenge to develop innovative approaches for providing health care professional students with the essential skills and competencies for effective chronic illness care. There must also be an economic benefit for providers to justify the necessary investment.

As the largest payer for health care for the elderly, Medicare must realize that it is in the chronic care business. It must realign its payments and incentive structure to encourage proactive primary care. If managed care is to fulfill its potential to improve chronic care, such care must be made profitable. Changes in the way the capitation rate is constructed must be introduced. These changes need to make it financially attractive to undertake chronic illness care. Ideally, they should be developed in such a way as to maximize the flexibility of how such care is delivered. At the same time, managed care organizations need to be held accountable for how well they provide chronic care and rewarded for doing it well. Although some of the current criteria developed by the National Committee for Quality Assurance under its Health Plan/Employer Data and Information Set, or HEDIS, program address chronic illnesses, they do not sufficiently address issues that reflect good chronic care management.

A similar emphasis of good chronic care management needs to be established for physician groups. As with other elements of care, information on the track records in achieving health outcome goals needs to be made publicly available to facilitate informed consumer choice. Although it is preferable to base these reports on outcomes information, it may be more feasible to begin by acknowledging physician groups that are at least taking steps toward developing the requisite competence. Acknowledging special training in chronic care, or even a certified commitment to chronic care management principles, may be worthwhile in the beginning.

Both the professional and lay communities must be convinced that an investment in better chronic care is worthwhile. To the extent that a new information infrastructure can accomplish this task, a source for technological development must be created. At present there are only a few sources to support the development of information tools for chronic disease. But there is no Institute for Chronic Care at the NIH, for example. The Agency for Healthcare Research and Quality has not established chronic care as a priority, and it certainly has not identified information support technology in that way. Only a few private foundations have taken up this cause. Private entrepreneurs may underwrite some development in this area in expectation of tapping a growing market, but some sustained support will likely be needed to move the field forward fast enough to prompt the level of experimentation and testing that will be needed to create the necessary sense of potential accomplishment.

11. Next Steps

The contemporary health care system is tragically incompatible with the needs of the predominant nature of disease problems today. The system is organized around a crisis-oriented acute model of care—emphasizing prompt and speedy diagnosis, treatment, and cure—that fails to address the long-term management needs of people with chronic conditions. The result is a mismatch between health problems and health care. Demographic changes will exacerbate this mismatch, compounding the urgency for refocusing the health care system to better meet the needs of people with chronic conditions. The nation's population is aging. The number of people with chronic conditions is rising. By 2020, a projected 157 million Americans, or nearly 50% of the total population, will have at least one chronic condition and about 81 million (25% of the population) will have multiple chronic conditions (Wolff, Starfield, & Anderson, 2002). The number of older adults in the United States with arthritis or chronic joint symptoms—already the leading cause of disability in the United States—is expected to double by 2030. America's population is also projected to become much more diverse, as the rate of growth among minority groups, who experience more problems in accessing health care services (Zuvekas & Taliaferro, 2003), continues to exceed the rate of growth in the total population. As a result, the patient population in the future will be more difficult to treat. Many individuals and organizations have issued a clarion call for reorganizing the current system, to align it better with the realities of chronic illness (Institute of Medicine, 2001; Martin et al., 2004; Wagner, Austin, & Von Korff, 1996b; World Health Organization, 2002). Progress, however, has been agonizingly slow.

The problem lies not so much in a lack of knowledge about what to do as in a failure to vigorously pursue techniques that have great promise. It seems obvious that we cannot continue on the way we are headed. Fortunately, models already exist for tackling the challenge for improving chronic illness care. They at least point the way.

Report Card on IOM Recommendations

One way to gauge the rate of progress in reforming the health care system toward chronic care is to revisit the landmark work of the Institute of Medicine's Committee on Quality of Health Care in America, which has been widely credited with refocusing the nation's attention on the deficiencies in the quality of our current system. Problems linked to quality fall most heavily on people with chronic conditions, who use a disproportionate share of health care services. In its second major report, *Crossing the Quality Chasm*, the Committee offered a roadmap for improving health care quality and safety through system change (Institute of Medicine, 2001). The Committee's roadmap includes a "set of simple rules to guide the redesign of the nation's health care system" for improved performance. The first steps in this redesigning, according to the Committee, should focus on systemic changes to improve care processes for a limited number of "common conditions that afflict many people and account for the majority of health care services." As the Committee notes, "nearly all of these conditions are chronic."

The Committee's "set of simple rules" thus forms the framework for a health care system fundamentally designed to better meet the needs of people with chronic conditions. Such a system must "serve the needs of patients, and . . . ensure that they are fully informed, retain control and participate in care delivery whenever possible, and receive care that is respectful of their values and preferences." It must also "facilitate the application of scientific knowledge to practice, and provide clinicians with the tools and supports necessary to deliver evidence-based care consistently and safely." Table 11.1 displays the Committee's 10 rules, which were developed to help private and public purchasers, health care organizations, clinicians, and patients to work together to redesign health care processes, in the format of a report card on how our health care system currently measures up, more than three years after the rules were issued (Institute of Medicine, 2001).

Tools to more rapidly implement these 10 rules are readily available in most instances. Clinical knowledge to effectively manage many chronic conditions now exists. For example, information exists on which lifestyle changes and health care interventions can reduce the risk of onset or complications of diabetes. New patient care technologies allow close monitoring and tight regulation of blood glucose levels. Advances in clinical knowledge and technologies have improved the care for other chronic conditions as well. Furthermore, studies across patients with different chronic conditions have identified fundamental components for a new system for chronic illness care. These components include disease management and other improved processes for care, more and better use of information technology, expanded roles for patient self-management, revised financial incentives, more and better trained health care professionals with new roles and responsibilities, and a renewed emphasis on prevention. These components comprise the "building blocks" that can be used to reorganize the health care system to more effectively respond to chronic conditions.

TABLE 11.1
Chronic Care Report Card

Rule	Grade	Comments
1. *Care based on continuous healing relationships.* Patients should receive care whenever they need it and in many forms, not just in face-to-face visits. This rule implies that the health care system should be responsive at all times (24 hours a day, every day) and that access to care should be provided over the Internet, by telephone, and by other means in addition to face-to-face visits.	C	Use of e-mail, the Internet, and other alternatives to face-to-face visits are slowly increasing. Some clinicians and patients remain wary of these alternatives. Concerns include confidentiality, liability, and timeliness. Reimbursement barriers remain.
2. *Customization based on patient needs and values.* The system of care should be designed to meet the most common types of needs but have the capability to respond to individual patient choices and preferences.	D	Any customization occurs only at the level of individual providers and patients. Some customization is reflected in the use of specialty clinics. Little is done on a systems level to encourage discussion and accommodation of patients' needs and values.
3. *The patient as the source of control.* Patients should be given the necessary information and the opportunity to exercise the degree of control they choose over health care decision that affect them. The health care system should be able to accommodate differences in patient preferences and encourage shared decision making.	D–	System's fragmentation and lack of coordination interferes with greater patient control over health care decisions. Although more patients are finding information from external sources, the health care system does not help them locate or evaluate it in a systematic way. Shared decision making between patients and clinicians is still more an ideal than a reality.
4. *Shared knowledge and the free flow of information.* Patients should have unfettered access to their own medical information and to clinical knowledge. Clinicians and patients should communicate effectively and share information.	C	Although HIPPA expands patients' access to their own medical information, its enactment (April 2003) is too recent to assess its impact. So far it seems to be fettering the free flow of information and hindering care.
5. *Evidence-based decision making.* Patients should receive care based on the best available scientific knowledge. Care should not vary illogically from clinician to clinician or from place to place.	D	The practice of evidence-based medicine is still in its infancy, hampered both by the lack of strong evidence in some instances and the failure to adopt best practices when such evidence exists. Substantial practice variations remain.
6. *Safety as a system property.* Patients should be safe from injury caused by the health care system. Reducing risk and ensuring safety require greater attention to systems that help prevent and mitigate errors.	C–	Despite unprecedented focus on medical errors, relatively few systemic changes have been implemented and the error rates remain high. Clinicians and patients believe the cause of errors lies with people, not systems.

TABLE 11.1
continued

Rule	Grade	Comments
7. *The need for transparency.* The health care system should make information available to patients and their families that allows them to make informed decisions when selecting a health plan, hospital, or clinical practice, or when choosing among alternative treatments. This should include information describing the system's performance on safety, evidence-based practice, and patient satisfaction.	D	Information about the health care system, including "report cards" on health plans, hospitals, nursing homes, and other health care organizations, is more readily available. But poor data, inconsistent criteria, and lack of objectivity often undercut its usefulness for patients.
8. *Anticipating needs.* The health care system should anticipate patient needs, rather than simply reacting to events.	F	System's core remains a reactive acute care model rather than a proactive chronic care model. Most care is in response to crisis or deterioration rather than focusing on preventing decline. Anticipatory management implies a willingness to invest in care; such willingness is rare under the current payment system.
9. *Continuous decrease in waste.* The health care system should not waste resources or patient time.	B–	Many efforts to reduce waste, primarily as a cost-saving measure. Any additional savings from waste reduction will be small. Efforts to improve satisfaction have included reducing wait times.
10. *Cooperation among clinicians.* Clinicians and institutions should actively collaborate and communicate to ensure an appropriate exchange of information and coordination of care.	C–	True collaboration among clinicians across practices and organizations remains rare. Limited use of information technologies in health care continue to make communication difficult.

Despite the growing body of clinical knowledge about the care and management of chronic conditions and the range of proven building blocks for reconfiguring the system, there is still no consensus on how to combine these tools into coherent and effective programs for improving chronic illness care. Prescriptions for improving chronic care differ in their emphasis on a narrowly focused condition-specific model, on the one hand, and more generic approaches, on the other. Much of the success to date in improving chronic care has relied on addressing individual chronic conditions, even specific points in the condition's natural history. A more generic approach is needed to make more headway. Research suggests that programs using a variety of approaches simultaneously are more likely to achieve substantial change (Casalino et al., 2003).

Models for Reform

Several organizations have successfully adopted a broader approach, focusing on the common elements that cut across more narrowly targeted strategies. One example is the Chronic Care Model, developed by researchers at the MacColl Institute for Healthcare Innovation at the Group Health Cooperative in Seattle. This model "identifies the essential elements of a system that encourages high-quality chronic disease management" and has been implemented by other health care organizations and used in a range of settings and for a variety of chronic conditions.[1] Other examples include the Geriatric Collaborative Practice Model, a comprehensive and integrated program for managing elderly adults with chronic conditions at the Carle Health Care System in Urbana, Illinois, and the range of chronic care programs and initiatives pursued by Kaiser Permanente. The Comprehensive Health Enhancement Support System (CHESS), developed by researchers at the University of Wisconsin, is an electronic system of integrated services, providing information, social support, and decision-making and problem-solving tools, designed to enhance chronic illness care. These models combine, in various configurations, the components of optimal chronic illness care discussed in this book. They provide a template for the shape of future care.

The "Chronic Care Model"

Edward Wagner and his colleagues at the Group Health Cooperative in Seattle, Washington, developed the Chronic Care Model (CCM)[2] in the early 1990s (Wagner, Austin, & Von Korff, 1996a). The CCM provides a framework for a multidimensional solution using what is known about promising strategies for improving chronic illness care. The model is not explanatory in nature; instead, it represents an organizational approach to care and is intended as a guide for activities to improve the quality and management of chronic illness care. It emphasizes the need for a multifaceted/multilevel approach. The model emphasizes health system leadership; regular, planned patient visits; instant access by clinicians to the latest evidence-based guidelines for care; use of information technology that tracks patients' health status; goal setting and self-management by patients; and involvement of community resources to keep patients well, involved, and active. Each element is interdependent: to ensure success, all must be aligned.

The Chronic Care Model (shown in fig. 11.1), which continues to be refined to reflect advances in the care of people with chronic conditions, employs a global strategy for improving care at the community, health care system, practice, and patient levels. The overall goal of strategies at each of these levels is to "foster productive interactions between patients who take an active part in their care and providers backed up by resources and expertise." More productive interactions between patients and provider teams are facilitated through coordinated changes in the model's six components. Specific strategies for change include:

- Self-management support: Empower and prepare patients to manage their health and health care.

  Emphasize patients' central role in managing their health.

  Use effective self-management support strategies that include assessment, goal setting, action planning, problem solving, and follow-up.

  Organize internal and community resources to provide ongoing self-management support to patients.

- Delivery system design: Assure the delivery of effective, efficient clinical care and self-management support.

  Define roles and distribute tasks among team members.

  Use planned interactions to support evidence-based care.

  Provide clinical case management services for patients with complex conditions.

  Ensure regular follow-up by the care team.

  Give care that patients understand and that fits with their cultural background.

- Decision support: Promote clinical care that is consistent with scientific evidence and patient preferences.

  Embed evidence-based guidelines in daily clinical practice.

  Integrate specialist expertise and primary care.

  Use proven provider education methods.

  Share evidence-based guidelines and information with patients to encourage their participation.

- Clinical information system: Organize patient and population data to facilitate efficient and effective care.

  Provide timely reminders for providers and patients.

  Identify relevant subpopulations for proactive care.

  Facilitate individual patient care planning.

  Share information with patients and providers to coordinate care.

  Monitor performance of practice team and care system.

- Health care organization: Create a culture, organization, and mechanisms that promote safe, high-quality care.

  Visibly support improvement at all levels of the organization, beginning with the senior leader.

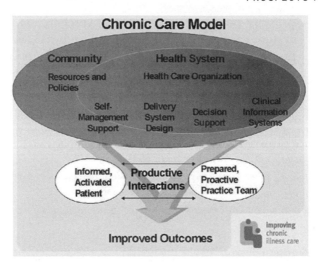

FIGURE 11.1.

The chronic care model.

Wagner, 1998; reprinted with permission from the American College of Physicians.

Promote effective improvement strategies aimed at comprehensive system change.

Encourage open and systematic handling of errors and quality problems to improve care.

Provide incentives based on quality of care.

Develop agreements that facilitate care coordination within and across organizations.

- Community: Mobilize community resources to meet needs of patients.

Encourage patients to participate in effective community programs.

Form partnerships with community organizations to support and develop interventions that fill gaps in needed services.

Advocate for policies to improve patient care.[3]

To date, several hundred health care organizations have adopted the Chronic Care Model as a guide to improving chronic illness care (Rothman & Wagner, 2003).[4] In 2002, the Rand Corporation initiated a four-year evaluation of the use of the Chronic Care Model in practice.[5]

Geriatric Collaborative Practice Model (Carle Clinic)

A multifaceted care management model to support care for patients with chronic diseases has been created and implemented at the Carle Healthcare

System in Urbana, Illinois. The Carle Healthcare System first developed and implemented its Geriatric Collaborative Practice Model[6] in 1998. It has since continually refined the model and in 2001, Carle was selected as one of 16 national sites for the Medicare Coordinated Care Demonstration (MCCD), a multiyear study of a range of programs aimed at chronically ill Medicare beneficiaries. The MCCD will assess the effectiveness of these programs on clinical outcomes, patient satisfaction, quality of life, and appropriate use and cost of Medicare-covered services.[7]

The Carle Healthcare System's Geriatric Collaborative Practice Model is an "integrated intervention system" designed to have an impact on mortality, preventive health practices, rates of health status and functional decline, hospitalizations, hospital bed days, total cost of care, patient satisfaction, and patient involvement in their health care. The Carle Healthcare System expanded the Geriatric Collaborative Practice Model for the MCCD to include the following eight components:

1. Collaborative Care Model. A collaborative team is led by a primary care physician (PCP) and includes a Nurse Partner (RN), who provides case management, and a Clinical Nurse Partner Specialist (an advanced practice nurse), who works with more acute needs (e.g., recently discharged patients and those with acute exacerbations). A Case Assistant provides patient monitoring, service arrangement, and office management. The Collaborative Care Model includes enhanced collaborative working relationships with and among physician specialists, hospital service providers, home and community care providers, and others working with the Collaborative Care Team to focus on (1) processes of care; (2) patient/family preparation for transitions in care settings and provider changes; (3) communication with and among providers across settings; (4) educational needs; and (5) self-management/self-efficacy skills. The Collaborative Care Team's responsibilities include:

• Conducting a standardized, comprehensive, joint (PCP/Nurse Partner) assessment with the patient/family to determine needs and resources

• Developing a mutually agreed upon plan of care based on disease management guidelines with the patient/family that ensures appropriate, high-quality, cost-efficient care

• Coordinating the sequence and types of care with the patient/family, health care providers, community agencies, and other supportive services

• Monitoring and evaluating the patient's progress within the guidelines and across the continuum of care

- Ensuring active patient/family decision making

- Enhancing patient self-management and coordination skill sets

- Ensuring patient and provider satisfaction

2. Research Guidelines. Guidelines to assist the clinicians and patients in making decisions about appropriate health care for specific clinical circumstances have been developed for each targeted chronic condition. The guidelines synthesize and incorporate national guidelines and clinical research. The degree of compliance with the guidelines is at the provider's discretion, in light of circumstances presented by the individual patient.

3. Education and Training. Coordinated education activities target physicians, nurse partners and case assistants, and patients and families. Education is geared toward use of the Research Guidelines and to assist patients and their families to participate in managing their chronic conditions, among other goals.

4. Supportive Care Services. These services, including homemaker, adult day care, respite care, and transportation, are offered on a selected basis to prevent avoidable, costly medical complications. Supportive care services are capped at $300 per year.

5. Pharmaceutical Consult Services. Services provided by pharmacists include review of medication regimes (e.g., for potential drug-drug interactions) for all patients with five or more drugs or by request.

6. Care Management Information and Clinical Alert System. This information system is a secure Web-based program that combines patient sociodemographic and clinical information into a comprehensive relational database. It includes the patient's initial assessment questionnaire, laboratory and x-ray results, medications, diagnoses, problems, signs/symptoms, interventions, activities, and contacts. The system is used to identify patients who need special assistance and higher levels of monitoring. It includes e-mail notification to the patient's Nurse Partner of any major use of health care services; an inpatient case coordinator and social service referral system; referrals to appropriate members of the Coordinated Care Team; and patient tracking, monitoring, and reporting.

7. Outcome Reporting. Reports at the patient-specific level, provider panel level, and population levels are generated at regular intervals. The reports include information on patient demographics; the clinical status of MCCD enrollees; contacts and interventions performed by Nurse Partners and Case Assistants with patient and panel; and emergency department and hospitalizations with nurse case manager's contacts prior to, during, and after

hospitalization. Reports support both clinical decision making and population-based interventions.

8. Health Care Management Committees (HCMC). A variety of HCMCs have been established at various organizational levels (e.g., clinical, administrative) within the structure of the program and the health care delivery system to facilitate and support communication and decision making for the program.

Kaiser Permanente

Kaiser Permanente (KP),[8] a group model, prepaid integrated delivery system, operates in eight states and the District of Columbia. Kaiser Health Plan (the insurer arm of KP) has exclusive arrangements with regional Permanente Medical Groups (the physician arm of KP) throughout the country to provide care for 8.4 million members. In California, Hawaii, and Oregon KP owns and operates hospital-based medical centers, which typically have their own home health care and hospice agencies. In other states KP contracts for all or many of these services. This structure provides a climate of aligned incentives, supports the physician/patient relationship, emphasizes primary and secondary prevention, and encourages measurement of clinical and process outcomes.

Kaiser Permanente has been developing and implementing strategies to accelerate improvement in the care of older adults and people with chronic diseases. These include targeting populations at risk, providing better coordination of existing resources and services, and altering basic traditional system characteristics and structure. Faced with increasing numbers of older members (880,000 members over 65 years of age and 68,000 over 85 years of age) and members with chronic diseases, KP is investing in new approaches to care and in the technological infrastructure required to support clinicians in their efforts to provide care that is evidence based and will improve outcomes for its members. KP's approach is to complement local efforts by identifying high-impact, systemwide opportunities for improved outcomes for specific conditions and populations.

Model of Care for Elders. About 15 years ago, KP leadership endorsed a conceptual model for population-based care of older adult members. Here, the population was defined not by a disease but by age. The model recognized the diversity of health and function in older adults and acknowledged the need to stratify older adults based on these characteristics, evaluate their needs, and then follow up with care ranging from immunization to ongoing care coordination. A project in Hawaii, for instance, placed social workers in primary care physicians' offices to assist them in assessing older adults and linking them to community and other needed KP services. Despite some increase in costs, the program continues today because of member satisfaction and physician perception that the social worker adds value as a member of the primary care team.

Variations of this model have been implemented in other parts of KP. A Colorado program, the Cooperative Care Clinic, has primary care physicians and their office teams meet monthly with groups of high-demand patients from their practices for the purpose of health education and promotion, as well as to draw on the group's collective experience in solving practical health care problems. The physician also sees patients individually during this time to address individual medical needs. This group care model has reduced overall cost, improved the delivery of preventive services, and raised physician and patient satisfaction (Scott et al., 2004). There are currently 40 ongoing cooperative clinics in Colorado, but the approach has not diffused widely throughout KP. The most commonly cited obstacles to dissemination include lack of meeting space and failure to allocate resources for support staff for coordinating the clinics and for ongoing physician training.

Team-Based Care. The "teaming" in team-based care is often virtual, without the traditional team meeting to review and discuss cases. One exception is in KP's approach to skilled nursing facility care, which uses physician/nurse practitioner teams to serve members who are long-term nursing home residents. Physicians' practices in these programs work exclusively with nursing home, hospice, and home health care patients. In a study of the primary care of nursing home residents in managed care and fee-for-service, all three managed care programs in the study utilized physician and nurse practitioner teams, but only KP used dedicated teams. All managed care programs provided more visits than fee-for-service, but KP was the only managed care site that demonstrated significantly fewer hospital admissions, emergency department visits, and a trend for better follow-up care after a reported fall or onset of a fever.

Community-Based Care. A 1997 geriatric initiative by KP turned outward toward families and community service organizations, establishing formal linkages and partnerships with local Alzheimer's Association chapters to ensure that the families of patients with dementia received an assessment and were reliably connected with the association. Several sites obtained patient or caregiver permission to fax referrals to the Alzheimer's Association rather than simply providing an 800 number. This resulted is a significant increase in contacts between patients/caregivers and the association.

Population Care Management. Also in 1997, Kaiser established a programwide Care Management Institute (CMI). CMI's mandate is to drive, fund, and catalyze care management activities within KP. Its express purpose is to improve the quality of care and health outcomes for members by creating, implementing, and evaluating effective and efficient care management programs. CMI has identified several priority diseases and populations, including asthma, diabetes, cardiovascular disease, depression, and elder care. Elder care areas of focus have included dementia, screening and follow-up action, high-risk medications, transitional and skilled nursing facility care, and the care of people with advanced, life-limiting illness. CMI annually conducts National Outcomes Studies in each of its clinical priority areas. Outcomes are typically process or "biological" indicators, but CMI also conducts quality-of-life surveys for people with diabetes and asthma.

CMI supports regional implementation of guidelines tailored at the local level by funding a network of CMI physician implementation managers, implementation specialists, and analysts in each KP region. An unanticipated outcome of CMI's elder care work was the formation of a new entity, the KP Aging Network (KPAN). KPAN is made up of clinicians and business leaders who are stakeholders in the care of older adults. KPAN has accountability for leveraging its national position to create, implement, and evaluate effective and efficient strategies and programs for KP's older adult membership. KPAN is working with stakeholders to set standards, empower local providers, and inform through the development of pilots.

CMI's Accomplishments. Most of CMI's work focuses on improving KP's performance in managing selected chronic diseases. For example, in 1998, a program for patients with coronary artery disease (CAD) was designed to improve all three areas of lipid management. By 2001, 80% of CAD patients had lipid screening (up from 66%), known low-density lipoprotein (LDL) control increased to 48% (up from 32.6%), and one-year post-myocardial infarction (post-MI) use of beta-blockers increased to 78% (from 62%).

What led to improved adherence to recommendations for care? Because developing and promulgating evidence-based guidelines have little impact by themselves, CMI has funded additional activities to support "making the right thing the easiest thing to do." It is working to assure that KP clinicians have advanced information technology tools so they can provide improved care. These tools include the use of laboratory and pharmacy databases along with population and disease registries for identifying populations, targeting interventions, and performance improvement measurement. There is an ongoing, programwide effort to decrease the use of high-risk medications such as long-acting benzodiazepines in older adults. Regional efforts have ranged from eliminating medications from local formularies to electronic alerts at point of service to prompt clinicians about prescribing appropriate medications, ordering needed tests, and following up when indicated.

CMI is playing an important role in building the evidence-based clinical content for KP's current initiative to implement a programwide electronic health record (EHR). One of the more powerful aspects of the EHR is its ability to provide decision support. For example, clinicians can use "Smartsets" that guide them in the diagnostic process and in treatment decisions by using best available evidence or strong clinician consensus. Alerts and prompts remind clinicians to consider recommended actions such as using a beta-blocker or discontinuing a high-risk medication. CMI issues an annual report that documents regional progress in decreasing the use of drugs that should be avoided in older adults. Another potential of the EHR is its ability to more easily measure processes considered indicators of quality care of geriatric syndromes, for example, incontinence, falls, and dementia. The EHR will allow for easier measurement of these quality indicators as well as outcomes at both patient and population levels.

Comprehensive Health Enhancement Support System (CHESS)

The Comprehensive Health Enhancement Support System (CHESS)[9] is a computer-based, interactive health communication system designed to improve health care for persons with selected chronic conditions. David Gustafson and his colleagues at the University of Wisconsin developed this computer support system in response to their research indicating that people facing a health crisis "often had difficulty finding good information about their condition, were hesitant or unable to attend support group meetings, and were being pressed to make and implement difficult decisions before they had adequate information, support and personal confidence about what decision might be best for them."

CHESS uses new computer tools to provide patients with chronic conditions and their families 14 distinct services in four categories: (1) present explicit health care information in a variety of ways; (2) provide human and emotional support; (3) offer help in making and implementing difficult decisions; and (4) provide skills training to promote more active and motivated patients. The CHESS program is designed to promote positive health behaviors and to enable individuals and families to "cope more effectively with their crisis, suffer less, and feel like they'd made better decisions as a result of using CHESS." The program's strength, relative to other information tools and the Internet itself, is that CHESS "provides a closed, guided universe of information and support options in an integrated package where everything points efficiently to everything else," insulating program participants from what can be lengthy, unfocused, and ultimately unproductive searches for relevant information, services, and support (Gustafson et al., 2002).

According to its Web site, CHESS "combines the best features of computers and human support" by:

- Providing timely, easily accessible resources (information, social support, decision-making and problem-solving tools) when needed most

- Combining various services and resources into one system, meeting the needs of various coping and information-seeking styles, and making use more likely and rewarding

- Tailoring and personalizing information and support to help users better manage their health and change behaviors that are harmful to their well-being

- Protecting privacy, encouraging openness and honesty in dealing with health concerns

- Presenting reliable, well-organized, detailed health information in language that is comprehensible to people at most educational levels

CHESS was initially a software-based program, installed on participants' personal computers. The program is now converting from software to the Internet, which allows information to be added and updated more easily and provides "carefully selected" links to some of the rapidly expanding base of health information on the Internet. Participants can access the program from their own home, by connecting to the Internet or using the software installed on their computer. For participants who do not have a computer, the CHESS program provides one on loan for up to a year. In addition, the CHESS program has been installed in computers in public settings, including community centers, health care centers, college dormitories, and the workplace.

CHESS has a limited number of condition-specific programs, or "modules," for persons with selected chronic conditions, such as breast cancer, asthma, and heart disease. CHESS also has a special module for caregivers of persons with memory disorders (e.g., dementia).

Computer-based peer support networks are a key component for advancing the CHESS program's goal of empowering patients. The program uses online bulletin board style "discussion groups" for families and patients to share information and support. This enables chronically ill patients to derive useful support from their peers. Additional online services allow CHESS users to share their personal stories about how they cope with the chronic conditions and provide them "a private place where [they] write their deepest thoughts and feelings about [their condition] in a timed, controlled environment" (Gustafson et al., 2002). Reflecting the program's "closed, guided universe" structure, participation in all of these online services is limited to CHESS participants.

CHESS is currently being used by several major health care organizations in the United States and Canada. Use of CHESS has been shown to:

- Improve patients' quality of life,

- Reduce demands on physician time,

- Reduce the cost of care in some cases, and

- Be used equally, although in different ways, by all types of people, including women, older people, low-income people, people with less education, and minorities.

Essential Issues for Chronic Care Reform

Although the puzzle is by no means complete, we now have most of the pieces. With information from recent advances in clinical knowledge for managing chronic conditions, the range of proven strategies and interventions for improving the structure and process for delivering chronic care, and the successful models for broad, comprehensive chronic care programs reviewed here, we know enough to reorganize chronic illness care. Exhibit 11.1 presents one clinician's view on how what we know about improving chronic illness care can be integrated into physician practices of the future.

Looking beyond physician practices to the health care system more broadly, a number of issues and developments will shape efforts at chronic care reform, regardless of the ultimate pace and direction of change. Some of these, including the quickening pace of advancements in information technology and the relentless efforts to contain health care costs, will affect the entire health care system; others, such as new or more expansive family support policies, will more narrowly influence chronic illness care.

EXHIBIT 11.1

A Clinician's Vision of the Future of Chronic Care

Future practices will be expected to manage the health care of patients more completely and efficiently than has been possible in the past. More of our new practices will be larger and have the infrastructure, staffing patterns, and experience to manage defined populations, report quality and efficiency indicators regularly, coordinate inpatient, outpatient, and telephonic care; and experiment with new models of management for patients with chronic illness while emphasizing prevention and health promotion at every opportunity. These practice and professional competencies will be a routine part of all future practices.

Knowing the illness burden of a defined population is the first step toward "managing" health and health care resources. How many patients have diabetes, hypertension, chronic lung disease, depression, and osteoarthritis? Who has all or several of these conditions? Which patients are seen most often? Are those visits improving measurable health outcomes? Which provider best manages all of that in collaboration with the patient, nurses, pharmacists, other health care professionals, and the patient's family? Who among all the people served is fully immunized? Which nurses can help with telephone-based educational "visits" adapted to the patient's learning style and "readiness for change?"

Practices will track the health-related interactions for this defined population to evaluate patterns that indicate a mismatch of needs versus care experiences of each patient. For example, does one frequently seen patient really understand his chronic medications? Is another satisfied with her care? Does she know that her physician and provider team actually understand and care about her? Are group visits more suited for this patient? Which community-based patient activation groups would be suitable for another patient? Is the practice properly "connected" to patient-led diabetes groups or asthma groups? Are frequent visits a sign of trouble for a subgroup of patients versus about right for managing their complex treatment plans? How do others on the multiprofessional care team know about this treatment plan? Practices will knowingly select phone contact from the nurse or health educator versus an actual office visit and will be paid for either.

Provider patterns of practice will be reviewed routinely. Those patterns will be tracked via electronic charting systems capable of showing individual and group data regarding pharmacy use, frequency of visits for common conditions, guideline "adherence," expense per patient visit, costs per patient visit and overall annual costs, rate of use of laboratory and diagnostic imaging, and patient satisfaction. These data will be available on a Web site for providers to review confidentially. Outcomes improvement teams will meet via virtual e-mail discussions as well as brief face-to-face meetings to address the most realistic path toward continually improved care.

Integrated medical and behavioral care teams will provide medical and behavioral health care and education. Therapists, psychologists, psychiatric nurses, case managers, and a few psychiatrists will have offices within the "medical" office environment to manage most common problems. Treatment of the more complex psychiatric issues will involve the patient seeing mental health team members in areas designed specifically for such long-term management.

The complexity of achieving the practice just described will add to the cost of care for some conditions. However, successful practices will find ways to improve care while lowering the net cost of overall care. Time- and dollar-efficient phone "visits" for minor illnesses will be about 30% of practice volume *and* income. Reimbursement barriers to this sensible and safe care will be overcome. The time gained will be used to manage medically complex and chronic problems. E-mail exchanges for medication refills, scheduling follow-up tests, obtaining feedback about new treatments, and just "checking in with the doctor" will be routine and included within the payment schedules. Patients and physicians will use mutually accessible Web sites to stay current. The time gained will be spent more actively teaching patients self-management skills, establishing rapport with new patients, and supervising other health care providers on the patient's team.

Hazardous transitions from clinic to hospital and hospital to home will be managed in an improved manner via team meetings, tele- and video-conferencing, and face-to-face sessions with providers, patients, and families. Reducing medical errors will involve a greater degree of teamwork and improved information exchange across boundaries among primary and specialty care, pharmacy, behavioral and medical care, and physician / nursing care. The practice of the future will move closer to meeting our expectations for "error-free care" at a cost shared by patients, health plans, and government. Providers and patients will be more satisfied with our future highly competent practices.

Macaran Baird, M.D., University of Minnesota

New Definitions

In the world of chronic care familiar terms assume new meanings. Prevention focuses less on avoiding conditions than on managing their consequences. This position does not mean that efforts to reduce risks should be abandoned. Immunizations, efforts to reduce smoking and the like should continue, but the emphasis shifts to providing better primary care in an effort to avoid functional catastrophes. Good care should reduce the rate of hospitalizations and emergency visits, which are clinically devastating and economically costly, by preventing exacerbations of the underlying conditions. The most preventable problems are iatrogenic. Overmedication or inappropriate medication may produce untoward consequences.

Patients' roles must change. They must become active partners in their care. The idea of presenting passively to the clinician for examination and instruction will no longer suffice. Patients are the only ones who experience chronic diseases 24 hours a day, seven days a week. They are in the best position to observe and report changes in their condition.

Patients must become actively involved in making decisions that will affect the courses of their lives. To make these decisions, they will need good information about the consequences of alternatives. They will need help in structuring the stages and components of these decisions and in sorting out just which outcomes they want to maximize. Once patients become joint decision makers, they must also be prepared to share the responsibility for the consequences of those decisions.

As monitors of their clinical conditions, patients will need structured tools to determine what to observe and how to communicate it. They will need to be taught how to recognize significant changes in their health status. They will need to have appropriate access to the health care professionals to provide this feedback. In some cases, this may simply mean a way to summarize the observations at the time of the next encounter. At other times it will mean knowing how to get access to the system in an emergency, or how to initiate a contact before the next scheduled one.

As the name implies, time plays a different role in chronic illness care. Chronic illness pays little attention to the artificial conventions of encounters. It continues regardless. Hence, the idea of assigning arbitrary dates for revisits seems anachronistic. Such appointments are based on some best guess about the patient's future clinical status. It makes more sense to use the actual clinical course as a guide. Patients who continue on their expected course need to be seen less frequently, but those who deteriorate more rapidly than expected need to be seen sooner.

Likewise, at a time when clinical encounters are brief, it no longer makes sense to expect that each encounter should be of equal length. Less time is needed with those who are staying on track, leaving longer visits for those whose clinical condition needs to be reevaluated. Much of the contact time with the former group can be given over to other personnel, leaving physicians free to concentrate more on those who need more attention.

Another implication of time is the payoff horizon for care investments. Under current payment schemes there is little incentive to provide intensive services at one point in the expectation that this investment will pay clinical dividends in the future. For example, the principles of geriatric evaluation and management are based on the evidence that spending substantial effort at one point in time will prevent later use of expensive hospital and nursing home care (Stuck et al., 1993).

The roles of health care workers need to be reassessed in the light of chronic illness care. There is growing evidence that nurse practitioners can perform many of the functions traditionally played by primary care physicians (Mundinger, 1994; Mundinger et al., 2000). At a time when the supply of primary care physicians is dwindling and the need for such people is increasing, some substitution seems imperative (Cooper, Laud, & Dietrich, 1998). Likewise, when nurses are also in short supply (Bednash, 2000), many nursing tasks can be performed by lesser trained personnel.

A question arises about who is best equipped to provide primary care for persons with chronic illnesses. In many cases all that is needed is competent primary care skills combined with an ability to remain aware of the impact of several simultaneous conditions, but in other cases the underlying nature of the dominant condition may make attention from a specialist paramount. However, many specialists are reluctant to move far from their organ system. A promising compromise may be to pair the specialist with a nurse practitioner. The former can treat the organ and the latter can attend to the person.

New Approaches

Expectations must change under the aegis of chronic disease. The concept of cure must yield to the emphasis on management to prevent exacerbations. Success must be redefined to recognize that the most frequent clinical course involves decline over time. Good care consists of slowing the rate of that decline, but such an achievement is invisible unless there is some way to capture the expected clinical course in the absence of that good care. Thus, the key to evaluating chronic care is comparing the actual with the expected course. As was shown in figure 1.1, the benefits reflected in the shaded area would not be apparent unless there was a means to display the expected course.

Clinical protocols, based on well-validated studies, may prove useful in managing some aspects of chronic disease, but much of this care involves working with several diseases simultaneously. Protocols work best when they can address a single predictable event. In those cases, such as care pathways for surgical recovery, they are extremely helpful to both practitioners and patients and their families. Armed with such clinical pathways, consumers know more about what to expect.

A variation on the concept of the clinical guideline or protocol is the clinical glidepath (Kane, Ouslander, & Abrass, 2003). This approach is based on the assumption that most practitioners will know what to do if they are aware of the problems. The clinical glidepath is similar to the information systems used to land an airplane. These devices tell the pilot when he or she is drifting out of the preplanned trajectory that will produce a smooth landing. They allow for minor course corrections to avoid major disturbances. Likewise, in clinical practice, by defining a limited number of salient clinical parameters for each chronic condition, monitoring them over time, and comparing the observed findings with the predicted clinical course, the clinician can determine when a patient is drifting off his clinical glidepath and intervene quickly to prevent unwanted exacerbations. Patients can collect and transmit most of the clinical observations needed to fuel the clinical glidepaths, giving them an active role in their own care.

New strategies to improve chronic disease care are already being tested. Many approaches fall under the general rubric of disease management. These approaches are usually layered onto existing care. Additional personnel, usually nurses, contact the patients to be sure that they are following their clinical regimens (Naylor et al., 1999). Some of these strategies are directed at specific populations, like patients with congestive heart failure discharged from hospital (Rich et al., 1995); others include everyone with a given diagnosis.

At the other end of the continuum are strategies designed to encourage patients to take a more active role in their own care through self-care (Lorig et al., 1999). Patients are taught both skills and ways to increase their sense of self-confidence and empowerment. A middle strategy seeks to create more effective partnerships between patients and their clinicians, enabling each to play amore effective role in the care process, but to do so in coordination.

Improving Linkages between Acute and Long-term Care

The vast extent of long-term care is linked to chronic disease. Effective long-term care (LTC) must rely on coordinating medical and social care. Historically, LTC has been torn between the so-called medical and social models of care. The medical model is usually depicted as focused on achieving some set of clinical goals, whereas the social model is more prone to addressing supportive measures that meet assessed needs. This conflict is unproductive. The first step in maximizing coordination is developing a set of shared goals. Collaboration and discussion among all parties are necessary to develop these mutual goals, which should reflect elements of both approaches.

In many systems, the payment for LTC is administered separately from that of acute care, impairing potential coordination. Merged payment may facilitate coordination, but it will not ensure it. More fundamental changes in practice patterns are needed. Case management may help to coordinate care, but it can also simply add another level of bureaucracy, unless it plays a proactive, hands-on role.

An important principle of LTC (and indeed of all chronic care) is the need to recognize the distinction between site of service and the nature of the services provided. Too often care is defined by where it is provided. Thus, home care is seen as an entity distinct from nursing home care. In truth, especially given the evolution of technology, the same patients can be served equally well in various locations. Patient-centered care should never be defined by the location of that care. Freed of that limitation, we can develop new packages of care that combine medical and social elements more creatively.

An overarching theme that must be constantly borne in mind when assessing old or new approaches to LTC is the need to focus on outcomes over process. Outcomes should be defined in terms of the contrast between observed and expected results.

Accountability

There is already a call for greater accountability in health care. To date most of the attention has been focused on looking at those issues that can be studied most readily. Recently, medical error rates and compliance with guidelines have been the predominant foci. With time the search will widen to include those conditions that affect the majority of patients in significant ways, namely chronic diseases and their management. The rate of this shift will depend in part on how quickly strong empirical evidence is developed to demonstrate which strategies are associated with the best outcomes. As health care organizations are held to a higher level of responsibility, they will be expected to open up the many "black boxes" of health care decision making. Patients and other recipients of health care services, but still more so, employers and other payers, will increasingly expect or even require health care organizations to report on what they do, explain their decisions, and justify their actions. For example, health plans and other organizations that make reimbursement decisions on whether to pay for new technologies to treat chronic conditions will be expected to make those decisions more visible and to provide rationales for their decisions.

Employers and other payers want assurance that they are getting "value" for their health care dollars and will ask for data to support providers' claim that they are providing high-quality care. This may promote the development of agreed-on ways to define and measure effective chronic care management. A model for such initiatives is the Health Plan/Employer Data and Information Set, or HEDIS, currently the most widely used measure of health plan performance. HEDIS was designed jointly by managed care plans and purchasers (i.e., large employers) to help assess the quality of the care being delivered and to encourage improvement. It contains a standardized performance measurement data set of 71 items in eight areas, such as use of services and patient satisfaction, to measure health plan quality.[10] Thus far, most of these have addressed fairly easy-to-measure items, which require minimal or no case mix adjustment, but the tide is turning. HEDIS items already address some chronic illnesses, such as congestive heart failure.

More managed care organizations and other health care insurers will inevitably shift toward paying health care providers on the basis of outcomes, putting the power of financial incentives behind their efforts to improve the quality of care. Quality and economic goals will coincide when it becomes cheaper to manage a problem well than to treat the consequences of poor management.

Information Technology

A key element in delivering modern chronic care will be better information systems. At present, clinicians must confront both too little and too much information when they see a patient. Salient information may be lost in a sea of irrelevant data. The multivolume chart is a clear signal that it will be hard to find a clear indication of the reasons for the current visit or the clinical history that preceded it. Under greater pressure to practice efficiently, clinicians need timely and focused information that will direct their attention to the salient data. In line with new modern shipping and manufacturing practices, clinicians need "just in time" information. And, just as much as airline pilots, they need warnings when things are not going according to plan. The goal of an information system should be to provide the right content and amount of information at the right time.

Structured data systems can assure that relevant information is recorded. By providing fields for items that address otherwise often ignored issues, like function and quality of life, these structured approaches can increase the likelihood clinicians will attend to them. Computerized flow sheets can display change in status over time. They can readily be transformed into graphs. Data that relate treatment and outcomes can be merged. Patient histories can be taken by computer before the patients see the clinicians. Computerized ordering of drugs can incorporate various fail-safe procedures that prevent drug-drug interactions or drug-disease interactions.

The pace of innovation in information technology will likely accelerate rather than slow down. Cutting-edge technologies will continue to reshape chronic illness care, beyond the impact of the innovations to create, store, and exchange information mentioned here and reviewed in the chapter on technology (see chapter 8). In one promising area, speech recognition (also called voice recognition) uses software to convert speech into text as a clinician, for example, dictates a report into a microphone attached to a computer. Speech recognition technologies can reduce the time and cost to prepare a report compared with traditional medical transcription services. With the traditional dictation method, the clinician dictates the report, a transcriptionist transcribes it, then the clinician reads the transcribed report and makes any necessary corrections before it is available as a finalized report. Although speech recognition software companies claim an accuracy rate as high as 95%, that hasn't been good enough to prompt many clinicians and other providers to buy and use speech recognition systems.

An alternative application of speech recognition technology is as a communication aid for people with chronic hearing loss. The technology enables people without hearing loss, be they health care professionals, teachers, co-workers, family members, or friends, to communicate with deaf or hard-of-hearing persons by converting speech into readable text or video-based sign language. Connecting speech recognition technology with the telephone could be a significant advancement over existing TTY (Telecommunications Devices for the Deaf) technology, which requires callers to type messages.

Interactive voice recognition (IVR) is a computer technology that can recognize spoken words and generate responses. Among IVR's many applications in health care settings, one allows patients with chronic conditions to obtain health information, report clinical information, and access a decision support system for making medication adjustments by using their telephone touch-tone keypad or speech recognition technology linked to their clinician. Patients have been found to be more likely to report sensitive information accurately in their interactions with IVR systems than they are during in-person interviews (Piette, 2000). Moreover, they can access IVR systems more frequently and conveniently than a doctor's office or outpatient clinic.

A major trend in information technology is toward wireless applications. Wireless refers to the transfer of information between computing devices (for example, a handheld computer and a central computer system) without a wired connection between them. Wireless technology can also provide computing devices with access to data on the Internet. Wireless Internet technology may be most useful outside of traditional health care delivery settings where wireless local area networks (the more common wireless data transfer method) are inconvenient or not available. In one sense, wireless technology extends the reach of electronic medical records, clinical decision support systems, and other forms of IT used in health care. It provides clinicians, regardless of their location, with documentation and access to patient data at the point of care. Expanded use of wireless technology in health care is currently hampered, in part, by concerns over data security. It is generally easier to safeguard confidential information from unauthorized users when the information is stored in hardwired networks.

Integrating IT with Patient Care Technologies

More patient care technologies will integrate information gathering, storage, and transmission into their function. This advance will permit patients and their clinicians to continuously monitor the patient's condition and adjust the therapy as needed. Some of that adjustment can be done using automated algorithms; other parts will require direct clinician or patient intervention, but from a position of knowledge about what has transpired and an early warning system to ensure timely actions. Through networks that link the patient care device with the clinician (e.g., using the Internet), clinicians will increasingly be able to monitor and manage the care of patients remotely, reducing the need for costly face-to-face visits.

For some chronic conditions, the perceived lack of patient compliance will continue to spark interest in developing patient-supplanting technologies. These devices (typically, but not necessarily, implantable) allow clinicians to monitor the patient's health and make adjustments in the device's functioning, if necessary, without the patient's involvement. The goal is to integrate these technologies into the management of the patient's chronic condition without interfering with the valuable goals and benefits of patient self-management.

Cost Containment

The pressures on health costs will continue to rise. We will become ever more sophisticated in managing the complications and end stages of illness, and these new technological developments will likely be more expensive. Cost pressures will be further exacerbated by the aging of the population. We will have to find ways to make care more efficient. Defining "efficiency" will be crucial. The current emphasis of event-based payment systems must yield to episode-based accounting. In that context aggressive primary care can be shown to be cost-effective.

New forms of chronic care management will need to prove their worth under this new regime. Some of the savings may come from shifting the burden from the formal health care system onto patients or their informal care providers, including family members and friends (who may opt to provide the needed care themselves or to hire surrogate caregivers), but most of it will need to derive from preventing acute exacerbations or other costly sequelae of chronic illnesses.

Ultimately, we will face some hard choices. Even if the push toward greater efficiency is successful, the total cost of health care will soon exceed society's ability to pay, presenting stark choices regarding the allocation of finite health care dollars. When resources are scarce relative to needs, which health care services or interventions, or features of the health care system (e.g., choice of clinician) are we willing to give up? Who decides who gets what when there is not enough to go around, and how should such decisions be made?

Family Support Policies

Cost containment pressures will likely conflict with proposals to provide more active financial and practical support to informal caregivers. With the overall shift toward placing more responsibility in the hands of individuals and their families, it seems unlikely that public dollars will be used to shore up family caregiving. On the other hand, prudent investments in preserving families from crisis (preventing them from pulling out of care) may be wise, especially in those situations where such care may be making a huge difference in patients' clinical trajectories. The challenge will lie in identifying where these investments in support can be best targeted. This task will fall to a new breed of case managers, who will be charged not only with authorizing such support but also with determining just what kind of support will work best. This support may range from practical advice and information (both in the form of formal teaching and through ongoing information support networks) to financial assistance and respite care.

Role of the Media

It seems unlikely that the news media will ever become a major venue for educating the public about either the policy or practical aspects of chronic illnesses and chronic care. (See Appendix A for a discussion of the news media's role in chronic care.) Indeed, the future of some forms of broadcast journalism may be in question. Various modes of continuously available streaming information may replace the traditional fixed-format shows. Other parts of the media may play more dominant roles in educating consumers about health and health care. The various talk shows on radio and television reach a wide audience and many of these personalities seem to have loyal followings. Perhaps they may be the vehicles to bring the chronic care message to a wider swath of the American public. Identifying champions and emphasizing real life stories of both success and failure may help to document and disseminate both the challenges and the power of good chronic care.

Developing a Chronic Illness Constituency

The majority of consumer-based, disease-focused organizations address diseases one at a time. These organizations compete with each other for public support and attention. Yet many in the general public complain about the "disease of the month" phenomenon. At some point it will become increasingly clear that there are large areas of common ground among disease-focused organizations and across patient groups, at least at the level of organizing patient care. Some form of coalition must evolve to pursue this common cause. Obvious partners are the organizations that reflect broader population groups, like the American Association of Retired Persons (AARP), most of whose members suffer from at least one chronic condition and hence have a natural stake in seeking ways to improve care delivery, but thus far these organizations have not taken up this political and social challenge. A model for such collaboration can be found in the United Patients' Organizations of the Chronically Ill in the Netherlands. This organization has succeeded in putting people suffering from chronic illnesses on the political agenda; indeed the organization receives substantial government funding (Wilson, 1999).

Furthermore, most disease-based groups have a natural coalition between the consumers who suffer from the chronic illness and their family members, and the health care professionals who treat that illness. Strong models exist for effective cooperation to raise money and focus public attention on their cause. A similar collaboration needs to develop around chronic illness in general. Because of its ubiquity, even stronger bonds are possible.

Anecdotal evidence suggests that many health care professionals involved in chronic health care have had to experience, either in coping with their own chronic conditions or those of families members, the very insults of an inadequate system for chronic care that form the agenda for reform. These professionals could provide an unusual and noteworthy basis for instigating change. Their personal testimonies could speak volumes about what needs to be revised, whereas their credibility would add weight to recommended reforms. A coalition of such professional consumers, using their own experiences in the health care system to formulate policy proposals for improving the delivery of chronic illness care, may help build consumer demand for improving chronic care.[11]

Apathy and satisfaction with the status quo are tough adversaries. It often takes a crisis to develop the momentum needed to accomplish real change, but by that time change will be disruptive and painful. Sometimes it seems like the science fiction movie where the hero scientist sees the asteroid coming toward earth but cannot get enough attention from anyone in power to institute evasive action or at least make preparations to manage the effects of the impact. Our asteroid is a combination of an aging population and enough medical success to permit many who would have died to survive with their chronic illnesses intact. Some people may cling to the hope that some clever scientist will find a cure for all these problems that will obviate the need to treat them, but it seems prudent, nonetheless, to start making preparations for the asteroid's impact. Maybe it's time we started looking upward.

APPENDIX A

Why Journalists Struggle with the Chronic Illness Story

Gary Schwitzer

Hopes of developing a strong public constituency to press for needed changes in chronic disease care will require the media to play an active role. Today's media come in many forms, but we still look to the news media to provide information on the pressing problems of our time. We therefore asked an expert in the news media, Gary Schwitzer, a professor of journalism at the University of Minnesota and a former journalist who worked on health stories, to offer his insights into how well the news media have risen to this challenge and what we can realistically expect. If the news media fail to respond to this need, as Professor Schwitzer's analysis suggests, we may need to look elsewhere for the dual task of educating and arousing the public. Other aspects of the media, often ones that are held in less regard by academics, such as the talk shows, may prove to be a more receptive forum. Clearly, relying on such venues raises some concerns, because they seem to like to sensationalize, but they also reach a large number of people and are constantly looking for issues and topics. If we hope to create a climate of constructive intolerance for the status quo, we may well find ourselves allied with such forces.

The spread of severe acute respiratory syndrome or SARS in 2003 provided journalists with one of their favorite types of stories. SARS became an epidemic in some places. The story had elements of mystery, frightening headline potential, and enticing photo opportunities (e.g., students stepping on a disinfectant mat before entering school, young Hong Kong ballerinas all wearing masks, SARS fashion masks, a Bangkok airport SARS-detecting thermal imaging camera). The SARS epidemic was new and hence newsworthy.

But news stories about the burden of chronic illness on Americans and the American health care system, or about policy changes required to address that burden, are rare. Chronic illness is endemic—so common that it

239

is perhaps not viewed as newsworthy. There is little mystery about chronic illness, and journalists may not see good headline or photojournalism potential in a story that is all around them. Endemic chronic diseases that kill continue to be pushed off the page and off the air by SARS and its other eye-catching public health risk competitors. Indeed, fears surrounding one Canadian cow with bovine spongiform encephalopathy became headline and lead story fodder. Then monkeypox-infected prairie dogs infecting a few humans grabbed the spotlight. Chronic illness is a prime example of how—in journalism—being important is different than being new and newsworthy.

The Harvard School of Public Health Center for Health Communication publishes an online news digest called *World Health News*.[1] For a 2002 year-ending report, the Web site reviewed 22 public health issues that shaped the year. The only chronic disease listed was chronic wasting disease in Wisconsin deer. Perhaps the strongest voice for improvement in health journalism is the five-year old Association of Health Care Journalists (AHCJ), based at the University of Minnesota's School of Journalism and Mass Communication.[2] More than 650 journalists have joined AHCJ. The association published a resource guide in 2002 to help journalists cover issues surrounding the quality of health care. One section covers chronic illness. But when AHCJ members exchanged thoughts informally on an e-mail listserv about the top health-medical stories of 2002, not one member mentioned any chronic illness issue.

Three dozen AHCJ members with responsibility for coverage of daily health or medical news responded to a short survey on the coverage of chronic illness issues. Respondents represented the top 100 newspapers, as listed in the *Editor & Publisher* Year Book. Cities served by these newspapers include Atlanta, Austin, Birmingham, Cleveland, Detroit, Louisville, Los Angeles, Minneapolis—St. Paul, New Orleans, Philadelphia, Providence, St. Louis, San Antonio, Tampa, Toledo, Washington, and Wichita. Smaller papers in the following states responded: Maine, Minnesota, Ohio, Pennsylvania, South Carolina, Texas, and Washington. Five broadcast journalists responded: two local and one network television journalist, and one local and one national radio journalist.

The survey asked:

1. Many health policy experts say we have a health care system that is geared to handle episodic acute care but not to handle chronic care. Have you ever done stories on this policy topic? (If so, please send copies.)

2. Chronic disease is the leading cause of disability in Americans. It is the main reason people seek health care. It accounts for 75 cents of every health care dollar spent in the United States. Do you think your coverage has adequately addressed the burden of chronic disease? (If yes, please send examples.)

3. If you answered "no" to question 2, or if you have had difficulty addressing chronic disease issues, can you identify any obstacles you face in trying to address these issues?

Only six journalists responded to question 1 with any evidence of anything close to what was described. No journalist answered question 2 affirmatively. The answers to question 3 provide much of the background for this essay.

The responses followed four main themes: transience in the job and lack of training for the health care beat; time restraints and work demands; news staff turf issues; and the topic itself is viewed as boring or too broad to address.

Obstacles Journalists Face

Transience and Training

Eight of the 34 journalists who responded to the survey said they were either too new to the beat to comment or they had recently left the health-medical beat to work on something else. A Pennsylvania writer who had begun work on the type of chronic disease management article the survey asked about wrote back a month later to say she was leaving the job and never wrote the article. An earlier survey of journalists in five Midwestern states found that nearly one quarter of those surveyed had less than two years experience covering health; nearly half had less than five years (Voss, 2002). The survey also showed that 83% of journalists covering health news had received no training for that type of coverage. Of those, 73% said that training would be helpful.

Time Restraints and Work Demands

One can gain a new appreciation for the demands placed on a daily health journalist by reading some of the comments sent in response to question 3. A Texas journalist wrote: "I'm the only health care writer at my paper, so I cover hospital construction projects, ambulance diversions, caring for the uninsured, nurse shortages, program cuts, public health, research, bioterrorism issues (smallpox vaccines), immunizations, mental health, disease outbreaks, stress on the health care system—just to name some major themes. So is my coverage of chronic disease adequate? I sincerely doubt it."

An East Coast journalist with a top 25 newspaper wrote: "I don't think we have covered chronic disease adequately, but then I don't think we cover anything adequately. Our staffing has been cut considerably in recent years and it makes it difficult to even skim the surface of a topic as broad as medicine plus all its accompanying financial and policy issues. We still have a larger medical reporting staff than most newspapers, but we cover an area with more than 60 hospitals and six medical schools. I think we would be far more likely to write about chronic problems in a smaller market with fewer hospitals and less high-quality research going on."

A national television correspondent responded: "As to whether we've adequately captured the burden of chronic disease on the system, I think the answer is no—not because we haven't done a number of stories on the topic, but because I think it would be tough to treat this issue in the fullness that it deserves while still managing to put on a few other types of health stories now and then!"

A local California television reporter wrote: "We are strapped for resources, which severely limits my ability to do these types of in-depth stories."

A Texas newspaper reporter wrote: "Time and competing demands (to cover everything else) are the major obstacles. I don't see that changing."

An Alabama reporter summarized: "Frankly the only problem is getting the time to do it."

A national television reporter who responded emphasized the time it takes to report these issues for television. "The only obstacle we face is time—both time to put together more stories on the subject amid all the other health issues we have to cover," she wrote. "Television is incredibly labor- and time-intensive and it can take us up to two to three weeks to produce a particular story. And getting enough time on our broadcast to air them. Otherwise, no problem!"

Turf Issues: Someone Else's Responsibility

In 1998–9, two University of Florida journalism professors worked with the Robert Wood Johnson Foundation and the Poynter Institute for Media Studies to conduct two seminars on improving health news coverage. Editors and journalists specializing in health issues discussed what works or doesn't work at their newspapers. One theme in those seminars was that "simply determining what 'health reporting' means is a daunting task at many papers because it requires reporters and their editors to define the basic elements of health care: personal health and fitness, medical research stories, clinical versus nonclinical subjects, health business, etc." (University of Florida Web site).

Our survey suggests that those definitions often leave out chronic illness. The most common of all the journalists' responses received was: "That's not my beat. Talk to someone on the (*insert one of varied responses*) beat."

From St. Louis: "I am a medical science writer and don't usually cover health policy. I cover chronic diseases such as obesity and diabetes from the science standpoint. I don't address insurance issues. That is covered by our business department."

From New Orleans: "I haven't. I focus more on insurance and business issues."

From Philadelphia: "I think you may need to differentiate among kinds of health reporters. I'm a business health reporter and cover health from a business point of view. So I've been much less concerned with chronic versus acute care and more about people getting denied access, huge CEO salaries, bankruptcies, system meltdowns, Medicare payments etc."

From Los Angeles: "This is a topic that's probably more geared to our health section. I cover health policy and public health—and much of my time is taken up with budget matters, bioterrorism, HIV/AIDS, nurses unions, emergency room overcrowding, etc."

From Tampa: "I cover consumer health, which means stories about how people can improve their health, lose weight, exercise, etc. I don't cover health policy, or focus on cost of care, per se."

From Minneapolis-St. Paul: "I cover health/fitness. Check with our medical reporter, or with the reporter who covers aging, or with the reporter who covers the business of health care."

From these responses it is possible to form an image of a topic that has no home. Perhaps it is a topic no one wants to tackle. These responses also provide a reminder of how overloaded many journalists are with wide-ranging responsibilities for a complicated beat that can be varyingly viewed as health, medicine, health policy, research, science, finance, politics, and other specialized areas of news. Some journalists are responsible for the entire range of topics. Some larger newspapers have individuals assigned to each topic type. Chronic illness—by the numbers one of the biggest issues in health care—hasn't yet found a home with any of these subspecialty areas.

Topic Is Too Boring or Too Broad

The following are excerpts of responses from reporters from around the country. (The state where the newspaper is published is listed in parentheses.)

"So many chronic diseases are so common, it's hard to write a feature on someone with, say, diabetes. The interest, I think, is for the dramatic or rare illnesses. Also, I think the chronic disease topic can be boring to readers; they already know what diabetes is and what causes it. What can I do to make it novel, interesting, or news?" (New Jersey)

"I've done stories on specific chronic diseases, such as heart disease, asthma, diabetes, etc., and pointed out in those stories the impact of the disease, and why doctors think we should pay attention to them because they have such a large impact. But I don't think I've done a story on the overall burden of chronic disease. To be honest, I doubt you'll get many journalists to bite-at least more than once on a broad topic like this. People can relate, for example, to heart disease because it's so common, but it's harder to relate to the broad topic of chronic disease." (Ohio)

"(Obstacles are) finding ways to make the coverage "sexy" for readers (and editors!), finding ways to spread and/or reinforce the message without having it sound like preaching." (Kansas)

"What I need help with is a way to explain the financial impact chronic diseases can have, in such a way that my editors will think it's a sexy story." (Ohio)

"Editors are slow to warm to these sorts of stories. My direct editor had particularly limited attention span for these sorts of stories." (Maine)

"I think one of the biggest obstacles might be that this can be a very depressing story to tell, given the current limitations in our health care system. And editors who assign/approve stories grow tired of the topic unless there's something new and different—and that's what the system sorely needs. . . . new and different" (national radio correspondent).

The response from a health journalist with a top-75 East Coast newspaper was too eloquent to shorten. "Like medicine itself, newspaper journalism is better suited to acute episodes—the individual with a gripping, heart-rending story, the protest rally, the black-and-white injustice, the clear problem with a clear solution. Chronic disease is a multifaceted, complex topic that is difficult to manage in the context of a newspaper story. It's mammoth. It's blurry around the edges, hard to bring into focus. In the crush of day-by-day, well-defined news events, few have the time to get their arms around such topics. Even finding a discrete piece of it to tackle is a time-consuming assignment. People suffering from chronic disease, numerous as they are, keep a low profile. They rarely even call the paper with their complaints. They're hard to find, and even when you find someone, his or her situation is likely to be complicated. I wanted to do a series on disability. I explained to my editors that care for the disabled eats up a surprising amount of our tax dollars, more than many other programs that get lots more attention in the press, and that we get pretty poor results from all that spending. I explained that even the people who oversee the program can't give me a good breakdown of who the disabled are, what their needs and disabilities are, and so forth. My editors yawned. Because it was nebulous, because there were so many unanswered questions and so much research required, because I could not, at the outset, provide details of a sexy result or even describe an individual who exemplifies the problem (as if it were one problem, as if anyone were typical), they would not allow me the time. To me, the potential for great journalism was obvious. To my editors, it was a black hole that would suck me away from the all-important task of filling the daily paper."

Survey Summary

The challenges health journalists face in covering chronic illness issues are not unique to this topic. They are the same challenges present in covering health policy issues, quality in medicine issues, safety net issues, health cost issues—indeed, any issue not coming out of a medical journal or a news release or a news conference. How can health reporters break out of the grind of daily journalism and the pressure placed on them to have the same stories their competition will have so that they can devote attention to "enterprise" stories that require more time and research? In today's newsroom environment, that can be an increasingly different task. Recent history has shown that the chronic illness "big picture" story is only told when there is special funding, when a journalist has a personal encounter with a chronic illness dilemma, or, rarely, when a journalist gets the inspiration to translate the statistics into a story of human costs and system failures.

Examples of Chronic Illness News Coverage

In recent years, there have been several examples of special journalism projects on the topic of chronic illness. In late 2001, more than 100 PBS (Public Broadcasting Service) television stations in the United States aired an hour-long special report, "Who Cares: Chronic Illness in America." The project was sponsored by the Robert Wood Johnson Foundation. The televised program was complemented by an outreach program and by a Web site that is still accessible.[3] This type of project is difficult to envision on any television network besides PBS, and difficult to envision without the foundation funding available in this case. In this program, Arthur Caplan, Ph.D., director of the Center for Bioethics at the University of Pennsylvania, criticized politicians and journalists. "Politicians and the media don't pay any attention. That's why policy hasn't changed in 20 years," Caplan claimed. "If (a person) could get a lung transplant for her asthma and couldn't pay, you guys in the media would be following her up her driveway. But if she goes every three months to the emergency room and doesn't get her medicine and the doctor in the ER has five minutes to see her, nobody cares."

Sound Partners, a program of the Benton Foundation, also funded by the Robert Wood Johnson Foundation, has brought chronic care issues to the radio airwaves in 27 communities. The local programs have covered such issues as diabetes among African-Americans, local resources for caregivers, and fighting chronic illness in Appalachian Kentucky.

Nationally syndicated columnist Judy Foreman addressed many aspects of the chronic illness dilemma in a 2001 column. The article profiled Helen Freeman, a woman with lung disease, diabetes, glaucoma, melanoma, and breast cancer. Foreman wrote:

> More and more Americans are finding that, like Helen Freeman, they must learn to cope with chronic illness. Half of all Americans today (20 million more than researchers had previously estimated) have at least one chronic illness and one in five has two or more, according to a recent analysis by researchers from the Johns Hopkins School of Public Health. Granted, for some of the 125 million people with chronic illnesses, the problems are minor, like allergies that can be stabilized with medications. But 60 million others have multiple chronic conditions such as heart disease, Alzheimer's disease, cancer, arthritis, epilepsy, mental illness and others that can be serious or life-threatening
>
> The toll of so much illness is enormous—$510 billion annually, said Jay Hedlund, deputy director of the Partnership for Solutions, a Johns Hopkins project aimed at improving the lives of people with chronic diseases. Indeed, chronic illnesses account for 77% of direct medical expenditures in America, he said. It leads to 70% of all deaths, according to the federal Centers for Disease Control and Prevention, and it accounts for one third of the years of potential life lost before age 65.

Journalist Madge Kaplan addressed chronic care issues after becoming a caregiver herself. "The Real-Life Education of a Health Care Reporter" was the title of an article she wrote in the *Columbia Journalism Review* after she became a long-distance caregiver for her father after he had a stroke. "I don't mind that I've been humbled into some new directions. Health care reporters need to be run over by the truth every now and then—even the awful truth."

Kaplan thought she would find story ideas in her experience with her father's condition, but says the ideas she gathered were not the ones she expected. "My experiences have put pressure on me as a journalist to connect more with people's every day encounters with the health care system," Kaplan wrote. "With all the change we hear about, it's been radicalizing to discover how much things have stayed the same. And that's big news and worthy of exploration by anyone on the health care beat." She added one other critique: "I think we journalists haven't done a good enough job getting to the bottom of who has a stake (financial stake?) in the status quo."

Kaplan's personal misfortune placed her in a situation where she had no problem seeing the news angle of what confronted her and her father. Editors who "are slow to warm to these types of stories," who yawn or are bored or need to be convinced of a "sexy" angle in chronic disease should hope that they or their loved ones avoid the trap of chronic illness—a trap that currently ensnares more than 125 million of their readers and viewers.

Different Drummers

At an increasing number of professional conferences, health care professionals and journalism professionals have discussed the state of health news dissemination in the United States. One such session—called a National Conference on Medicine and the Media—was held at the Mayo Clinic in Rochester, Minnesota, in September 2002 (Lantz & Landier, 2002). Journalists, physicians, researchers and public relations or other communications professionals attended the three-day conference. One of the clearest messages at the conclusion of the conference was that journalists have a different mission than the one physicians and researchers envision for them. Repeatedly, physicians, researchers, and consumer health advocates at the conference stated that they expect reporting to contain an educational element. Repeatedly, journalists stated that they consider themselves primarily reporters rather than public educators. Peggy Girshman of National Public Radio said, "Medical professionals encourage journalists to assume a more educational role. Media people obviously disagree."

But not all journalists agreed with Girshman. *Time* magazine medical writer Christine Gorman said, "There's an element of education in addition to reporting the news and I think there has to be with medical coverage." And Judy Peres of the *Chicago Tribune* said, "I actually see a great part of my job as education." These different viewpoints on how to cover this beat may help explain why coverage of chronic illness can be a tough sell. If journalists don't have some responsibility for educating Americans about the burden of chronic disease, it is easier to see why they may leave this complicated issue alone. Educating is not the same thing as advocacy journalism, and journalists are not health educators. Advocacy and health education are not roles for journalists. But educating readers and viewers about issues of national importance when evidence shows these issues fail to gain attention—and not just reporting today's news—clearly falls within the guidelines of ethical journalism. The code of ethics of the Society of Professional Journalists states "that public enlightenment is the forerunner of justice and the foundation of democracy. The duty of the journalist is to further those ends by seeking truth and providing a fair and comprehensive account of events and issues." An argument could be made that the public is not enlightened about the burden of chronic illness on this society and that U.S. journalists have not provided a fair and comprehensive account of this burden.

Associated Press medical editor Daniel Haney was described by one colleague at the Mayo conference as one of the most influential health care journalists in the country because newsrooms across the country subscribe to the AP newswire service that carries his stories. Haney's view of his responsibility on this beat is worth reviewing. "We are reporters at the AP," Haney explained. "And we get up in the morning and we're looking for stories. And we're covering medicine like a political reporter covers elections." That quote may also explain why chronic illness is chronically abandoned by many journalists. A medical reporter who covers medicine like a political reporter covers elections may run with the best quote, the best controversy du jour, and the best headline. A political reporter covering a political campaign often has his/her agenda dictated by the politician being covered. Political news stories aren't necessarily about the most important issues; they tend to be about the issues the candidates want to discuss. One analysis showed that "despite rising health care costs and the growing number of uninsured Americans, health care played a relatively modest role as an issue in the 2002 congressional elections" (Blendon et al., 2002).One way of looking at this finding is that the electorate showed little interest in health issues because politicians did not discuss them and journalists did not write about them.

Questions about journalism's performance on health policy issues come at a time of unprecedented self-scrutiny within the profession. In their 2002 book, *The News about the News: American Journalism in Peril*, Downie and Kaiser wrote: "Bad journalism—failing to report important news, or reporting news shallowly, inaccurately or unfairly—can leave people dangerously uninformed." They asserted, "In an information age, when good journalism should be flourishing everywhere, it isn't" (Downie & Kaiser, 2002). In *The Elements of Journalism*, Kovach and Rosensteil listed two principles that could be applied to the coverage of chronic illness. They wrote that journalism "must strive to make the significant interesting and relevant . . . (and) must keep the news comprehensive and proportional" (Kovach & Rosensteil, 2001). Editors who are bored by chronic illness topics would fail under the scrutiny of these standards.

Summary

This essay will not conclude with any tips about how to use the media to improve the discussion of chronic illness issues in this country. Respectable journalists will not and should not allow themselves to be "used." But the responses to our survey point to several clear gaps that journalists should contemplate about the way in which chronic illness is covered. Those who promote more in-depth news coverage of chronic illness issues could engage newspaper publishers and broadcast news directors in a discussion of the following questions.

1. Are editors, news directors, producers, and reporters aware of the current burden of chronic illness in the United States, much less the health policy implications of aging Baby Boomers with increasing chronic illness?

2. Have reporters and editors or news directors discussed priorities for health news coverage? Are they comfortable with the mix of news they've been reporting? Has there been too much news on clinical medicine or on new drugs or devices? Is coverage driven by publicity events or journal publications more than by independent analysis of issues important to the readers and viewers being served?

3. Are journalists who are assigned to the health care beat being asked to cover too much, yet with no time to address policy issues such as this?

4. Have specific beats been adequately defined? Which beat reporter owns responsibility for covering the policy issues affecting chronic illness care?

5. Have reporters and editors or news directors explored the issues covered earlier in this book—a discussion of which reveals what is novel, interesting, important, and even "sexy" about this topic?

What would it look like if journalists did a good job covering this story? First, the challenges journalists mentioned in our survey must be addressed so that health journalists have the environment in which to do this work properly. The health journalism beat would be established as one that is vital and supported by the news organization—one with a future and with growth potential—a place journalists want to stay. Reporters would be given the time and training needed to do their research and to report a multifaceted story on chronic illness. Editors would assign clear responsibility for chronic illness issues to a given reporter. Editors and reporters would cast aside any biased perspectives about what is too broad and too boring to find what is newsworthy about an increasingly important health policy issue.

Second, adequate coverage of this issue would not be an isolated story. The issues outlined in this book should be the backbone of a multipart series, or a special project that is revisited every six months, and/or a newspaper or television station Web site that is updated regularly with new policy discussions, new human interest stories, and new clinical and technological developments in the management and treatment of chronic illnesses.

Third, the ideal coverage would cover the gamut of issues from broad system failure questions to local-regional attempts to establish best practices in chronic illness management to individual stories of success and failure in navigating the system and coping with chronic illness. Ideal coverage would avoid any possibility of losing readers and viewers in a "policy wonk" story by making it relevant to individuals—as the issue became relevant to journalist Madge Kaplan when misfortune entered her life, or as journalist Judy Foreman showed the relevance in one woman's life.

Finally, this special journalistic effort deserves promotion. News organizations have no difficulty promoting their sports coverage or their Doppler radar. Attention to this issue—if it is ever given—deserves to be trumpeted. Television stations, which several times each year devote extra preparation, air time, and promotion to topics during ratings "sweeps" periods, should consider covering the chronic illness story in their communities rather than stories about Botox, alleged cures for cancer and the common cold, and claims of fountain of youth discoveries (Schwitzer, 2003).

At a 2003 University of Minnesota Center on Aging conference entitled, "Caring for Chronic Illness: Can It Be Done?" one of the nation's thought leaders on chronic disease delivered the keynote address. Ed Wagner, M.D., M.P.H., director of the MacColl Institute for Healthcare Innovation at Group Health Cooperative in Seattle, said that in today's typical chronic illness care the patient's role in self-management is not emphasized. The interaction between patient and doctor is often not productive and is frustrating for both parties. But in models of improved chronic illness care, "informed, activated patients have the motivation, information, skills and confidence necessary to effectively make decisions about their health and to manage it" (Wagner, presentation at the University of Minnesota, June 5, 2003). But he also said he has been surprised by the "absence of patients' and families' voices advocating for change" in chronic illness care.

For more than 30 years, scholars have reflected on the "agenda-setting" role of the mass media (McCombs & Shaw, 1972). Throughout this book, a case has been made that the burden of chronic illness in the United States has not been adequately discussed on the nation's health policy agenda. The "informed, activated" patients that Wagner calls for would benefit from journalism's increased attention to chronic illness issues. They would benefit from journalism demonstrating the best practices that have been established in chronic disease management around the world. Perhaps an informed electorate would not be so silent about health policy change. Perhaps 125 million Americans and more than that number of caregiving family members would find an "informed, activated" form of journalism useful. It might sell more newspapers and bolster the dwindling trust Americans have expressed in television health news (Lantz & Lanier, 2002). The story of chronic illness and chronic care in the United States has its place in many journalism beats. It can be a political or public policy story, a business story, a technology story, an education story, a quality in medicine story, a controversial story, and a human interest story. It is a story of systems of financing and delivery of care out of step with the complexities of caring for individuals with chronic illness. Journalists should reflect on the job they have done in reporting on these issues, which are endemic in our society.

Lessons from the United Kingdom

David Colin-Thome, Sue Roberts, and Ian Philp

The care and management of chronic disease has developed differently in the United Kingdom than in the United States. Because the United Kingdom provides most of its health care through a National Health Service (NHS), it does not have to contend with many of the problems faced in the diverse American scene. Ideally, it provides a more effective means to translate public policy into action. Several articles have contrasted the NHS with American managed care (Dixon et al., 2004; Feachem, Sekhri & White, 2002; Klein, 2004; Lewis & Dixon, 2004). In light of these developments and because the NHS has specifically identified chronic disease management as a central part of its strategy to address health care improvement, we thought it would be enlightening to examine how chronic care management is evolving in the context of the NHS. We asked several experts working within the NHS to undertake this task: David Colin-Thome (National Clinical Director for Primary Care, NHS), Sue Roberts (National Clinical Director for Diabetes Care, NHS, and Ian Philp (National Clinical Director for Older People's Services, NHS). The analysis by Drs. Colin-Thome, Roberts, and Philp suggests that developments in chronic care in each of the two countries may hold valuable lessons for the other.

The shape of the National Health Service (NHS) in the United Kingdom is changing radically. There has been increased devolution of health care policy at two levels: (1) nationally, in the four countries of the United Kingdom (Scotland, Northern Ireland, Wales, and England); and (2) locally. The "national" health service will increasingly be delivered by diverse, locally appropriate services, set in a framework of national standards and accountability. The NHS has established overarching priority areas in primary care, the care of older people, diabetes care, cancer, heart disease, mental health, children's services, emergency care and patient experience, with a national director or health "Czar" from the field, appointed to lead each of these programs.

England's health policy, the focus of this essay, is framed by The NHS Plan: a 10-year strategy to put the patient back at the center of the health service.[1] The vision is for prompt, convenient, and high-quality services built around the needs of the patient rather than the system. Three developments illustrate the importance of this vision for people with chronic illnesses. First, recent changes in health policy in England create a new opportunity to deliver effective chronic illness care through a strengthened role of primary care organizations[2] in commissioning services across the whole care system. Second, new approaches to the care of older people with age-related needs are being developed which encompass chronic illness care, but with subtle differences from established models, to accommodate the management of people with multiple illnesses. Finally, new models for care of people with diabetes that combine the strength of primary and secondary care position such models at the forefront of good practice in chronic illness care.

Developments in Primary Care

The abolition of general practitioner (GP) fundholding in 1999 marked the start of the fundamental reshaping of primary care structures. The GP fundholding system, which allocated budgets to general practices to purchase community and nonemergency hospital services, was a voluntary scheme that was criticized for causing fragmentation and creating inequities in NHS services. For example, it was often true that the patients of fundholding practices had better access to services, in particular, to specialist services, as a consequence of practice-based commissioning. Nevertheless, the GP fundholding system had demonstrated the benefits of concentrating much of the power for commissioning health services with primary care providers. The new incoming structures in England primary care groups (PCGs) maintained the role of primary care commissioning; but, by bringing together providers, including GPs and social and community services, they emphasized integration, patient centeredness, and a new strategic approach to meeting the needs of the whole health economy.[3]

Primary Care Trusts

The PCG model evolved into 303 primary care trusts (PCTs).[4] Primary care trusts are characterized by stronger accountability mechanisms, an even more powerful commissioning role, and an altered but central management role for local providers such as GPs. Responsible for arranging the provision of all primary and community care services and the majority of specialist care, and spearheading the development of partnerships with social care providers, PCTs are the evolving heart of health service planning in England's modern NHS.

Their formation devolves power to the frontline. PCTs control 75% of the entire NHS budget and virtually all of the local health care budgets. Though still in their relative infancy, their combined role as providers and commissioners makes them powerful agents to improve the care of patients. They represent the move to a more flexible and responsive local structure where clinicians and other health care professionals have greater freedom and stronger incentives to shape services around the needs of their local communities.

Clearly a lot of these community "needs" will center on the better management of chronic disease and the enhancement of self-care. The power available to PCTs as commissioners of a wide range of health services will be central in building the integrated services the NHS needs to improve outcomes for these patients and to reduce the levels of demand for hospital inpatient and outpatient services.

All PCTs have three clear key roles or responsibilities:

- to improve the health of their population and reduce inequalities in health care;

- to secure the totality of services; and

- to bring primary, secondary (i.e., specialist), and social care closer together.

Modern disease management relies on the integration of the primary, secondary, and, in many cases, social care functions. Other NHS organizations had been developing integrated partnership approaches to chronic disease management well before the creation of PCTs. The model of diabetes care in Northumbria described later in this essay is one such example. This model uses multidisciplinary teams and is built on the principles of patient centeredness, empowerment of patients and staff, a systematic approach to care, and quality assurance. But the PCTs provide structure and impetus to the wider adoption of integrated chronic disease care across the NHS. It is likely, for instance, that the increasing number of PCTs will encourage the provision of more specialist care in the community setting. This could be realized through:

- The further development of GPs with a special interest. Currently, over 1,200 GPs carry out procedures in areas such as ophthalmology, orthopedics, dermatology, and ear nose and throat surgery; however, they remain predominantly generalists.[5]

- The development of other clinical practitioners with a similar special clinical interest, such as nurses, hospital-based scientists, and optometrists. The Department of Health has an ongoing program to develop these practitioners with a specialized clinical interest, including developing the role of community-based dentists and pharmacists.

- The commissioning of clinical specialists to work in primary care settings

- The potential for the employment of such specialists in areas like diabetes and asthma

The three key roles are as relevant at the practice level as they are at the PCT level. Their realization of better systems to manage chronic disease in the community will depend heavily on the primary care team working innovatively and flexibly and forging stronger working relationships with their partners in secondary (specialist) and social care settings.

General Medical Services Contract

The new General Medical Services (GMS) contract between PCTs and primary care practitioners, which will apply across the entire NHS, should be a central lever for motivating primary care teams to align their efforts more closely with better services and outcomes for chronically ill patients. Essentially, the relevance of the new contract to the better management of chronic disease falls into two main areas:

- the promotion of greater freedoms and flexibilities for general practices to decide how to design services to better meet local needs; and

- the clearer focus on meeting clinical quality standards linked to the care of chronic disease sufferers and substantial rewards to recognize achievements in these areas.

For the first time in any health care system the new contract will establish systematic payments to the general practitioner's practice on the basis of how well they care for patients, rather than simply on the basis of the number of patients they treat or the services they provide. In essence, the income for primary care practices will depend in part on the outcomes they achieve.

The contract will effectively put quality improvement at the center of primary care. Under the existing arrangements, less than 4% of total spending on GP fees and allowances is allocated to rewarding high standards. In contrast, as much as 40% of the new funding for practices will depend on meeting these quality standards, which are fundamentally about ensuring that excellent management of a wide range of chronic disease becomes the norm in primary care. This funding will be allocated through a new quality and outcomes framework, which sets out a range of evidence-based national standards and indicators linked to 10 categories of chronic disease. Demographic factors such as age and gender and the population's needs relating to morbidity and mortality will also be accounted for in the new GMS funding allocation formulae.

Paying for Results

The system of incentives embodied in the new primary care contracts is further reinforced by reforms to the way funding flows through the NHS. The new system of "financial flows" will mean providers are paid for the activity they undertake. If they fail to deliver agreed-on levels of activity, PCTs can use their powers as commissioners to reallocate funds so patients can be treated elsewhere. By introducing a "payment by results" system, PCTs are effectively gaining another powerful lever for securing service improvements. The incentive will be on providers not only to be more responsive to PCTs and patients and meet agreed levels of activity, but to gain more funding by carrying out additional work. Providers are paid for what they do, but the local PCT can also introduce a result-based local contract if it wishes. For chronic disease, an increasing amount of this activity will need to be used to encourage hospital staff to work more flexibly in integrated, multidisciplinary teams.

Local Delivery, National Standards

With PCTs leading the commissioning process and the new GMS contract empowering and motivating primary care teams to work across organizational boundaries and seek new and better ways to integrate services, delivery has become a local issue for the NHS. But although this is appropriate in a system that needs plurality of provision to support choice and drive up standards for patients, it is also appropriate that quality standards and accountability remain in the national domain. The quality and outcomes framework will be one important iteration of these national standards. In terms of assuring quality, a crucial role belongs to the Commission for Health Improvement (CHI), soon to become the Commission for Healthcare Audit and Inspection (CHAI). This body has direct responsibility for inspecting all NHS health care providers and ensuring that national standards are met. The National Institute of Clinical Excellence (NICE)[6] provides patients, health care professionals, and the public with authoritative guidance on current best practice in medicines and management for specific conditions.

A key example of national standards delivered through local initiatives is the promotion and facilitation of self-care. Self-care initiatives in the NHS are still largely fragmented and have not benefited in the past from robust central support in terms of policy, but this is about to change. We already have "NHS Direct," a nurse-led service giving health advice and support to patients. This service handled more than five million telephone calls between 2001 and 2002. Its online service receives thousands of hits a day. Demonstration projects testing the potential of offering similar services via digital television have been sufficiently encouraging for NHS ministers to sanction further development of these technologies.

Given that between 100 million and 150 million GP consultations a year in the United Kingdom are for potentially self-treatable conditions, a clear imperative exists for practices and their PCTs to encourage self-care for minor conditions. Local initiatives include diverting patients with minor ailments from GP surgeries to community pharmacies, such as in Newcastle-upon-Tyne.[7]

Self-care interventions for chronic diseases, including self-management and collaborative care, are other major growth areas for primary care. Research has shown that generic self-management interventions across a range of long-term conditions, including asthma, diabetes and coronary heart disease, can reduce visits to GPs by more than 40% (Fries & McShane, 1998), cut hospital admissions by half (Montgomery, Lieberman, Singh & Fries, 1994), and significantly reduce outpatient visits (Lorig, Kraines, Brown & Richardson, 1985).

The progress to date has been encouraging. The "expert patient" program, for instance, is training patients to help fellow sufferers manage their disease in the long term.[8] This program, based on the work of Lorig, has been introduced recently in approximately half of all PCTs for patients with many types of chronic disease (Lorig et al., 1999). The Medicines Partnership is a Department of Health (DH)-funded program[9] designed to involve patients as partners and works closely with two other DH-funded organizations, the National Collaborative Medicines Management Programme and the National Prescribing Centre, an NHS body. The Collaborative has a program to work with PCTs and some of their general practices to improve medicine management, whereas the Centre promotes high-quality, cost-effective prescribing. The Medicines Partnership program helps patients achieve the maximum benefit from their medication by emphasizing "concordance," that is, where the patient and clinician work as partners to reach an agreement about the illness and the treatment, rather than the patient's compliance with the clinician's orders.

Information Technology Investment

The national IT program for the NHS[10] is bringing massive investment to the Service's IT infrastructure with up to £2.3 billion committed for the next three years. It focuses on four key areas: electronic appointment booking, electronic patient records, electronic prescribing, and an underpinning IT infrastructure that will link different parts of the NHS to give health care professionals access to information about patients from different locations. Because better management of all health care but, in particular, chronic disease care is predicated on a more robust whole-systems approach, the role of IT in helping the NHS dismantle institutional boundaries and streamline patient care is paramount—an issue the new linking infrastructure will address technologically. The electronic patient record, in particular, is a valuable vehicle for engendering greater patient involvement in managing chronic conditions because patients will have ownership and hence access to their own health information, which ties in well with concepts of self-care and self-management. However, patient health records, even in hard copy, are rare in the NHS and so the widespread introduction of the electronic record will require both the IT investment and cultural change.

Enhanced information, e.g., the new OSCAR (Online System for Comparative Analysis and Reporting)[11] system, providing online benchmarking (initially of comparative information on aspects of hospital-based care) and performance analysis to PCTs and to general practices, will support improved local NHS care in general practices, PCT-based community services, and PCT-commissioned specialist services. This information will be crucial in developing better applications for managing chronic disease in the community. Such systems will support anticipatory care that incorporates prevention, screening, chronic disease management, and case management, thereby helping registered list-based general practices, and other NHS organizations who serve geographically based populations, to identify and target those patients at greatest risk. The potential of general practice demonstrated by the work at Castlefields Health Centre in Runcorn is attached as a case study. (See exhibit B.1.)

National Service Frameworks

The national service frameworks (NSFs)[12] also play a vital role in setting national standards and in giving the local NHS operational units an evidence-based, systematic and structural basis on which to build services in priority areas. The NSFs set national standards; define service models; outline strategies to support implementation; and establish performance measures. In essence they offer the NHS—and, in particular, primary care organizations to whom they all apply—evidence-based clinical guidelines for systematically

TABLE B.1.
The National Service Framework Standards for Older People

Standard	Aim
1. Rooting out age discrimination	To ensure that older people are never unfairly discriminated against in accessing NHS or social care services as a result of their age.
2. Person-centered care	To ensure that older people are treated as individuals and they receive appropriate care and timely packages of care which meet their needs as individuals, regardless of health and social services boundaries.
3. Intermediate care	To provide integrated services to promote faster recovery from illness, prevent unnecessary acute hospital admissions, support timely discharge, and maximize independent living.
4. General hospital care	To ensure that older people receive the specialist help they need in hospital and that they receive the maximum benefit from having been in hospital.
5. Stroke	To reduce the incidence of stroke in the population and ensure that those who have had a stroke have prompt access to integrated stroke care services.
6. Falls	To reduce the number of falls which result in serious injury and ensure effective treatment and rehabilitation for those who have fallen
7. Mental health in older people	To promote good mental health in older people and to treat and support those older people with dementia and depression
8. The promotion of health and an active life in older age	To extend the healthy life expectancy of older people

improving all aspects of care. There are currently NSFs for mental health, coronary heart disease, cancer, older people, and diabetes, with others for children, renal, and long-term medical conditions on their way.

Although the new PCT-led commissioning framework and the new GMS contract will help accelerate integration and a systems approach, the NSFs have a particular relevance in promoting the integration of personal care over the lifetime of an individual. They focus not just on treatment, but also on prevention, diagnosis, self-care (in particular, the self-management of long-term conditions), and rehabilitation. The standards for older people's services are summarized in table B.1.

Care for People with Multiple Health Problems

Service issues and the self-management tasks in chronic disease management differ according to which population is being dealt with. The main groups are those with disease-specific chronic conditions and those with multiple health problems (see table B.2).

Patients with multiple health problems often have associated features that create additional challenges, such as polypharmacy, resulting in in-

TABLE B.2.
Chronic Disease Management for Two Groups

| Groups | Elements of Care | |
	Preventive Health	Acute Exacerbations
Disease specific	Service needs • Ongoing systematic care Self-management tasks • Day-to-day lifestyle change: usually unpleasant tasks for long-term gain; motivation hard; may choose not to comply	Service needs • "Fix it" by the acute service Self-management tasks • Rapid rehabilitation to previous state; motivation to follow instructions high, short term • Opportunity to motivate for prevention
Multiple health problems	Service needs • Promoting independence (service models embryonic at present) Self-management tasks • Developing social networks, using community heath resources; generally rapid positive feedback: motivation potentially high	Service needs • "Fix it" by acute service but less perfect outcome (stepped deterioration) • Immediate care for rehabilitation • Caregiver support Self-management tasks • Carrying out specific relevant tasks to aid realistic recovery—motivation can be high Combined • Realistic adaptation to end of life issues

creased drug interactions, side effects, and poor compliance; diagnostic challenge due to atypical disease presentation; reduced physiological reserve leading to rapid loss of homeostasis after minimal challenge; sensory and cognitive impairments; and complex and sometimes fragile social networks.

To some extent, the English health care system is well suited to caring for people with complex problems. Primary health care is well developed, with patients benefiting from easy access to a range of professionals, including general medical practitioners, community nurses, pharmacists, dentists, opticians, etc. Patients shop around when they move to an area but then tend to build long-term relationships with a small number of trusted practitioners for their health care. Apart from the inner cities, where there are problems of recruitment and retention and more mobile populations, primary care practitioners often remain in one locality for many years.

Another strength of the English system has been the development of effective partnerships between health and social care, despite the fact that health care is managed as a national service, and social care is managed through local government. Partnerships will be improved further with the introduction of a shared-records system in health and social care for the identification of needs and planning care. This development is part of a plan to provide consistent standards of health and social care for people with age-related needs (Philp, 2003).

The English system also benefits from having long-established specialties in geriatric medicine and old-age psychiatry, which are among the biggest specialties in internal medicine and psychiatry, respectively. Both have a focus on treating people with multiple health problems and have influenced mainstream work in hospital and mental health services, respectively. They have, for example, pioneered the development of multidisciplinary stroke, falls, and dementia care services.

However, a gap has opened between specialist practice in hospitals and primary care. By international standards, acute hospital stays in England have comparatively long lengths. Intermediate care services are being developed to support earlier discharge (post-acute care), avoid unnecessary hospital admission (hospital at home), and provide care closer to or in the patient's home. Intermediate care services blur the boundary between primary and secondary care. When developed well, they bring together the different strengths of primary care practitioners and hospital secondary-care specialists. Integrating these levels of care is of particular benefit to people with complex health needs, who frequently move between primary and secondary care. Nursing staff play a central role in the care of these patients, ensuring appropriate use of primary, intermediate, and secondary care services.

A Model for Nurse-Led Chronic Disease Management: Castlefields

Castlefields is a group practice serving an area of social deprivation in a town called Runcorn situated in the North West of England. Many years ago, health care professionals in Runcorn recognized that good chronic disease management is essential to maintain people's health and to help manage their workload.

In a joint project with social services, Castlefields Health Centre was able to show that systematic care of individual patients with chronic illness, if underpinned by good information and preferably led by nurses with the active support of doctors and social care workers, leads to better quantitative and qualitative outcomes of care. (See exhibit B.1.) Patients prefer to be in their homes, and in this project hospital utilization was reduced and clinical measurements improved. List-based general practice enabled better accountability of the clinicians and a population and individual patient focus to care.

Castlefields has also pioneered chronic disease management for patients with more clearly defined diseases, using easily available information to identify and track their progress; including heart disease, cancers, hypertension, asthma, chronic obstructive pulmonary disease, hypothyroidism, epilepsy, and rheumatoid arthritis. Patient outcomes have improved, for example, with a re-

EXHIBIT B.1

Case Management at Castlefields Health Centre

An urban, deprived practice, Castlefields Health Centre, participated in a joint project with Halton Social Services designed to reduce admissions and length of stay among people older than 65 years of age with poor health status in Runcorn, Cheshire, a city of approximately 65,000. The practice population was 11,900, of whom 1170 were over 65 years of age and 471 were over 75. Targeted case management, proactive discharge planning, and close working on the ground between a practice-based social worker and a nominated district nurse were the project's three key elements. Practices in Runcorn not participating in the project area continued to deploy community nursing in the usual manner and accessed social services and community mental health services through normal channels.

A qualified social worker, managed by Halton Social Services, was appointed Social Care Manager. He was responsible for the day-to-day management of the project and had an office in the practice building with computer access to both the medical and social records. He was also responsible for all the elderly social work input to the Castlefields registered population. One of the district nurses was appointed nursing care manager to work with the project half-time while remaining a part of the district nurse team. A community psychiatric nurse provided seven hours per week to address functional mental health issues that arose in the project.

A close working relationship was forged between the social care manager and the district nurse. They worked together to coordinate care and deploy packages of support, usually after a joint assessment, including both medical and social services. Referrals were accepted from any member of the primary health care team or from consumers or their caregivers.

Links were established with the three local acute care hospitals that dealt with the overwhelming majority of the acute admissions. They provided information on admissions and accident and emergency attendances, so that the discharge-planning element of the project could begin on admission.

For inclusion in the case management element of the project, consumers must be registered at Castlefields Health Centre, be 65 years of age or older and have at least three of the following:

- Four or more active chronic diagnoses
- Four or more medications for more than six months
- Two or more hospitalizations in the past 12 months
- Two or more accident and emergency attendances in the past 12 months
- Significant impairment in one or more major Activity of Daily Living (ADL)
- Significant impairment in one or more instrumental ADLs, particularly where there is no support system in place
- Consumers in the top 3% of frequent visitors to the practice

- Consumers who have had two or more outpatient appointments
- Consumers whose total hospital stay exceeds four weeks in a year
- Consumers whose social work contact exceeded four assessment visits in each three-month period
- Consumers whose pharmacy bill exceeds £100 per month

Consumers meeting the criteria were contacted by the case management nurse for follow-up, health education, practical advice, support, and referral to other services. The fundamental aim was for consumers to manage their chronic conditions better.

The most significant result was improved communication among professionals within the health center and with outside agencies. Social work assessments were carried out on the day of referral for 97% of cases and within two working days for the rest. Previously, an "urgent" visit took three weeks. The case management nurse visited the wards to begin discharge planning within two working days of admission, in most cases. Previously, discharge planning began toward the end of the inpatient stay if at all.

The level of awareness improved in Castlefields Health Centre about the support mechanisms available within the community and the locality. Access to services was easier for consumers who have a low level need for intervention, as all professionals, especially district nurses, were able to point them in the right direction.

Forty-eight individuals (4% of the over 65-year-olds) were identified for case management. The case management nurse managed nine exclusively. The case management nurse and social care manager jointly managed 35. The management of four patients also included input from the mental health nurse. The district nurse's caseload was reduced because of more efficient discharge planning and better chronic disease management.

After the project had been running a year, comparisons were made with the rest of Runcorn. Castlefields saw a 14% reduction in hospital admissions, whereas the rest of Runcorn followed the national trend by increasing 9%. All three elements of the project played a part in these results. The length of stay declined 31%, compared with the rest of Runcorn, which fell by only 6%. This was the most dramatic change and is accounted for by the hospital discharge planning.

The hospital received the most benefits, experiencing less pressure on its acute beds from Castlefields residents. An average cost for an elderly acute bed is at least £342 per day. The bed days saved were 930 compared with the previous year, amounting to at lease £318,060 for one practice in one year.

Castlefields Health Centre and Halton Social Services experienced no extra costs. The Castlefields registered population remained within their social services budget, even though the rest of Runcorn was overspent. There was no flood of cases needing expensive social services packages. The numbers entering residential and nursing care remained within expected levels.

This project demonstrates that the barriers between health and social care at "street level" can be broken down. Social services and district nurses share the same clientele. It thus makes perfect sense to integrate and coordinate their activity so that assessments can be made together and packages of care can be designed and implemented jointly. In this project each consumer was referred only once but was exposed to the services of both organizations. There was no need for further written referral between the services and both responded equally quickly.

The notion of case management also has benefits. People were identified as having high risk for a further breakdown of care requiring an emergency admission. They were pro-actively managed by both organizations. This aspect of the project seems to have contributed to the reduction of individuals being admitted.

Jayne Penney, National Primary Care Development Team, England
David Lyon, M.D., National Clinical Director for Primary Care, England

duction of incidence and death from myocardial infarction of more than 50%. However, to illustrate best practice in chronic disease management of a single disease entity, we turn now to an example from another setting in England.

A Model for Disease-Specific Care

The management of care for people with diabetes is a particularly important example of disease-specific care. The model of diabetes care in Northumbria offers a case study of best-practice chronic care in the United Kingdom. Northumbria is the largest geographical health care area in the United Kingdom. It covers 500,000 people, 94 general practices, and 3 general and 6 community hospitals. There are areas of affluence and extreme rural and postindustrial poverty. The ethnic minority population is small. The model of diabetes care developed in one part of the area, North Tyneside, during the past 15–20 years. The approach has been transferred rapidly to the larger area of Northumberland.

Nature of the Model

The secondary care service has changed its focus and working practices fundamentally to become a "specialist" service. It acts as an expert resource and coordinator of services, offering proactive support for others providing direct diabetes care everywhere in the patch, including primary care, hospitals, and other institutions.

Diabetes care is acknowledged as being a primary care-based responsibility. The target of "85% of all clinical care will take place within primary care" is being achieved rapidly. Care is based in individual primary care practices. All practices have received increased funding in the last two years to enable them to provide an increasingly structured multidisciplinary approach on site. Several localities use a formal capitation scheme for the work done.

The Specialist Service is responsible for providing, coordinating, and developing all support services within the practices and throughout the patch. It also provides all the clinical care for children, young adults, pregnant women, and 15% of the clinical episodes involving complex multidimensional problems.

There is a unified management led by a clinical director-general manager and a service budget. Day-to-day the service is run by a small team of senior staff representing the main specialist functions and with appropriate geographical spread (education, training, administration, social services, psychology, hospital care, primary care coordination, clinical care, and heads of dietetics and podiatry).

The service is delivered by many multidisciplinary teams based in or around primary care localities or the main hospitals. Individual staff all have roles that extend beyond their conventional specialist training. Most have an additional locality link and an area of specialist responsibility. Everyone is expected to look beyond the individual patient encounter to facilitate care for the individual and to seek opportunities or gaps for service improvement, to take action or report back for help. Staff are part of a "matrix" or "system" of care and everyone is responsible for sustaining or improving it.

The specialist service manages (and holds the budget for) doctors (currently consultants and specialist registrars), all specialist nurses, services facilitators and coordinators, administration (including register and eye-screening support), all specialist, primary care, and "Healthy Hearts" dietetics, specialist podiatrists, and psychologists. The service has links with and manages much of the Healthy Hearts program (vascular nurses, physical education advisors and liaison staff, psychologists and facilitators).

This coordinated approach provides immense flexibility in working practices, skill development, and training, offers consistency of approach across all traditional institutional sectors, and builds day-to-day trust among staff. For instance, specialist-trained dieticians work as part of primary care diabetes teams, the skill mix of clinics can be changed according to varying referral patterns, and new problems arising anywhere can have a targeted solution found quickly.

The key determinates of success include:

- The specialist service has a formal management structure that differs from the loose coordination of consultant-led services more common in the United Kingdom.

- The service is based on a clear vision set out as aims and principles and developed by a wide range of stakeholders, including people with diabetes. It is signed up for by senior members of all the participating organizations and modeled in the approach to staff management. The principles are regularly reviewed and used as an operational checklist.

- Integrated clinical, operational, and budgetary accountability supports a rapid and flexible response to need.

- Patient-centered principles are applied, i.e., care is organized around the needs of patients and not traditional service structures.

- A multipronged approach is taken to developing and maintaining service improvement.

Principles of the Service

All aspects of the Service are developed from and evaluated against these principles.

- Patient centeredness: A high priority is put on responding to individual needs, not just in terms of access and service responsiveness. All staff are trained in active listening and a range of helpful responses by involving their individual skills, accessing the skills and expertise of other team members, and using their knowledge of the Service to facilitate a rapid and tailored response.

- Empowerment: Building on these principles, the Service uses every opportunity to help people with diabetes feel confident in making appropriate choices and managing their own diabetes. In a similar way the Service works to help primary care (and others) to be and feel confident in delivering high-quality diabetes services. Both people with diabetes and health care professional service users should be able to influence the strategic and operational direction of the overall service and the parts that apply to them.

- Structured care across a system: Every aspect of the Service is planned (organized) to include the development and maintenance of patient centeredness and user empowerment. This includes the evaluation of new evidence and its dissemination, clinical care and consultation, patient education, staff training, and quality assurance. The local health-diabetes economy is a complex interrelated system in which each part can influence and support all others in achieving excellent outcomes.

- Teamwork: It is accepted that medical and nonmedical aspects of care for an individual should be integrated. All clinical care is multidisciplinary at the point of delivery. This not only avoids multiple appointments but also enables the person with diabetes and the health care professionals to work together to develop a truly integrated "holistic" care plan. Thus, teamwork is at the heart of every aspect of the Service from direct clinical care to organization. The fundamental principles of this (that everyone should be clear about the aims of the activity, their role within it, and how they work together) are thus reviewed regularly.

- Quality assurance, evaluation, and monitoring: Quality assurance methods include audit, routine monitoring, and involvement in internal and external self-assessment and benchmarking. Information from the primary and specialist services is shared, coordinated, and used for service improvement.

Comparisons with the United States

It is instructive to consider how far this approach to care is unique to the United Kingdom and how much is similar to the Chronic Care Model in the United States.[13] Both have common antecedents in the literature and European experience of the 1980s(Wagner, Austin & von Korff, 1996b). Both have the same essential elements of chronic care: these are self-management, decision support, delivery system redesign, clinical information systems, health care organization, and community resources. In the United Kingdom the aim has been equality of input using a complex, multifaceted approach (Bradley, Wiles, Kinmonth, Mant, & Gantley, 1999). In Northumbria this has been associated with sustained levels of process performance and outcomes equal to those in a major, highly resourced trial, the UKPDS (Whitford, Roberts, & Griffin, 2004). The United States, in contrast, has used the Chronic Care Model to apply the principles in a targeted approach built on case management of high-risk or high-cost cases with demonstrable improvement in costs and reduction in the use of hospital beds.

Summary

The National Health Service remains a service that responds to need irrespective of the patient's ability to pay. Equity has been achieved sometimes at the expense of responsiveness and choice compared with health care systems in other developed countries. However, there has recently been a drive in the United Kingdom to reduce waiting times for investigations and treatment. There is a risk that this will increase the focus of health service activity toward episodic care and away from the traditional strengths in chronic illness care. Nonetheless, health policy is also encouraging a strengthening of chronic illness care, increasing capacity for timely response and choice in acute and procedure-based services. In part, this is driven by an expectation that the demand for acute services will be reduced. This is supported by international research about the impact of self-management across a range long-term conditions (Montgomery et al., 1994), and by our own experience described in the preceding case studies. The new powers of primary care organizations to commission the whole system of local health care services in England and incentives to improve quality have created new opportunities to improve chronic illness care in the United Kingdom. Getting services right for people with single disease entities such as diabetes and people (mostly very old) with multiple chronic illnesses will provide two contrasting tests of the new care systems.

Notes

Introduction

1. President's New Freedom Commission on Mental Health. Final Report to the President. July 2003. www.mentalhealthcommission.gov/reports/reports.htm (accessed July 30, 2003).

2. For a good review of the problems besetting the treatment of chronic mental illness see Improving Chronic Illness Care, a national program of the Robert Wood Johnson Foundation. www.improvingchroniccare.org/change/model/components.html

Chapter 2. The Dimensions of Chronic Illness

1. Global disease burden is measured by using disability-adjusted life years, or DALY. One DALY is considered one lost year of "health and the burden of disease is considered the gap between a person's current health status and the health status that one could expect with old age, perfect health, and no disability" (WHO, 2002).

2. "Out-of-pocket expenditures" in this section do not include health insurance premiums.

Chapter 3. How the Current System Fails People with Chronic Illness

1. Pathology is defined as the damage or abnormal processes that occur within an organ or organ system inside the body, whereas pathophysiology is the functional changes that accompany a particular syndrome or disease.

2. Self-efficacy can be defined as people's belief in their own ability to succeed at something they want to do.

3. Underuse is defined as the failure to provide health care services where the expected benefits to the patient clearly outweigh the risks of harm. Overuse refers to the use of health care services where the risks of harm to the patient exceed the expected benefits. Misuse occurs when appropriate or recommended treatments are provided in an inferior manner (e.g., failure to follow up on a positive test result).

4. The Dartmouth Atlas of Health Care. 2000. Center for the Evaluative Clinical Sciences at Dartmouth Medical School. www.dartmouthatlas.org/99US/chap_7_sec_1.php (accessed July 28, 2003).

5. The Dartmouth Atlas of Health Care. 2000. Center for the Evaluative Clini-

cal Sciences at Dartmouth Medical School. www.dartmouthatlas.org/99US /chap_7 _sec_1.php (accessed July 28, 2003).

6. With understatement, the researchers conclude that "the gap between what we know works and what is actually done is substantial enough to *warrant attention*" (McGlynn et al., 2003). (Emphasis added.)

Chapter 4. Reorganizing Care in the Face of Chronic Illness

1. Medicare's "Voluntary Chronic Care Improvement" program, an element of the Medicare Prescription Drug, Improvement, and Modernization Act of 2003, is discussed in exhibit 4.1.

2. The Expert Patient: A New Approach to Chronic Disease Management for the 21st Century. http://www.doh.gov.uk/healthinequalities/ep_report.pdf (accessed July 24, 2003).

3. Thus, not an "interdisciplinary" team as defined above.

4. The Disease Management Association of America (DMAA) was formed in 1999 as the national trade association for DM organizations. The professional journals include *Disease Management and Health Outcomes* www.adis.com/page.asp?objectID=43) and *Disease Management,* the official publication of the DMAA (www.dmaa. .org/dmho.html) (accessed July 24, 2003).

5. The Disease Management Association of America (DMAA). www.dmaa.org/ (accessed July 30, 2003).

6. This approach is the underlying model for the new Medicare pilot project, "Voluntary Chronic Care Improvement"; see exhibit 4.1.

7. "Case management" is the most widely used term, although "care management" may be a more accurate alternative because the management process at issue is designed to improve an individual patient's *care.*

8. This broad definition excludes so-called "case management" programs that are either designed only reduce hospital length of stay or to identify the least costly alternative among covered treatments.

Chapter 5. The Right Health Care Workers with the Right Skills

1. We use the term "health care professionals" to refer to all workers trained and licensed to provide health care services to patients including, for example, nurses, pharmacists, dentists, all types of therapists, physicians, chiropractors, and social workers. We reserve the term "clinicians" to refer to all health care professionals who are responsible for the direct observation and treatment of patients. Thus, as used here, "clinicians" include physicians, advanced practice nurses, and other health care professionals who are responsible for patient care. The term does not include health care professionals, such as pharmacists, technicians, and aides, who carry out the orders of those responsible for a patient's care.

2. The Institute of Medicine defines primary care as "the provision of integrated, accessible health care services by clinicians who are accountable for addressing a large majority of personal health care needs, developing a sustained partnership with patients, and practicing in the context of family and community."

3. The ten disciplines include four nursing disciplines (nurse practitioners, certified nurse-midwives, certified registered nurse anesthetists, and clinical nurse specialists), physician assistants, chiropractors, naturopaths, optometrists, podiatrists, and practitioners of acupuncture and herbal medicine

4. Another source of primary care is physician assistants, who generally go through a two- to four-year training program and work under the supervision of a physician. They can extend the physician's productivity by caring for many routine problems, but they are not generally viewed as bringing new skills to bear.

5. Registered nurses (RNs) provide professional nursing care to patients, assessing patient health problems and needs; developing and implementing nursing care plans; maintaining medical records; assisting patients in complying with the prescribed medical regimen; and supervising licensed practical nurses (LPNs) and nursing assistants. Registered nurses can be licensed following a two-year associate degree program, a four-year baccalaureate program, or a (less common) three-year diploma program.

6. U.S. Department of Health and Human Services, Health Research and Services Administration, Bureau of Health Professions. *Health workforce analysis: Projected supply, demand and shortages of Registered Nurses 2000–2020.* http://bhpr.hrsa.gov/healthworkforce/rnproject/default.htm (accessed July 28, 2003).

7. Physician training combines four years of medical school training, termed "undergraduate medical education," and a subsequent period of training in a medical specialty varying in length from three to seven years, depending on the specialty, termed "graduate medical education" or GME. Graduate medical education is sometimes referred to as residency training.

8. The core competencies are part of the ACGME "Outcomes Project" to enhance residency education through outcomes assessment. See the Accreditation Council of Graduate Medical Education's Outcomes Project at www.acgme.org/outcome/comp/compFull.asp (accessed July 28, 2003).

9. The Cochrane Library is a collection of evidence-based medical databases on the effects of health care interventions.

10. Ironically, the arguments now used to differentiate the care provided by advanced practice nurses from physician care mirror those used several decades ago to highlight the unique nature of family practice. Publications from the American Academy of Family Practice characterize family physicians as "specialists whose training focuses on the whole person, not just body systems or specific diseases. The family physician's care utilizes knowledge of the patient in the context of the family and community. Family physicians encourage their patients' participation in achieving good health. They emphasize prevention of problems and teach patients to take more responsibility for staying well" (Flanagan, 1998).

Chapter 7. Innovative Technology

1. The terminology in this area is confusing and in flux. Among the terms that have been used to describe the application of information, computer, and communication technology to health and health care are *medical informatics, consumer health informatics, telemedicine, telehealth,* and *eHealth.* These terms are defined differently by experts in the field and some terms overlap, except for "telemedicine," which has a relatively clear consensus definition. This chapter avoids these terms and focuses instead on the various applications of information technology in health care.

2. A tablet PC, roughly the size of a clipboard, combines the computing power of a PC with the mobility and ease of use of a personal digital assistant (PDA).

3. The barriers that restrain increased use of IT in health care are discussed later in this chapter.

4. See, Executive Order 13335, issued April 27, 2004.

5. These are also referred to as the electronic medical record (EMRs) or computerized patient records (CPRs).

6. PND (paroxysmal nocturnal dyspnea) is when one wakes up during the night suddenly short of breath. Orthopnea is the plight of a person who can breathe easily only when sitting straight or standing erect. Edema is the presence of abnormally large amounts of fluid in the intercellular tissue spaces of a person's body. BPV (benign positional vertigo) is when one feels the room spinning when moving one's head because of a small stone in the inner ear.

7. The Decade of Health Information Technology: Delivering Consumer-centric and Information-rich Health Care. Framework for Strategic Action. July 21, 2004. www.hsrnet.net/nhii/materials/strategic_framework.pdf

8. The Leapfrog Group's other two initial methods to improve patient safety are evidence-based hospital referral and intensive care unit physician staffing. See: The Leapfrog Group, www.leapfroggroup.org/safety1.htm (accessed July 29, 2003).

9. In October 1999, in what is thought to be the first malpractice verdict nationwide to rest on a doctor's illegible handwriting, a jury in Odessa, Texas, ordered Ramachandra Kolluru, M.D., to pay $225,000 to the family of Ramon Vasquez, who died after a pharmacist misread Dr. Kolluru's writing. The 42-year-old heart patient was given the wrong medication at eight times the recommended dosage. Two weeks later, he was dead from an apparent heart attack. See: www.ama-assn.org/sci-pubs/amnews/pick_99/pr121122.htm

10. Survey conducted in January 2003 by CIGNA, "Net Effect: Online Health-Care Tools Still Missing the Mark for Consumers." www.prnewswire.com/cgi-bin/micro_stories.pl?ACCT=149478&TICK=CI20&STORY=/www/story/03-102003/0001904988&EDATE=Mar+10,+2003

11. In April 2003, researchers at the University of Pittsburg reported the development of a noninvasive method to test blood sugar levels in patients with diabetes. Instead of the common method of drawing blood from a finger prick—which is uncomfortable and depends on patient skill and compliance—the new method would embed the sensing material into contact lenses worn in the patient's eyes. Patients will then determine glucose levels by looking in a mirror and comparing the color of the sensing material with a color chart to indicate glucose concentrations.

12. Ken Riff, M.D., Medtronic. June 5, 2003. University of Minnesota Center on Aging Summer Institute, Minneapolis, MN.

13. Assistive Technology Act of 1998 (S.2432).

14. For more information on the ILSA project, see: www.htc.honeywell.com /projects/ilsa/about_introduction.html

15. Andrew Wiesenthal, The Permanente Federation. May 22, 2003. University of Minnesota. HIMSS (Healthcare Information and Management Systems Society) Conference. Minneapolis, MN.

Chapter 8. Prevention

1. Changes in the environment and the use of adaptive equipment account for the rest of the decline

2. Paradoxically, eliminating certain chronic diseases may actually increase, in some instances, the numbers of persons with disabilities because many common chronic diseases are fatal. For example, preventing cancer or heart disease may allow people who survive to then develop another chronic disease. Preventing or curing nonfatal chronic diseases such as arthritis would reduce disability more than eliminating fatal chronic conditions.

3. Establishing the effectiveness of such screening programs is difficult because of "detection bias." Uncovering a disease earlier in its course may make survival appear longer. Establishing the effectiveness of screening requires either randomized trials or large-scale epidemiological studies, which compare mortality rates in populations in which the screening test is used aggressively with those in which it is used less.

Chapter 9. Paying for Chronic Care

1. There is some provision for very long stays.

2. British general practitioners have long been paid on a capitation basis, but their most recent contract includes performance standards that are linked to payment.

Chapter 10. The Context for Reform

1. For information on the IOM's Health Care Quality Initiative, see www.iom .edu/focuson.asp?id=8089

2. Medicare has two parts: part A is for hospital services and part B is for physician services. All eligible beneficiaries are automatically enrolled in part A; although part B is voluntary, it is subsidized (about 75% of costs are paid by the government), and the vast majority of those eligible sign on.

3. A controversial new drug benefit has been authorized to go into effect in 2006.

4. The National Bipartisan Commission on the Future of Medicare. http: //medicare.commission.gov/medicare/ (accessed July 28, 2003).

Chapter 11. Next Steps

1. Improving Chronic Illness Care, a national program of the Robert Wood Johnson Foundation. www.improvingchroniccare.org/change/model/components .html (accessed July 30, 2003).

2. This section is based on a description of the Chronic Care Model at the Web site of "Improving Chronic Illness Care." www.improvingchroniccare.org/change/index.html (accessed July 30, 2003).

3. Improving Chronic Illness Care, a national program of the Robert Wood Johnson Foundation. www.improvingchroniccare.org/change/ICIC%20Chronic%20Care%20Model%20refinements%20July%202003.doc (accessed July 30, 2003).

4. Profiles of programs using the Chronic Care Model in a variety of diverse health care organizations are recorded at: www.improvingchroniccare.org/ACT_Report_May_2002_Curing_The_System.pdf

5. RAND Health. Improving Chronic Illness Care Evaluation. www.rand.org/health/ICICE/about.html (accessed July 30, 2003).

6. The Carle Health Care System (Carle Foundation Hospital and Carle Clinic Association) is a vertically integrated system in Urbana, Illinois. The Carle Healthcare System serves as the regional medical center for over 1.2 million in the predominantly rural area of east-central Illinois and west-central Indiana. The system includes a 295–bed hospital, a 240 bed skilled nursing facility, home care services, retail pharmacies, and other health care services. Carle Clinic Association is a multispecialty, physician group practice with approximately 300 practicing physicians. The Foundation Hospital is the primary teaching hospital for the University of Illinois College of Medicine.

7. The description of the Carle System's model in this section is based on the Carle Foundation Hospital's 2002 grant proposal to the Research Retirement Foundation.

8. This section on Kaiser Permanente's chronic care initiatives was written by Richard Della Penna, M.D., Director, Kaiser Permanente Aging Network, The Permanente Federation.

9. This description of the CHESS program is based on information on their Web site. University of Wisconsin—Madison. Center for Health Systems Research and Analysis. Comprehensive Health Enhancement Support System (CHESS): http://chess.chsra.wisc.edu/Chess/abtchess/abtchess_whatis.htm (accessed July 30, 2003).

10. National Committee for Quality Assurance (NCQA). The Health Plan Employer Data and Information Set (HEDIS) program. www.ncqa.org/Programs/HEDIS/index.htm (accessed July 30, 2003).

11. A national organization of such professionals, Professionals with Personal Experience with Chronic Care (PPECC), operates a Web site that shares stories: www.ppecc.org/.

Appendix A

1. www.WorldHealthNews.harvard.edu

2. Disclaimer: The author of this essay is a member of the AHCJ Board of Directors.

3. www.pbs.org/fredfriendly/whocares/index.html

Appendix B

    1. See *The NHS Plan—A Plan for Investment, a Plan for Reform* at www.doh.gov.uk /nhsplan/index.htm

    2. "Primary care organization" is a generic phrase that includes primary care groups (PCGs), primary care trusts (PCTs), and also the equivalent but structurally and functionally different organizations of the other U.K. countries. PCTs have far more primary care clinical input than any previous NHS organization. In one sense, a PCT is a misnomer because they have the funding not only for primary care but for all the local NHS. Local means the local geographically based population of a PCT, groups of PCTs, or of the larger Strategic Health Authorities—but still part of the NHS.

    3. Primary care groups (PCGs) were the predecessors of Primary Care Trusts. They were subcommittees of the now-defunct Health Authorities; thus, they did not have their own budget but had GPs and other primary care clinical professionals in management and leadership positions.

    4. Primary care trusts (PCTs) have replaced Health Authorities as the "commissioner" of health care for a defined geographically based population. They control health spending for a defined geographic area. PCTs also provide community-based nursing and therapy services. They are statutory NHS organizations with primary care clinicians in leadership positions on a Professional Executive Committee. The PCT has a chief executive, a management team, and a nonexecutive board of a majority of lay people as do other NHS organizations.

    5. General practitioners (GPs) work in general practices with a varying number of GPs; the average is three GPs. These practices have a registered population of patients and staff employed by the GPs, which often includes nurses. That team is often known as the primary care team. But an extended team, including PCT-employed nurses and other staff and even hospital and social care staff, can be organized to provide care for a general-practice patient population and they also can be referred to as a primary care team. Any other community-based team can be referred to as a primary care team but the term usually applies to a GP patient population.

    6. For more details, see www.nice.org.uk

    7. For more details, see Blenkinsop (2003) "Community Pharmacy Minor Ailments Scheme" at www.rpsgb.org.uk/nhsplan/pdfs/minailmat.pdf

    8. For more details, see www.ohn.gov.uk

    9. For more details, see www.medicines-partnership.org

    10. For more details, see "Delivering IT in the NHS" at www.doh.gov.uk/ipu /programme/index.htm

    11. For more details, see OSCAR (Online System for Comparative Analysis & Reporting) Avoca Systems at www.avoca.co.uk

    12. For more details, see National Service Frameworks at www.doh.gov.uk/nsf /index.htm

    13. The Chronic Care Model is discussed in chapter 11.

References

ABIM Foundation (2002). Medical professionalism in the new millennium: A physician charter. Ann Intern Med, 136(3), 243–246.

Adams, K., & Corrigan, J. (2003). Priority areas for national action: Transforming health care quality. Washington, DC: National Academy Press.

Adams, W. L., McIlvain, H. E., Lacy, N. L., Magsi, H., Crabtree, B. F., Yenny, S. K., et al. (2002). Primary care for elderly people: Why do doctors find it so hard? Gerontologist, 42(6), 835–842.

Agostini, J., Baker, D., & Bogardus, S. (2001). Geriatric evaluation and management units for hospitalized patients. Agency for Healthcare Research and Quality. Retrieved July 29, 2003, from www.ahcpr.gov/clinic/ptsafety/chap30.htm

Aiken, L. H. (2003). Achieving an interdisciplinary workforce in health care. N Engl J Med, 348(2), 164–166.

Alcecxih, L., Zeruld, S., & Olearczyk, B. (2001). Characteristics of caregivers based on the survey of income and program participation. National Family Caregiver Support Program. Retrieved July 31, 2003, www.aoa.gov/carenetwork/AlecxihMonograph.pdf

Anderson, G. F. (1997). In search of value: An international comparison of cost, access, and outcomes. Health Aff (Millwood), 16(6), 163–171.

Anderson, G., & Knickman, J. R. (2001). Changing the chronic care system to meet people's needs. Health Aff (Millwood), 20(6), 146–160.

Applebaum, R., & Phillips, P. (1990). Assuring the quality of in-home care: The "other" challenge for long-term care. Gerontologist, 30(4), 444–450.

Arno, P. S., Levine, C., & Memmott, M. M. (1999). The economic value of informal caregiving. Health Aff (Millwood), 18(2), 182–188.

Aubert, R. E., Herman, W. H., Waters, J., Moore, W., Sutton, D., Peterson, B. L., et al. (1998). Nurse case management to improve glycemic control in diabetic patients in a health maintenance organization. A randomized, controlled trial. Ann Intern Med, 129(8), 605–612.

Bach, P. B., et al. (2004). Primary care physicians who treat blacks and whites. N Engl J Med, 351(6), 575–584.

Baker, L., Wagner, T. H., Singer, S. & Bundorf, M. K. (2003). Use of the Internet and e-mail for health care information: Results from a national survey. JAMA, 289(18), 2400–2406.

Baldwin, D. (1994). The role of interdisciplinary education and teamwork in primary care and health care reform. Washington, DC: U.S. Department of Health and Human Services, Health Resources and Services Administration, Bureau of Health Professions.

Barlow, J., Wright, C., Sheasby, J., Turner, A. & Hainsworth, J. (2002). Self-management approaches for people with chronic conditions: A review. Patient Educ Couns, 48(2), 177–187.

Bates, D. W., Leape, L. L., Cullen, D. J., Laird, N., Petersen, L. A., Teich, J. M., et al. (1998). Effect of computerized physician order entry and a team intervention on prevention of serious medication errors. JAMA, 280(15), 1311–1316.

Bates, D. W., Teich, J. M., Lee, J., Seger, D., Kuperman, G. J., Ma'Luf, N., et al. (1999). The impact of computerized physician order entry on medication error prevention. J Am Med Inform Assoc, 6(4), 313–321.

Baumgarten, M., Hanley, J. A., Infante-Rivard, C., Battista, R. N., Becker, R. & Gauthier, S. (1994). Health of family members caring for elderly persons with dementia. A longitudinal study. Ann Intern Med, 120(2), 126–132.

Beck, A., Scott, J., Williams, P., Robertson, B., Jackson, D., Gade, G., et al. (1997). A randomized trial of group outpatient visits for chronically ill older HMO members: The Cooperative Health Care Clinic. J Am Geriatr Soc, 45(5), 543–549.

Bednash, G. (2000). The decreasing supply of registered nurses: Inevitable future or call to action. JAMA, 283(22), 2985–2987.

Beisecker, A. E., Murden, R. A., Moore, W. P., Graham, D. & Nelmig, L. (1996). Attitudes of medical students and primary care physicians regarding input of older and younger patients in medical decisions. Med Care, 34(2), 126–137.

Belleville, J. (2002). The French paradox: Possible involvement of ethanol in the protective effect against cardiovascular diseases. Nutrition, 18(2), 173–177.

Berenson, R., & Horvath, J. (2003). Confronting the barriers to chronic care management in Medicare [web exclusive]. Health Aff. Retrieved July 31, 2003 from www/healthaffairs.org/WebExclusives/Berenson_Web_Excl_012203 .htm

Berland, G. K., Elliott, M. N., Morales, L. S., Algazy, J. I., Kravitz, R. L., Broder, M. S., et al. (2001). Health information on the Internet: Accessibility, quality, and readability in English and Spanish. JAMA, 285(20), 2612–2621.

Berwick, D. (2002). Escape fire: Lessons for the future of health care. New York: Commonwealth Fund.

Billings, J., Anderson, G. M., & Newman, L. S. (1996). Recent findings on preventable hospitalizations. Health Aff (Millwood), 15(3), 239–249.

Blendon, R. J., DesRoches, C. M., Brodie, M., Benson, J. M., Rosen, A. B., Schneider, E., et al. (2002). Views of practicing physicians and the public on medical errors. N Engl J Med, 347(24), 1933–1940.

Blendon, R. J., Brodie, M., Altman, D. E., Benson, J. M., Pelletier, S. R., & Rosenbaum, M. D. (2002, May 29, 2003). Where was health care in the 2002 election [web exclusive]. Health Aff. Retrieved December 11, 2002, from www.healthaffairs.org/WebExclusives/Blendon_Web_Excl_121102.pf.htm

Bodenheimer, T. (1999). Disease management—Promises and pitfalls. N Engl J Med, 340(15), 1202–1205.

Bodenheimer, T. (2000). Disease management in the American market. BMJ, 320(7234), 563–566.

Bodenheimer, T., & Grumbach, K. (2003). Electronic technology: A spark to revitalize primary care? JAMA, 290(2), 259–264.

Bodenheimer, T., Lorig, K., Holman, H. & Grumbach, K. (2002). Patient self-management of chronic disease in primary care. JAMA, 288(19), 2469–2475.

Bodenheimer, T., Wagner, E. H., & Grumbach, K. (2002a). Improving primary care for patients with chronic illness. JAMA, 288(14), 1775–1779.

Bodenheimer, T., Wagner, E. H., & Grumbach, K. (2002b). Improving primary care for patients with chronic illness: The chronic care model, Part 2. JAMA, 288(15), 1909–1914.

Boult, C., Boult, L., & Pacala, J. T. (1998). Systems of care for older populations of the future. J Am Geriatr Soc, 46(4), 499–505.

Boult, C., Boult, L. B., Morishita, L., Dowd, B., Kane, R. L. & Urdangarin, C. F. (2001). A randomized clinical trial of outpatient geriatric evaluation and management. J Am Geriatr Soc, 49(4), 351–359.

Boyd, M. L., Fisher, B., Davidson, A. W. & Neilsen, C. A. (1996). Community-based case management for chronically ill older adults. Nurs Manage, 27(11), 31–32.

Bradley, F., Wiles, R., Kinmonth, A. L., Mant, D. & Gantley, M. (1999). Development and evaluation of complex interventions in health services research: Case study of the Southampton heart integrated care project (SHIP). The SHIP Collaborative Group. BMJ, 318(7185), 711–715.

Brown, R. S., Clement, D. G., Hill, J. W., Retchin, S. M. & Bergeron, J. W. (1993). Do health maintenance organizations work for Medicare? Health Care Financ Rev, 15(1), 7–23.

Brown, S. A., & Grimes, D. E. (1995). A meta-analysis of nurse practitioners and nurse midwives in primary care. Nurs Res, 44(6), 332–339.

Buerhaus, P. I., Staiger, D. O., & Auerbach, D. I. (2000). Implications of an aging registered nurse workforce. JAMA, 283(22), 2948–2954.

Canadian Association on Gerontology. (2000). Policy Statement: Health Promotion for Individual Seniors [Web page]. Retrieved March 20, 2003, from www.cagacg.ca/english/554_e.html

Caplan, A. L., Englehardt, H., & McCartney, J. (1981). Concepts of health and disease: Interdisciplinary perspectives. Reading, MA: Addison-Wesley.

Carter, B., & McGoldrick, M. (1988). The changing family life cycle. New York: Gardner Press.

Casalino, L., Gillies, R. R., Shortell, S. M., Schmittdiel, J. A., Bodenheimer, T., Robinson, J. C., et al. (2003). External incentives, information technology, and organized processes to improve health care quality for patients with chronic diseases. JAMA, 289(4), 434–441.

Cassell, E. (1991). The nature of suffering and the goals of medicine. New York: Oxford University Press.

Centers for Disease Control and Prevention. (2002). Annual smoking-attributable mortality, years of potential life lost, and economic costs—United States, 1995–1999. MMWR Morb Mortal Wkly Rep, 51(14), 300–303.

Centers for Disease Control and Prevention. (2003). Preventing heart disease and stroke. Retrieved October 2003, from www.cdc.gov/nccdphp/pe_factsheets/pe_cvh.htm

Chin, T. (2003, February 17). Doctors pull plug on paperless system. AMNews. Retrieved from www.ama-assn.org/sci-pubs/amnews/pick_03/bi120217.htm

Chmielewski, C. M., Holechek, M. J., McWilliams, D., Powers, K. & Tu, A. (1996). Advanced practice in nephrology nursing. Dial Transplant, 25, 260–270.

Chobanian, A. V., Bakris, G. L., Black, H. R., Cushman, W. C., Green, L. A., Izzo, J. L., Jr., et al. (2003). The seventh report of the Joint National Committee on Prevention, Detection, Evaluation, and Treatment of High Blood Pressure: The JNC 7 report. JAMA, 289(19), 2560–2572.

Christianson, J., Riedel, A., Abelson, D., Hamer, R., Knutson, D. & Taylor, R. (2001). Managed care and the treatment of chronic illness. Thousand Oaks, CA: Sage Publications.

Cintron, G., Bigas, C., Linares, E., Aranda, J. M. & Hernandez, E. (1983). Nurse practitioner role in a chronic congestive heart failure clinic: In-hospital time, costs, and patient satisfaction. Heart Lung, 12(3), 237–240.

Clark, N. M. (2003). Management of chronic disease by patients. Annu Rev Public Health, 24, 289–313.

Clark, N. M., & Gong, M. (2000). Management of chronic disease by practitioners and patients: Are we teaching the wrong things? BMJ, 320(7234), 572–575.

Cohen, A. J. (1998). Caring for the chronically ill: A vital subject for medical education. Acad Med, 73(12), 1261–1266.

Cohen, H. J., Feussner, J. R., Weinberger, M., Carnes, M., Hamdy, R. C., Hsieh, F., et al. (2002). A controlled trial of inpatient and outpatient geriatric evaluation and management. N Engl J Med, 346(12), 905–912.

Coleman, E. A., Eilertsen, T. B., Kramer, A. M., Magid, D. J., Beck, A. & Conner, D. (2001). Reducing emergency visits in older adults with chronic illness. A randomized, controlled trial of group visits. Eff Clin Pract, 4(2), 49–57.

Cooper, B., & Fishman, E. (2003). The interdisciplinary team in the management of chronic conditions: Has its time come? Baltimore: Partnership for Solutions.

Cooper, R. A. (2001). Health care workforce for the twenty-first century: The impact of nonphysician clinicians. Annu Rev Med, 52, 51–61.

Cooper, R. A., Laud, P., & Dietrich, C. L. (1998). Current and projected workforce of nonphysician clinicians. JAMA, 280(9), 788–794.

Cooper, S., & Coleman, P. (2001). Caring for the older person: An exploration of perceptions using personal construct theory. Age Aging, 30(5), 399–402.

Coye, M. J. (2001). No Toyotas in health care: Why medical care has not evolved to meet patients' needs. Health Aff (Millwood), 20(6), 44–56.

Cutler, D. M. (2001). Declining disability among the elderly. Health Aff (Millwood), 20(6), 11–27.

Dahle, K. L., Smith, J. S., Ingersoll, G. L. & Wilson, J. R. (1998). Impact of a nurse practitioner on the cost of managing inpatients with heart failure. Am J Cardiol, 82(5), 686–688, A688.

Davis, B. E., Nelson, D. B., Sahler, O. J. Z., McCurdy, F. A., Goldberg, R. & Greenberg, L. W. (2001). Do clerkship experiences affect medical students' attitudes toward chronically ill patients? Acad Med, 76(8), 815–820.

Davis, J., & Barnes, M. (1997). "More than giving out the pills": Changing attitudes to aged care through continuing education. Geriaction, 15(2), 9–12.

DeBusk, R. F., Miller, N. H., Superko, H. R., Dennis, C. A., Thomas, R. J., Lew, H. T., et al. (1994). A case-management system for coronary risk factor modification after acute myocardial infarction. Ann Intern Med, 120(9), 721–729.

Department of Health. (2000). National Beds Enquiry: Shaping the future NHS: Long-term planning for hospitals and related services. London: Department of Health.

Dick, R., Steen, E., & Demeter, D. (Eds.). (1997). The computer based patient record: An essential technology for healthcare. Washington, DC: National Academy Press.

Dickstein, L. (2001). Educating for professionalism: Creating culture of humanism in medical education. JAMA, 285(24), 3147–3148.

Dimeo, F. C., Stieglitz, R. D., Novelli-Fischer, U., Fetscher, S. & Keul, J. (1999). Effects of physical activity on the fatigue and psychologic status of cancer patients during chemotherapy. Cancer, 85(10), 2273–2277.

DiPollina, L., & Sabate, E. (2003). Adherence to long-term therapies in the elderly. In E. Sabate (Ed.), Adherence to long-term therapies: Evidence for action. Geneva: World Health Organization.

Dixon, J., Lewis, R., Rosen, R., Finlayson, B. & Gray, D. (2004). Can the NHS learn from US managed care organisations? BMJ, 328, 223–225.

Doherty, W. J., & Carroll, J. S. (2002). The families and democracy project. Fam Proc, 41, 579–590.

Donaldson, M., Yordy, K., Lohr, K. & Vanselow, N. (1996). Primary care: America's health in a new era. Washington, DC: Institute of Medicine.

Doolan, D. F., & Bates, D. W. (2002). Computerized physician order entry systems in hospitals: Mandates and incentives. Health Aff (Millwood), 21(4), 180–188.

Downie, L., & Kaiser, R. (2002). The News About the News: American Journalism in Peril. New York: Alfred A. Kopf.

Drinka, T., & Clark, P. (2000). Health care teamwork interdisciplinary practice and teaching. Westport, CT: Auburn House.

Druss, B. G., Marcus, S. C., Olfson, M., Tanielian, T. & Pincus, H. A. (2003). Trends in care by nonphysician clinicians in the United States. N Engl J Med, 348(2), 130–137.

Dudley, R. A., & Luft, H. S. (2001). Managed care in transition. N Engl J Med, 344(14), 1087–1092.

Elasy, T. A., Ellis, S. E., Brown, A. & Pichert, J. W. (2001). A taxonomy for diabetes educational interventions. Patient Educ Couns, 43(2), 121–127.

Ellison, R. C. (2002). Balancing the risks and benefits of moderate drinking. Ann N Y Acad Sci, 957, 1–6.

Eng, T. (2001). The eHealth landscape: A terrain map of emerging information and communication technologies in health & health care. Princeton, NJ: The Robert Wood Johnson Foundation.

Englehardt, H. (1995). Health and disease: Philosophical perspectives (2nd ed.). New York: Macmillan.

Etzwiler, D. D. (2003). Self-management of chronic disease. JAMA, 289(12), 1508; author reply 1509.

Evans, R. G., & Stoddart, G. L. (2003). Consuming research, producing policy? Am J Public Health, 93(3), 371–379.

Eysenbach, G., Powell, J., Kuss, O. & Sa, E. R. (2002). Empirical studies assessing the quality of health information for consumers on the World Wide Web: A systematic review. JAMA, 287(20), 2691–2700.

Feachem, R. G., Sekhri, N. K., & White, K. L. (2002). Getting more for their dollar: a comparison of the NHS with California's Kaiser Permanente. BMJ, 324(7330), 135–141.

Fiatarone, M. A., O'Neill, E. F., Ryan, N. D., Clements, K. M., Solares, G. R., Nelson, M. E., et al. (1994). Exercise training and nutritional supplementation for physical frailty in very elderly people. N Engl J Med, 330(25), 1769–1775.

Fichtenberg, C. M., & Glantz, S. A. (2000). Association of the California Tobacco Control Program with declines in cigarette consumption and mortality from heart disease. N Engl J Med, 343(24), 1772–1777.

Firshein, J. (1999). Filling the geriatric gap: Is the health system prepared for an aging population? (National Health Policy Forum Issue Brief 729). Washington, DC: George Washington University.

Fisher, L., & Weihs, K. L. (2000). Can addressing family relationships improve outcomes in chronic disease? Report of the National Working Group on Family-Based Interventions in Chronic Disease. J Fam Pract, 49(6), 561–566.

Flanagan, L. (1998). Nurse practitioners: Growing competition for family practice? Fam Pract Manag, 5(9), 34–36, 41–43.

Flegal, K. M., Carroll, M. D., Ogden, C. L. & Johnson, C. L. (2002). Prevalence and trends in obesity among US adults, 1999–2000. JAMA, 288(14), 1723–1727.

Fletcher, A. E., Price, G. M., Ng, E. S. W., Stirling, S. L., Bulpitt, C. J., Breeze, E., et al. (2004). Population-based multidimensional assessment of older people in UK general practice: A cluster-randomised factorial trial. Lancet, 364(9446), 1667–1677.

Foote, S. M. (2004). Chronic care improvement in Medicare FFS: Cosmetic or transforming? Washington, DC: George Washington University Press.

Fox, S., & Rainie, L. (2000). The on-line health care revolution: How the web helps Americans take better care of themselves. Pew Internet & American Life Project. Retrieved from www.pewinternet.org/reports/pdfs/PIP_Health_Report.pdf

French, S. A., Story, M., & Jeffery, R. W. (2001). Environmental influences on eating and physical activity. Annu Rev Public Health, 22, 309–335.

Fries, J. F. (1980). Aging, natural death, and the compression of morbidity. N Engl J Med, 303(3), 130–135.

Fries, J. F., & McShane, D. (1998). Reducing need and demand for medical services in high-risk persons. A health education approach. West J Med, 169(4), 201–207.

Fries, J. F., Koop, C. E., Beadle, C. E., Cooper, P. P., England, M. J., Greaves, R. F., et al. (1993). Reducing health care costs by reducing the need and demand for medical services. The Health Project Consortium. N Engl J Med, 329(5), 321–325.

Fries, J. F., Bloch, D. A., Harrington, H., Richardson, N., & Beck, R. (1993). Two-year results of a randomized controlled trial of a health promotion program in a retiree population: The Bank of America Study. Am J Med, 94(5), 455–462.

Fries, J. F., Koop, C. E., Sokolov, J., Beadle, C. E. & Wright, D. (1998). Beyond health promotion: Reducing need and demand for medical care. Health Aff (Millwood), 17(2), 70–84.

Fulmer, T. (2002). Elder mistreatment. Annu Rev Nurs Res, 20, 369–395.

Gagnon, A. J., Schein, C., McVey, L. & Bergman, H. (1999). Randomized controlled trial of nurse case management of frail older people. J Am Geriatr Soc, 47(9), 1118–1124.

Gallagher, D., Rose, J., Rivera, P., Lovett, S. & Thompson, L. W. (1989). Prevalence of depression in family caregivers. Gerontologist, 29(4), 449–456.

Glasgow, R. E., Funnell, M. M., Bonomi, A. E., Davis, C., Beckham, V. & Wagner, E. H. (2002). Self-management aspects of the improving chronic illness care breakthrough series: Implementation with diabetes and heart failure teams. Ann Behav Med, 24(2), 80–87.

Glasgow, R. E., Orleans, C. T., Wagner, E. H., Curry, S. J., & Solberg, L. I. (2001). Does the chronic care model serve also as a template for improving prevention? Milbank Q, 79(4), 579–612, iv–v.

Goins, R. T., Kategile, U., & Dudley, K. C. (2001). Telemedicine, rural elderly, and policy issues. J Aging Soc Policy, 13(4), 53–71.

Goldman, J., & Hudson, Z. (2000). Virtually exposed: Privacy and e-health. Health Aff (Millwood), 19(6), 140–148.

Goldsmith, J., Blumenthal, D., & Rishel, W. (2003). Federal health information policy: A case of arrested development. Health Aff (Millwood), 22(4), 44–55.

Graber, D. R., Bellack, J. P., Musham, C. & O'Neil, E. H. (1997). Academic deans' views on curriculum content in medical schools. Acad Med, 72(10), 901–907.

Grant, R., & Finocchio, L. (1995). Interdisciplinary collaborative teams in primary care: A model curriculum and resource guide. San Francisco: Pew Health Professions Commission.

Greenfield, S., Kaplan, S. H., Ware, J. E., Jr., Yano, E. M. & Frank, H. J. (1988). Patients' participation in medical care: Effects on blood sugar control and quality of life in diabetes. J Gen Intern Med, 3(5), 448–457.

Greenfield, S., Kaplan, S., & Ware, J. E., Jr. (1985). Expanding patient involvement in care. Effects on patient outcomes. Ann Intern Med, 102(4), 520–528.

Griffith, C. H., & Wilson, J. F. (2001). The loss of student idealism in the 3rd-year clinical clerkships. Eval Health Prof, 24(1), 61–71.

Griffiths, C., Kaur, G., Gantley, M., Feder, G., Hillier, S., Goddard, J., et al. (2001). Influences on hospital admission for asthma in south Asian and white adults: Qualitative interview study. BMJ, 323(7319), 962–966.

Grimshaw, J. M., & Russell, I. T. (1993). Effect of clinical guidelines on medical practice: A systematic review of rigorous evaluations. Lancet, 342, 1317–1322.

Grimshaw, J. M., Shirran, L., Thomas, R., Mowatt, G., Fraser, C., Bero, L., et al. (2001). Changing provider behavior: An overview of systematic reviews of interventions. Med Care, 39(8 Suppl. 2), II-2–II-45.

Gross, P. A., Greenfield, S., Cretin, S., Ferguson, J., Grimshaw, J., Grol, R., et al. (2001). Optimal methods for guideline implementation: Conclusions from Leeds Castle meeting. Med Care, 39(8), II-85–II-92.

Grumbach, K., & Bodenheimer, T. (2002). A primary care home for Americans: Putting the house in order. JAMA, 288(7), 889–893.

Gurwitz, J. H., Field, T. S., Harrold, L. R., Rothschild, J., Debellis, K., Seger, A. C., et al. (2003). Incidence and preventability of adverse drug events among older persons in the ambulatory setting. JAMA, 289(9), 1107–1116.

Gustafson, D. H., Hawkins, R. P., Boberg, E. W., McTavish, F., Owens, B., Wise, M., et al. (2002). CHESS: 10 years of research and development in consumer health informatics for broad populations, including the underserved. Int J Med Inform, 65(3), 169–177.

Hanlon, J. T., Schmader, K. E., Boult, C., Artz, M. B., Gross, C. R., Fillenbaum, G. G., et al. (2002). Use of inappropriate prescription drugs by older people. J Am Geriatr Soc, 50(1), 26–34.

Harris Interactive Inc. (2001). Chronic illness and caregiving: Survey of the general public, adults with chronic conditions and caregivers. Rochester, NY: Harris Interactive Inc.

Headrick, L. A., Wilcock, P. M., & Batalden, P. B. (1998). Interprofessional working and continuing medical education. BMJ, 316(7133), 771–774.

Hersh, W. R. (2002). Medical informatics: Improving health care through information. JAMA, 288(16), 1955–1958.

Hill, J. O., & Peters, J. C. (1998). Environmental contributions to the obesity epidemic. Science, 280(5368), 1371–1374.

Hodgson, T. A., & Cohen, A. J. (1999). Medical expenditures for major diseases, 1995. Health Care Financ Rev, 21(2), 119–164.

Hoenig, H., Taylor, D. H., Jr., & Sloan, F. A. (2003). Does assistive technology substitute for personal assistance among the disabled elderly? Am J Public Health, 93(2), 330–337.

Hoffman, C., Rice, D., & Sung, H. Y. (1996). Persons with chronic conditions. Their prevalence and costs. JAMA, 276(18), 1473–1479.

Holman, H., & Lorig, K. (2000). Patients as partners in managing chronic disease. Partnership is a prerequisite for effective and efficient health care. BMJ, 320(7234), 526–527.

Hughes, D. A., Bagust, A., Haycox, A. & Walley, T. (2001). The impact of non-compliance on the cost-effectiveness of pharmaceuticals: A review of the literature. Health Econ, 10(7), 601–615.

Hunink, M. G., Goldman, L., Tosteson, A. N., Mittleman, M. A., Goldman, P. A., Williams, L. W., et al. (1997). The recent decline in mortality from coronary heart disease, 1980–1990. The effect of secular trends in risk factors and treatment. JAMA, 277(7), 535–542.

Hunt, D. L., Haynes, R. B., Hanna, S. E. & Smith, K. (1998). Effects of computer-based clinical decision support systems on physician performance and patient outcomes: A systematic review. JAMA, 280(15), 1339–1346.

Hunter, D. J. (2000). Disease management: Has it a future? It has a compelling logic, but needs to be tested in practice. BMJ, 320(7234), 530.

Hurley, R. E., Freund, D. A., & Gage, B. J. (1991). Gatekeeper effects on patterns of physician use. J Fam Pract, 32(2), 167–174.

Hwang, W., Weller, W., Ireys, H. & Anderson, G. (2001). Out-of-pocket medical spending for care of chronic conditions. Health Aff (Millwood), 20(6), 267–278.

Iglehart, J. K. (1999). The American health care system—Medicare. N Engl J Med, 340(4), 327–332.

Iglehart, J. K. (2003). The dilemma of Medicaid. N Engl J Med, 348(21), 2140–2148.

Institute for Clinical Systems Improvement. (1998). Technology assessment: Case management for chronic illness, the frail elderly, and acute myocardial infarction. Minneapolis, MN: Institute for Clinical Systems Improvement.

Institute for Clinical Systems Improvement. (2001). Technology assessment: Computerized physician order entry (ICSI). Minneapolis, MN: Institute for Clinical Systems Improvement.

Institute of Medicine. (2001). Crossing the quality chasm: A new health system for the 21th century (Vol. 2001). Washington, DC: National Academy Press.

Jennings, B., Callahan, D., & Caplan, A. L. (1988). Ethical challenges of chronic illness. Hastings Cent Rep, 18(1, Suppl.), 1–16.

Johnson, H., & Broder, D. (1996). The system: The American way of politics at the breaking point. Boston: Little Brown and Company.

Johnston, B., Wheeler, L., Deuser, J. & Sousa, K. H. (2000). Outcomes of the Kaiser

Permanente Tele-Home Health Research Project. Arch Fam Med, 9(1), 40–45.

Juniper, E. F., Guyatt, G. H., Feeny, D. H., Ferrie, P. J., Griffith, L. E. & Townsend, M. (1996). Measuring quality of life in children with asthma. Qual Life Res, 5(1), 35–46.

Kamerow, D. B. (2003). How should Medicare cover preventive services?: A policy analysis, a better Medicare for healthier seniors: Recommendations to modernize Medicare's prevention policies (pp. 35–53). Washington, DC: Partnership for Prevention.

Kane, R. A., & Kane, R. L. (1987). Long-term care: Principles, programs, and policies. New York: Springer.

Kane, R. L. (1998). Managed care as a vehicle for delivering more effective chronic care for older persons. J Am Geriatr Soc, 46, 1034–1039.

Kane, R. L., Ouslander, J. P., & Abrass, I. B. (2003). Essentials of clinical geriatrics (5th ed.). New York: McGraw Hill.

Kaplan, B. (2001). Evaluating informatics applications—clinical decision support systems literature review. Int J Med Inform, 64(1), 15–37.

Kapur, K., Joyce, G. F., Van Vorst, K. A. & Escarce, J. J. (2000). Expenditures for physician services under alternative models of managed care. Med Care Res Rev, 57(2), 161–181.

Kedziera, P., & Levy, M. H. (1994). Collaborative practice in oncology. Semin Oncol, 6, 705–711.

Kessler, R. C., Berglund, P., Demler, O., Jin, R., Koretz, D., Merikangas, K. R., et al. (2003). The epidemiology of major depressive disorder: Results from the National Comorbidity Survey Replication (NCS-R). JAMA, 289(23), 3095–3105.

Kickbusch, I. (1992). Enhancing health potential. In A. Kaplun (Ed.), Health promotion and chronic illness: Discovering a new quality of health (pp. 8–10). Geneva: World Health Organization.

Kiecolt-Glaser, J. K., Dura, J. R., Speicher, C. E., Trask, O. J. & Glaser, R. (1991). Spousal caregivers of dementia victims: Longitudinal changes in immunity and health. Psychosom Med, 53(4), 345–362.

Klein, R. (2004). Britain's national health service revisited. N Engl J Med, 350(9), 937–942.

Kohn, L. T., Corrigan, J. M., & Donaldson, M. S. (Eds.). (2000). To err is human: Building a safer health system. Washington, DC: National Academy Press.

Kolata, G. (2004, August 11). Health plan that cuts costs raises doctors' ire. New York Times, pp. A1.

Kosecoff, J., Kanouse, D. E., Rogers, W. H., McCloskey, L., Winslow, C. M. & Brook, R. H. (1987). Effects of the National Institutes of Health Consensus Development Program on physician practice. JAMA, 258(19), 2708–2713.

Kovach, B., & Rosensteil, T. (2001). The elements of journalism. New York: Crown Publishers.

Kramer, B. J. (1997). Gain in the caregiving experience: Where are we? What next? Gerontologist, 37(2), 218–232.

Kutner, N. G. (1978). Medical students' orientation toward the chronically ill. J Med Educ, 53(February), 111–118.

Kuttner, R. (1998). The risk-adjustment debate. N Engl J Med, 339(26), 1952–1956.

Lantz, J. C., & Lanier, W. L. (2002). Observations from the Mayo Clinic National Conference on Medicine and the Media. Mayo Clinic Proc, 77, 1306–1311.

Lawrence, D. (1997). Quality lessons for public policy: A health plan's view. Health Aff (Millwood), 16(3), 72–76.

Lawrence, D. (2002). From chaos to care—The promise of team-based medicine. Cambridge, MA: Da Capo Press.

Leatherman, S., Berwick, D., Iles, D., Lewin, L. S., Davidoff, F., Nolan, T., et al. (2003). The business case for quality: Case studies and an analysis. Health Aff (Millwood), 22(2), 17–30.

Lerner, M. J., & Simmons, C. H. (1966). Observer's reaction to the "innocent victim": Compassion or rejection? J Pers Soc Psychol, 4(2), 203–210.

Leveille, S. G., Wagner, E. H., Davis, C., Grothaus, L., Wallace, J., LoGerfo, M., et al. (1998). Preventing disability and managing chronic illness in frail older adults: A randomized trial of a community-based partnership with primary care. J Am Geriatr Soc, 46(10), 1191–1198.

Levin, A. (1975). Talk back to your doctor: How to demand and recognize high quality health care. New York: Doubleday.

Levit, K., Smith, C., Cowan, C., Lazenby, H., Sensenig, A. & Catlin, A. (2003). Trends in U.S. health care spending, 2001. Health Aff (Millwood), 22(1), 154–164.

Lewin, B., Robertson, I. H., Cay, E. L., Irving, J. B. & Campbell, M. (1992). Effects of self-help post-myocardial-infarction rehabilitation on psychological adjustment and use of health services. Lancet, 339(8800), 1036–1040.

Lewin, S. A., Skea, Z. C., Entwistle, V., Zwarenstein, M. & Dick, J. (2002). Interventions for providers to promote a patient-centred approach in clinical consultations (Cochrane Review). The Cochrane Library, 2002(2).

Lewis, K. S. (1998). Emotional adjustment to a chronic illness. Lippincotts Prim Care Pract, 2(1), 38–51.

Lewis, R., & Dixon, J. (2004). Rethinking management of chronic diseases. BMJ, 328, 220–222.

Lomas, J., Enkin, M., & Anderson, G. M. (1991). Opinion leaders versus audit and feedback to implement practice guidelines. JAMA, 265, 2202–2207.

Lomas, J., Anderson, G. M., Domnick-Pierre, K., Vayda, E., Enkin, M. W. & Hannah, W. J. (1989). Do practice guidelines guide practice? The effect of a consensus statement on the practice of physicians. N Engl J Med, 321(19), 1306–1311.

Lomas, J., Sisk, J., & Stocking, B. (1993). From evidence to practice in the United States, the United Kingdom, and Canada. Milbank Q, 71(3), 405–410.

Lorig, K. R., & Holman, H. R. (1989). Long-term outcomes of an arthritis self-management study: Effects of reinforcement efforts. Soc Sci Med, 29(2), 221–224.

Lorig, K. R., Kraines, R. G., Brown, B. W., Jr. & Richardson, N. (1985). A workplace health education program that reduces outpatient visits. Med Care, 23(9), 1044–1054.

Lorig, K. R., Sobel, D. S., Stewart, A. L., Brown, B. W., Jr., Bandura, A., Ritter, P., et al. (1999). Evidence suggesting that a chronic disease self-management program can improve health status while reducing hospitalization: A randomized trial. Med Care, 37(1), 5–14.

Lorig, K. R., Ritter, P., Stewart, A. L., Sobel, D. S., Brown, B. W., Jr., Bandura, A., et al. (2001a). Chronic disease self-management program: 2–year health status and health care utilization outcomes. Med Care, 39(11), 1217–1223.

Lorig, K. R., Sobel, D. S., Ritter, P. L., Laurent, D. & Hobbs, M. (2001b). Effect of a self-management program on patients with chronic disease. Eff Clin Prac, 4(6), 256–262.

Lorig, K. R., Mazonson, P. D., & Holman, H. R. (1993). Evidence suggesting that health education for self-management in patients with chronic arthritis has sustained health benefits while reducing health care costs. Arthritis Rheum, 36(4), 439–446.

Lynne, J. (2004). Sick to death and not going to take it anymore! Berkeley, CA: University of California Press.

Martin, J. C., Avant, R. F., Bowman, M. A., Bucholtz, J. R., Dickinson, J. R., Evans, K. L., et al. (2004). The future of family medicine: A collaborative project of the family medicine community. Ann Fam Med, 2(Suppl. 1), S3–S32.

McCain, J. (2001). Predictive modeling holds promise of earlier identification, treatment. Manag Care, 10(9).

McCombs, M., & Shaw, D. (1972). The agenda-setting function of mass media. Public Opin Q, 36, 176–187.

McGinnis, J. M., & Foege, W. H. (1993). Actual causes of death in the United States. JAMA, 270(18), 2207–2212.

McGlynn, E. A., Asch, S. M., Adams, J., Keesey, J., Hicks, J., DeCristofaro, A., et al. (2003). The quality of health care delivered to adults in the United States. N Engl J Med, 348(26), 2635–2645.

McNutt, R. A. (2004). Shared medical decision making: problems, process, progress. JAMA, 292(20), 2516–2518.

Mechanic, D. (2003). Physician discontent: Challenges and opportunities. JAMA, 290(7), 941–946.

Mechanic, D., McAlpine, D. D., & Rosenthal, M. (2001). Are patients' office visits with physicians getting shorter? N Engl J Med, 344(3), 198–204.

Mendenhall, T. J., & Doherty, W. J. (2003). Partners in diabetes: A collaborative, democratic initiative in primary care. Fam Syst Health, 21, 329–335.

Mezey, M., & Ebersole, P. (2001). The future geriatric medicine: A national crisis looms. Aging Today. Retrieved June 23, 2003, from www.asaging.org/at/at-220/Nurses.html

Miller, R. H., & Sim, I. (2004). Physicians' use of electronic medical records: Barriers and solutions. Health Aff (Millwood), 23(2), 116–126.

Milz, H. (1992). Healthy ill people: Social cynicism or new perspectives? In A. Kaplun (Ed.), Health promotion and chronic illness: Discovering a new quality of health (pp. 32–40). Geneva: World Health Organization.

Mokdad, A. H., Bowman, B. A., Ford, E. S., Vinicor, F., Marks, J. S. & Koplan, J. P. (2001). The continuing epidemics of obesity and diabetes in the United States. JAMA, 286(10), 1195–1200.

Mokdad, A. H., Marks, J. S., Stroup, D. F. & Gerberding, J. L. (2004). Actual causes of death in the United States, 2000. JAMA, 291(10), 1238–1245.

Montgomery, E. B., Jr., Lieberman, A., Singh, G. & Fries, J. F. (1994). Patient education and health promotion can be effective in Parkinson's disease: A randomized controlled trial. PROPATH Advisory Board. Am J Med, 97(5), 429–435.

Montgomery, R., & Kosloski, K. (2001). Continuity and diversity among caregivers. National Family Caregiver Support Program. Retrieved June 23, 2003, from *www.aoa.gov/carenetwork.Fin-Montgomery.pdf*

Moyers, P. A. (1999). The guide to occupational therapy practice. American Occupational Therapy Association. Am J Occup Ther, 53(3), 247–322.

Mundinger, M. (1994). Advanced-practice nursing—Good medicine for physicians? N Engl J Med, 330(3), 211–214.

Mundinger, M., Kane, R. L., Lenz, E. R., Totten, A. M. (2000). Primary care outcomes in patients treated by nurse practitioners or physicians. JAMA, 283(1), 59–68.

National Asthma Education and Prevention Program. (2002). Expert panel report: Guidelines for the diagnosis and management of asthma update on selected topics—2002. J Allergy Clin Immunol, 110(5, Suppl.), S141–S219.

National Research Council. (1997). For the record: Protecting electronic health information. Washington, DC: National Academy Press.

Naylor, M. D., Brooten, D., Campbell, R., Jacobsen, B. S., Mezey, M. D., Pauly, M. V., et al. (1999). Comprehensive discharge planning and home follow-up of hospitalized elders: A randomized clinical trial. JAMA, 281(7), 613–620.

Neumann, P. J., Sandberg, E. A., Bell, C. M., Stone, P. W. & Chapman, R. H. (2000). Are pharmaceuticals cost-effective? A review of the evidence. Health Aff (Millwood), 19(2), 92–109.

Norris, S. L., Nichols, P. J., Caspersen, C. J., Glasgow, R. E., Engelgau, M. M., Jack, L., et al. (2002). Increasing diabetes self-management education in community settings. A systematic review. Am J Prev Med, 22(4, Suppl.), 39–66.

Ogawa, M., Suzuki, R., & Otake, S. (2002). Long-term remote behavioral monitoring of the elderly using sensors installed in domestic houses. Paper presented at the Second Joint EMBS/BMES Conference, Houston, TX, October 23–26, 2002.

Partnership for Solutions. (2002a). Chronic conditions: Making the case for ongoing care. Baltimore: The John Hopkins University.

Partnership for Solutions. (2002b). Physician concerns: Caring for people with chronic conditions. Baltimore: The Johns Hopkins University.

Partnership for Solutions. (2002c). Public concerns: Caring for people with chronic conditions. Baltimore: The Johns Hopkins University.

Pearlin, L. I., Mullan, J. T., Semple, S. J. & Skaff, M. M. (1990). Caregiving and the stress process: An overview of concepts and their measures. Gerontologist, 30(5), 583–594.

Pestotnik, S. L., Classen, D. C., Evans, R. S. & Burke, J. P. (1996). Implementing antibiotic practice guidelines through computer-assisted decision support: Clinical and financial outcomes. Ann Intern Med, 124(10), 884–890.

Peyriere, H., Cassan, S., Floutard, E., Riviere, S., Blayac, J. P., Hillaire-Buys, D., et al. (2003). Adverse drug events associated with hospital admission. Ann Pharmacother, 37(1), 5–11.

Philp, I. (2003). The development and implementation of the National Service Framework for Older People's Services. Generations Rev, 13, 24–25.

Picker Institute. (1996). Eye on patients report. Washington, DC: Picker Institute and American Hospital Association.

Piette, J. D. (2000). Interactive voice response systems in the diagnosis and management of chronic disease. Am J Manag Care, 6(7), 817–827.

Pittman, J. (2003). The chronic wound and the family. Ostomy Wound Manage, 49(2), 38–46.

Pope, A., & Tarlov, A. (1991). Disability in America: Toward a national agenda for prevention. Washington, DC: National Academy Press.

Rankin, S. H., & Weekes, D. P. (2000). Life-span development: A review of theory and practice for families with chronically ill members. Sch Inq Nurs Pract, 14(4), 355–373; discussion, 375–358.

Rehm, J., Sempos, C. T., & Trevisan, M. (2003). Alcohol and cardiovascular disease—more than one paradox to consider. Average volume of alcohol consumption, patterns of drinking and risk of coronary heart disease—a review. J Cardiovasc Risk, 10(1), 15–20.

Renders, C. M., Valk, G. D., Griffin, S. J., Wagner, E. H., Eijk Van, J. T. & Assendelft, W. J. (2001). Interventions to improve the management of diabetes in primary care, outpatient, and community settings: A systematic review. Diabetes Care, 24(10), 1821–1833.

Retchin, S. M., & Brown, B. (1991). Elderly patients with congestive heart failure under prepaid care. Am J Med, 90(2), 236–242.

Retchin, S. M., Clement, D. G., Rossiter, L. F., Brown, B., Brown, R. & Nelson, L. (1992). How the elderly fare in HMOs: Outcomes from the Medicare competition demonstrations. Health Serv Res, 27(5), 651–669.

Retchin, S. M., Brown, R. S., Yeh, S. J., Chu, D. & Moreno, L. (1997). Outcomes of stroke patients in Medicare fee for service and managed care. JAMA, 278(2), 119–124.

Retchin, S., & Brown, B. (1990). Quality of ambulatory care in Medicare health maintenance organizations. Am J Public Health, 80(4), 411–415.

Retchin, S., Clement, D., & Brown, R. (1994). Care of patients hospitalized with strokes under the Medicare risk program. In H. Luft (Ed.), HMOs and the elderly (pp. 167–194). Ann Arbor, MI: Health Administration Press.

Rezler, A., & Flahertly, J. (1985). The interpersonal dimensions of medical education. New York: Springer.

Rich, M. W., Beckham, V., Wittenberg, C., Leven, C. L., Freedland, K. E. & Carney, R. M. (1995). A multidisciplinary intervention to prevent the readmission of elderly patients with congestive heart failure. N Engl J Med, 333(18), 1190–1195.

Robert Wood Johnson Foundation. (1996). Chronic care in America: A 21st century challenge. Princeton, NJ: Robert Wood Johnson Foundation

Robert Wood Johnson Foundation. (2002). A portrait of informal caregivers in America, 2001. Princeton, NJ: Robert Wood Johnson Foundation and Foundation For Accountability.

Robinson, J. C. (2001). The end of managed care. JAMA, 285(20), 2622–2628.

Rothman, A. A., & Wagner, E. H. (2003). Chronic illness management: What is the role of primary care? Ann Intern Med, 138(3), 256–261.

Rukeyser, J., Steinbock, C., & Agins, B. D. (2003). Self-management of chronic disease. JAMA, 289(12), 1508–1509; author reply, 1509.

Ryan, C. E. (2002). Clinical and research issues in the evaluation and treatment of families. Med Health R I, 85(9), 278–280.

Saadine, J. B., Engelgau, M. M., Beckles, G. L., Gregg, E. W., Thompson, T. J. & Narayan, K. M. (2002). A diabetes report card for the United States: Quality of care in the 1990s. Ann Intern Med, 136, 565–574.

Sackett, D. L., Rosenberg, W. M., Gray, J. A., Haynes, R. B. & Richardson, W. S. (1996). Evidence based medicine: What it is and what it isn't. BMJ, 312(7023), 71–72.

Safran, C., Rind, D. M., Davis, R. B., Ives, D., Sands, D. Z., Currier, J., et al. (1995). Guidelines for management of HIV infection with computer-based patient's record. Lancet, 346(8971), 341–346.

Safran, D.G. (2003). Defining the future of primary care: What can we learn from patients? Ann Intern Med, 138(3), 248–255.

Sarti, C., Stegmayr, B., Tolonen, H., Mahonen, M., Tuomilehto, J. & Asplund, K. (2003). Are changes in mortality from stroke caused by changes in stroke event rates or case fatality? Results from the WHO MONICA Project. Stroke, 34(8), 1833–1840.

Schofield, R. F., & Amodeo, M. (1999). Interdisciplinary teams in health care and human services settings: Are they effective? Health Soc Work, 24(3), 210–219.

Schulz, R., O'Brien, A. T., Bookwala, J. & Fleissner, K. (1995). Psychiatric and physical morbidity effects of dementia caregiving: Prevalence, correlates, and causes. Gerontologist, 35(6), 771–791.

Schulz, R., Visintainer, P., & Williamson, G. M. (1990). Psychiatric and physical morbidity effects of caregiving. J Gerontol, 45(5), P181–P191.

Schwitzer, G. (2003). Merely lights and wires? Minn Med. Retrieved June 12, 2003, from www.mmaonline.net/publications.MNMed2003/April/Schwitzer.html

Scott, J. C., Conner, D. A., Venohr, I., Gade, G., McKenzie, M., Kramer, A. M., et al. (2004). Effectiveness of a group outpatient visit model for chronically ill older health maintenance organization members: A 2–year randomized trial of the cooperative health care clinic. J Am Geriatr Soc, 52(9), 1463–1470.

Segal, R., Evans, W., Johnson, D., Smith, J., Colletta, S., Gayton, J., et al. (2001). Structured exercise improves physical functioning in women with stages I and II breast cancer: Results of a randomized controlled trial. J Clin Oncol, 19(3), 657–665.

Segar, M. L., Katch, V. L., Roth, R. S., Garcia, A. W., Portner, T. I., Glickman, S. G., et al. (1998). The effect of aerobic exercise on self-esteem and depressive and anxiety symptoms among breast cancer survivors [comment]. Oncol Nurs Forum, 25(1), 107–113.

Shapiro, E. R. (2002). Chronic illness as a family process: A social-developmental approach to promoting resilience. J Clin Psychol, 58(11), 1375–1384.

Simpson, R. J., Jr., Weiser, R. R., Naylor, S., Sueta, C. A. & Metts, A. K. (1997). Improving care for unstable angina patients in a multiple hospital project sponsored by a federally designated quality improvement organization. Am J Cardiol, 80(8B), 80H–84H.

Smith, L. E., Fabbri, S. A., Pai, R., Ferry, D. & Heywood, J. T. (1997). Symptomatic improvement and reduced hospitalization for patients attending a cardiomyopathy clinic. Clin Cardiol, 20(11), 949–954.

Smith, V., DesJardines, T., & Peterson, K. (2000). Exemplary practices in primary care case management: A review of state Medicaid PCCM Program. Princeton, NJ: Center for Health Care Strategies.

Spillman, B. C. (2004). Changes in elderly disability rates and the implications for health care utilization and cost. Milbank Q, 82(1), 157–194.

Spillman, B. C., & Pezzin, L. E. (2000). Potential and active family caregivers: Changing networks and the "sandwich generation." Milbank Q, 78(3), 347–374, 339.

Starr, P. (1983). The social transformation of American medicine. New York: Basic Books.

Stoline, A., & Weiner, J. (1993). The new medical marketplace: A physician's guide to health care economics in the 1990's. Baltimore: John Hopkins University Press.

Strunk, B., Ginsberg, P., & Gabel, J. (2002, September 25). Tracking health care costs: Growth accelerates again in 2001 [web exclusive]. Health Aff. Retrieved from www.healthaffairs.org/WebExclusives/Strunk_Web_Excl_092592.htm

Stuck, A. E., Siu, A. L., Wieland, G. D., Adams, J. & Rubenstein, L. Z. (1993). Comprehensive geriatric assessment: A meta-analysis of controlled trials. Lancet, 342(8878), 1032–1036.

Summer, L. (1999). Chronic conditions. Washington, DC: National Academy on an Aging Society.

Surgeon General. (2001). Surgeon General's call to action to prevent and decrease overweight and obesity. Washington, DC: Public Health Service, Office of the Surgeon General.

Thomas, L. (1974). The lives of a cell: Notes of a biology watcher. New York: Viking Press.

Thompson, B., Coronado, G., Snipes, S. A. & Puschel, K. (2003). Methodologic advances and ongoing challenges in designing community-based health promotion programs. Annu Rev Public Health, 24, 315–340.

Tinetti, M. E., & Fried, T. (2004). The end of the disease era. Am J Med, 116(3), 179–185.

Tone, B. (1999, March 29, 1999). Looking for a job: Think about moving to the country. Nurseweek. Retrieved January 6, 2005, from www.nurseweek.com/features/99–3/rural.html

Toombs, S. K. (1987). The meaning of illness: A phenomenological approach to the patient-physician relationship. J Med Philos, 12(3), 219–240.

Tran, B. (2002). Home care technologies for promoting successful aging in elderly populations. Paper presented at the Second Joint EMBS/BMES Conference, Houston, TX, October 23–26, 2002.

van der Waal, M. A., Casparie, A. F., & Lako, C. J. (1996). Quality of care: A comparison of preferences between medical specialists and patients with chronic diseases. Soc Sci Med, 42(5), 643–649.

Vedhara, K., Cox, N. K., Wilcock, G. K., Perks, P., Hunt, M., Anderson, S., et al. (1999). Chronic stress in elderly carers of dementia patients and antibody response to influenza vaccination. Lancet, 353(9153), 627–631.

Veen, M., Finkelstein, S. M., Speedie, S., & Lundgren, J. M. (2002). Patient satisfaction with TeleHomeCare. Paper presented at the Second Joint EMBS/BMES Conference, Houston, TX, October 23–26, 2002.

Villagra, V. (2004). Strategies to control costs and quality: A focus on outcomes research for disease management. Med Care, 42(4, Suppl.), III24–III30.

Von Korff, M., Gruman, J., Schaefer, J., Curry, S. J. & Wagner, E. H. (1997). Collaborative management of chronic illness. Ann Intern Med, 127(12), 1097–1102.

Von Korff, M., Glasgow, R. E., & Sharpe, M. (2002). Organising care for chronic illness. BMJ, 325(7355), 92–94.

Voss, M. (2002). Checking the pulse: Midwestern reporters' opinions on their ability to report health care news. Am J Public Health, 92(7), 1158–1160.

Wagner, E. H. (1998). Chronic disease management: What will it take to improve care for chronic illness? Eff Clin Pract, 1(1), 2–4

Wagner, E. H. (2000). The role of patient care teams in chronic disease management. BMJ, 320(7234), 569–572.

Wagner, E. H. (2001). Meeting the needs of chronically ill people. BMJ, 323(7319), 945–946.

Wagner, E. H., Austin, B. T., & Von Korff, M. (1996a). Improving outcomes in chronic illness. Manag Care Q, 4(2), 12–25.

Wagner, E. H., Austin, B. T., & Von Korff, M. (1996b). Organizing care for patients with chronic illness. Milbank Q, 74(4), 511–544.

Walker, J., Gerard, P. S., Bayley, E. W., Coeling, H., Clark, A. P., Dayhoff, N., et al. (2003). A description of clinical nurse specialist programs in the United States. Clin Nurse Spec, 17(1), 50–57.

Warshaw, G. A., & Bragg, E. J. (2003). The training of geriatricians in the United States: Three decades of progress. J Am Geriatr Soc, 51(7, Suppl.), S338–S345.

Warshaw, G. A., Bragg, E. J., Shaull, R. W. & Lindsell, C. J. (2002). Academic geriatric programs in US allopathic and osteopathic medical schools. JAMA, 288(18), 2313–2319.

Weingarten, S. R., Henning, J. M., Badamgarav, E., Knight, K., Hasselblad, V., Gano, A., Jr., et al. (2002). Interventions used in disease management programmes for patients with chronic illness-which ones work? Meta-analysis of published reports [comment]. BMJ, 325(7370), 925.

Wellington, M. (2001). Stanford Health Partners: Rationale and early experiences in establishing physician group visits and chronic disease self-management workshops. J Ambul Care Manage, 24(3), 10–16.

Whitford, D., Roberts, S., & Griffin, S. (2004). Sustainability and effectiveness of comprehensive diabetes care to a diabetes population. Diabet Med, 21(11), 1221–1228.

Wilson, J. (1999). Acknowledging the expertise of patients and their organisations. BMJ, 319(7212), 771–774.

Wolff, J. L., Starfield, B., & Anderson, G. (2002). Prevalence, expenditures, and complications of multiple chronic conditions in the elderly. Arch Intern Med, 162(20), 2269–2276.

Wolpert, H. A., & Anderson, B. J. (2001). Management of diabetes: Are doctors framing the benefits from the wrong perspective? BMJ, 323(7319), 994–996.

Woolf, S. H., Grol, R., Hutchinson, A., Eccles, M. & Grimshaw, J. (1999). Potential benefits, limitations, and harms of clinical guidelines. BMJ, 318, 527–530.

World Health Organization. (2002). Innovative care for chronic conditions: Building blocks for action (WHO/MNC/CCH/02.01). Geneva: World Health Organization.

Wu, S., & Green, A. (2000). Projections of chronic illness prevalence and cost inflation. Washington, DC: RAND Health.

Young-McCaughan, S., Mays, M. Z., Arzola, S. M., Yoder, L. H., Dramiga, S. A., Leclerc, K. M., et al. (2003). Research and commentary: Change in exercise tolerance, activity and sleep patterns, and quality of life in patients with cancer participating in a structured exercise program. Oncol Nurs Forum Online, 30(3), 441–454; discussion, 441–454.

Zarit, S. H. (1996). Behavioral disturbances of dementia and caregiver issues. Int Psychogeriatr, 8(Suppl. 3), 263–268; discussion, 269–272.

Zuvekas, S. H., & Taliaferro, G. S. (2003). Pathways to access: Health insurance, the health care delivery system, and racial/ethnic disparities, 1996–1999. Health Aff (Millwood), 22(2), 139–153.

Index

Robert L. Kane, M.D., holds an endowed Chair in Long-term Care and Aging at the University of Minnesota's School of Public Health, where he directs the University's Center on Aging and the Clinical Outcomes Research Center, as well as an AHRQ-funded Evidence-based Practice Center. He has written widely on long-term care issues—at both the clinical and policy levels—managed care, and the medical care of older persons. His most recent book, *It Shouldn't Be This Way,* describes his experience in trying to get the health care system to provide adequate care for his mother.

Reinhard Priester, J.D., is a Coordinator at the University of Minnesota's School of Public Health, where he manages an interdisciplinary research project in long-term care and aging policy. He has held research positions with the University of Minnesota's Center for Biomedical Ethics, the Minnesota Center for Health Care Ethics, and the Minnesota Department of Health. His primary work is in long-term care reform, coverage and reimbursement issues, and health care system reform. He is the coeditor of *Ethical Challenges in Managed Care: A Casebook,* and the author of more than 40 articles on health and long-term care issues.

Annette M. Totten, Ph.D., recently completed her doctorate in Health Services Research with a minor in Gerontology at the University of Minnesota. Her prior experiences include directing studies of primary care for chronic illnesses, developing geriatric interdisciplinary team training initiatives, and studying outcomes across different types of long-term care. She has worked as a legislative aide in state government and as staff for private foundations;